The Reality Diet

The Reality Diet

Lose the Pounds for Good
with a Cardiologist's Simple,
Healthy, Proven Plan

Steven A. Schnur, M.D.

Recipes developed by chef Andrew Hunter

AVERY
A MEMBER OF PENGUIN GROUP (USA) INC. ✳ NEW YORK

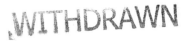

Published by the Penguin Group

Penguin Group (USA) Inc., 375 Hudson Street, New York, New York 10014, USA · Penguin Group (Canada), 90 Eglinton Avenue East, Suite 700, Toronto, Ontario M4P 2Y3, Canada (a division of Pearson Penguin Canada Inc.) · Penguin Books Ltd, 80 Strand, London WC2R 0RL, England · Penguin Ireland, 25 St Stephen's Green, Dublin 2, Ireland (a division of Penguin Books Ltd) · Penguin Group (Australia), 250 Camberwell Road, Camberwell, Victoria 3124, Australia (a division of Pearson Australia Group Pty Ltd) · Penguin Books India Pvt Ltd, 11 Community Centre, Panchsheel Park, New Delhi—110 017, India · Penguin Group (NZ), Cnr Airborne and Rosedale Roads, Albany, Auckland 1310, New Zealand (a division of Pearson New Zealand Ltd) · Penguin Books (South Africa) (Pty) Ltd, 24 Sturdee Avenue, Rosebank, Johannesburg 2196, South Africa · Penguin Books Ltd, Registered Offices: 80 Strand, London WC2R 0RL, England

Most Avery books are available at special quantity discounts for bulk purchase for sales promotions, premiums, fund-raising, and educational needs. Special books or book excerpts also can be created to fit specific needs. For details, write Penguin Group (USA) Inc. Special Markets, 375 Hudson Street, New York, NY 10014.

An application has been submitted to catalogue this book in the Library of Congress.
ISBN 1-58333-250-2

Printed in the United States of America
10 9 8 7 6 5 4 3 2 1

Book design by Lovedog Studio

Acknowledgments

Writing this book has been an amazing journey. In addition to thanking all my friends, family, research participants, and colleagues, I must express special gratitude to the core group of individuals who helped make it possible.

Shirley DeLeon, Registered Dietitian, head of the South Florida Cardiology Associates Wellness Program, whose dedication to the project was paramount. When she walked into my office two years ago, the journey began. Together we have shaped the Reality Diet into what it is today.

Gail Schnur, marketing manager, whose excitement about the project was infectious and whose knowledge of nutrition and marketing has greatly benefited the book.

Dr. Jose Rios, my good friend and colleague for more than twenty years, whose assistance in reviewing the book and valuable contributions to it are greatly appreciated.

Dr. Perry Krichmar, my friend and cofounder of South Florida Cardiology Associates more than fifteen years ago, who is a true expert in the field of preventive medicine.

Dr. Handre Hurwit and Donna Hurwit, who guided many patients to the Wellness Program and helped build the practice to what it is today. Handre's work ethic should be a model for medical students.

Dr. Steven Strumwasser, who provided welcome expertise in the field of medical and behavioral psychology and had an unwavering faith in this project's success.

Carole Bidnick, my literary agent, who believed in me and in my vision and put together what I call "The Dream Team."

Linda Kahn, the most fantastic writer and a true friend with an unbelievable devotion to putting out the best book possible.

Andrew Hunter, recipe developer, who provided delicious menus for all of us to enjoy.

My exceptional office staff at Mount Sinai Medical Center in Miami Beach, who have always been so supportive, especially Kimberly Hernandez, Johanna Johnson, Xi Zhu, Jackie Ferrer, Ken Tucker, and Vivian Baldizon.

All of the doctors at South Florida Cardiology Associates, in particular Dr. Manuel Abella, Dr. Lou Fernandez, Dr. Francesca Gallarello, Dr. Lewis Elias, and Dr. Islon Woolf, who offered patient support.

The dedicated staff at Pembroke Pines medical office, especially dietitians Carissa Kline-Vega and Shana Leird.

Ariel Soffer, M.D., president and CEO of Healthworx, for his support and friendship throughout the years.

Eric Welber, CEO of South Florida Cardiology Associates, whose encouragement and support never wavered.

Candice Lederman, marketing director for South Florida Cardiology Associates, who provided much positive feedback and expertise.

Gonzalo Acevedo, senior vice president at HSBC Private Bank, whose initial introduction to Mitch Kaplan started the journey.

Mitch Kaplan, owner of Books & Books in Coral Gables, Florida, who led me down the right path and helped me make the right connections.

Atif Khan, President of Timeous Systems, who has been a good friend and great sounding board throughout the process.

Steven Sonenreich, CEO at Mount Sinai Medical Center, Miami, who has given me the freedom to pursue my vision.

Marc Auerbach, who has always provided me with sound advice.

David Glanz, whose ideas were terrific.

Ethel Slater at Mount Sinai Medical Library, who pulled hundreds of articles for me on a timely basis.

Berkeley Heart Labs, Liposcience, and DiaDexus, the makers of the Plac test, for their collaboration.

The amazing staff at Avery, including Megan Newman, Kate Stark, and Lucia Watson, who went above and beyond their duties to make this book a success.

Mayte Prida, author of A *Difficult Journey: My Battle with Cancer*, a good friend who provided me with much inspiration.

All of my friends, especially Charles Valenti, Mario Louis, Michael Rose, Jimmy and Nancy Diaz, Kayvan Amini, and Jeffrey Weissner.

My tennis and exercise buddies Mike Gyarmaty, Clinton Nossel, Tony Antunes; my tennis instructor, Iphton Louis; and my personal trainer, Teofilo Hernandez.

And most of all, I'd like to thank my loving family: My wife, Eliane, who has given me all of her love, support, patience, and motivation. My amazing daughter, Samantha, who woke up with me at five in the morning and made me breakfast while I worked. My son, Dylan, who, even at fourteen months, made me laugh when I was ready to pull my hair out while writing the book. And my mom and dad, my brother Mark, and my cousin Adam, whose input at work with the patients was invaluable.

To all, *bon appétit!*

P.S. If I forgot to mention anyone, I promise to catch you in the next book.

To Eliane, Sami, Dylan, Mark, Mom, and Dad

Contents

Part III. Living with Reality

Part IV. Meal Plans and Recipes

The Reality Diet

Introduction

Welcome to Reality!

Perhaps you've struggled with weight issues your whole life. Or maybe you've found yourself steadily putting pounds on since middle age. Perhaps it's leftover pregnancy weight that you just never got around to losing. Or maybe you've developed a habit of eating under stress. Whatever the reason, you realize that you need to lose weight and are looking for a diet that works.

But how do you choose? There are thousands of diet books out there, plus hundreds of other programs that claim astounding results. Is it really possible to lose thirty pounds in thirty days? Or to feel satisfied substituting meals with shakes? Or to lose ten pounds of belly fat in two weeks? Or to lose weight and improve your health without counting calories, worrying about portions, or even exercising? Beware the money-back guarantees and promises of effortless weight loss. The only guarantees in life are death and taxes.

If dieting were easy, we would be a nation of supermodels. Instead, 60 percent of American adults are currently overweight, and half of those are clinically obese. And this is in spite of how often we hear about the very serious health risks of obesity: heart disease, diabetes, cancer, depression, and infertility. Clearly, the weight-loss industry has not lived up to its promises.

Most of the fad diets out there are calorie restrictive. They don't tell you that because they want you to believe they know some special secret. There's no miracle ingredient in their shakes or patented weight-loss ingredient in their prepared foods. By telling you certain foods are "bad" for you, they're just forcing you to eat less by limiting your choices. Besides, is it realistic never to eat a potato, a piece of watermelon, a bunch of grapes, or a carrot stick again? Last time I checked, Bugs Bunny was very skinny. Are we that gullible as a society?

I'm not a nutritionist—I'm a cardiologist. As president of one of South Florida's largest cardiology practices, I see patients every day who are experiencing the life-threatening effects of excess weight: diabetes, clogged arteries, hypertension, high cholesterol, heart attack, and stroke. I also see patients who are suffering side effects from fad diets—dizziness, irregular heartbeat, high cholesterol, even life-threatening cardiovascular events. You don't have to be an M.D. to realize that a diet of unlimited bacon, eggs, and heavy cream will clog your arteries. If I were in medicine purely for the money, I'd be grateful to all these trendy weight-loss plans for sending so many sick patients my way. But I'm not—what gets me through my day is helping my patients live longer, healthier lives. Seeing more and more of them compromising their health when they honestly believed they were doing something good for themselves made me mad. So I hit the books, reading everything I could get my hands on about human nutrition, metabolism, and obesity.

Like Indiana Jones in search of buried treasure, I searched the medical literature for clues that would lead me to my holy grail—weight loss without hunger and with plenty of energy to exercise. The pathway was clear—calorie restriction—but how could I achieve that without sacrificing my patients' health? I wanted my patients to feel so full that they could pass up the fried dough at the state fair or walk by a Pizza Hut and keep on walking. To feel their stomachs turn at the thought of a double bacon cheeseburger with fries. And then, out of the blue, I hit on the answer.

What keeps you full is fiber, and when you're full, you really don't want to eat a lot of high-calorie junk. Plus, fiber is naturally found in foods that are high in vitamins, minerals, and phytonutrients (nutrients from plants). Other diets talk about the importance of fiber, but none of them—especially those that restrict carbohydrate-containing foods, which are your main source of fiber—provides a foolproof way to guarantee that you get enough. The Reality Diet is the only diet that ensures you get enough heart-healthy, fat-fighting fiber. All you need to do is learn one simple rule for choosing the carbohydrates you eat, and in a matter of weeks you'll be able to throw your fat clothes away for good.

What You Can Expect

In the following pages, you'll find that I am up-front and honest about how the Reality Diet works, putting you, the reader, in the driver's seat. I also refuse to sacrifice nutrition and exercise standards that are essential for good health. Yes, the recommended meal plans are devised to meet specific caloric and nutritional requirements. Yes, they are portion-controlled. And, yes, you will have to exercise. But you'll have plenty of energy—not only to exercise, but also to go to work and function normally without any side effects.

On the Reality Diet, you will not feel hungry, light-headed, constipated, or guilty about having a beer or a baked potato. You will also not lose thirty pounds in thirty days—guaranteed. And I will let you in on a secret: You don't want to. Trust me, I've seen people who've tried it—in the emergency room. Rather, you will lose eight to ten pounds of mostly fat in the first month—not water or lean muscle, but weight that will stay off. That's more than thirty pounds in four months!

Furthermore, I will explain to you exactly what your body's nutritional requirements are, and why, so that you will be equipped with the knowledge necessary to cook up your own simple recipes, make healthy choices when you eat out, and compensate for now-and-again indulgences on holidays or special occasions. When you understand how the diet works, you'll realize that if you stray, you won't need to abandon ship altogether—you'll have all the facts you need to get right back on board and continue losing fat.

The Reality Diet ensures that you eat the right carbohydrates, the right proteins, and the right fats and, unlike any other diet out there, plenty of satisfying, healthy fiber. All you need to do is to eat from seven basic food groups each day and follow one simple rule. Enjoy waffles, bananas, hamburgers, hot dogs, potatoes—all the foods you enjoy. Even easier than keeping track of your servings, just follow the menu plans in the back of the book—we've done the work for you! Part III contains eight weeks of menus for both men and women, developed and tested by award-winning food writer Andrew Hunter, in conjunction with my cardiology practice's head dietitian, Shirley DeLeon. You don't have to do a thing but follow the basic plan. You can also mix and match—if you like Monday's breakfast, Wednesday's lunch, and Sunday's dinner, that's fine. If you're feeling adventurous, you can even create your own recipes using the lists of equivalent substitutions at the back of the book.

The Reality Diet is for real people leading real lives. If you're trying to get three kids out of the house to meet the school bus and make it to work on time, you can eat the same simple breakfast every day of the week. Prepare your kitchen in advance with our "Stock Your Pantry" list and you'll find it a snap to fix a nutritious meal after a long day on the job. Too busy to cook? Eat out or order in, using the guidelines for various ethnic cuisines.

Livability and flexibility are the acid tests for a successful long-term diet. If you're not satisfied, feel tired or weak or uncomfortable, get bored of eating the recommended food, or feel deprived because there are foods you can't touch, you'll eventually rebel and go off whatever diet you're on, usually undoing weeks or months of hard work. It's nothing to feel bad about— it's human nature. We're designed to eat from all food groups, and to eat until we're full. We're also designed to actively use our bodies, not to sit in cars, at desks, or in front of television sets and computer screens all day. Therefore, if you eat a variety of healthy foods that keep your taste buds satisfied and your stomach full, and you exercise enough to burn just slightly more calories than you eat, you'll lose weight. It's that simple.

The Basics

Imagine your body is a bank. You make a deposit every time you eat, and you make a withdrawal every time you use your body. To maintain your weight, your deposits need to equal your withdrawals. To lose weight, you need to spend more than you put in. Not a great model where money is concerned, but an ideal scenario for dropping pounds and keeping them off.

Calories in vs. calories out—I'm sure you've heard it before. It's not a new idea, but it's one we've gotten away from in recent years as fad diets have tried to convince us that there's other magic involved in weight loss. The "magic," however, is really just smoke and mirrors designed to distract you from the basic truth.

A pound of fat equals 3,500 calories, so if you can use up 500 calories a day more than you consume, you should lose a pound a week. To lose two pounds a week, you'll need a deficit of 1,000 calories a day. The Scarsdale Diet, an early low-carb diet that promised rapid weight loss, promoted daily menus that *totaled* less than 1,000 calories! Long term, this kind of dieting is neither sustainable nor desirable—it's impossible to get adequate nutrition, and you can actually slow down your metabolic rate by putting your body into starvation mode. Instead, it's much wiser to reduce your intake by a few hundred calories a day and "spend" a few more calories through exercise.

That's it, as far as calories are concerned. Honestly. There's no magic to it, just simple math. If you're an average woman, you need approximately 1,900 calories a day to maintain your weight. You can eat 1,400 calories worth of M&M's a day and lose at least a pound a week. If you also burn an extra 500 calories a day through exercise, you will lose at least two pounds a week. If your preference is Oreos, fine—same difference. You can jog a half-hour to the nearest McDonald's, consume a Quarter Pounder, large fries, and a twelve-ounce chocolate shake (total calories eaten = 1,380), jog home (total calories burned = 500), and sit in front of the TV for the rest of the day and you'll still lose weight.

So why don't I recommend the Mars/Nabisco/McDonald's free-for-all diet? Because, as I said earlier, losing weight at all costs is not always good for your health. *How* you lose the weight is equally important. While shedding pounds is simply a numbers game, when it comes to protecting your most vital asset—your health—the quality of the calories you consume matters as much as the quantity.

To maintain optimal health, your body requires energy from three different types of food: proteins, which provide essential amino acids; fats, which transport certain vitamins and are good for your blood and brain; and carbohydrates, which are often nutrient- and fiber-rich and contribute the energy required for your most basic bodily functions. A diet rich in M&M's is nutrient poor. A diet rich in fruits, vegetables, complex carbohydrates, lean meat, fish, poultry, eggs, low-fat dairy, and unsaturated fats, by contrast, is just what this doctor orders.

And if you do indulge in those M&M's once in a while? I'm not going to beat you up—and you shouldn't beat yourself up, either. Life's too short to obsess over the occasional junk-food foray. Clearly, I don't recommend making a habit of it. But if you do digress, just make up for it the next day, either by cutting back what you eat or doing extra exercise. Remember, you're in control.

Proof Positive
That the Reality Diet Works

If you ask most people how they know if their diet is working, they'll reply, "Because I'm losing weight." If you ask most scientists, they'll say, "Because participants keep the weight off long-term." If you ask most cardiologists, they'll answer, "Because the patient's blood profile has improved." Being a scientist, a cardiologist, and a former dieter, I say that for a diet to be successful, all three requirements have to be met: weight loss, maintenance, and a healthier blood profile. What good is it to lose a lot of weight quickly, as you do on a low-cal or low-carb diet, only to gain it back when you go off? And what good is it to lose weight by eating lots of fat and protein, only to see your cholesterol skyrocket and end up in the hospital?

The Reality Diet works because people lose fat, keep it off, and reduce all significant blood markers for heart disease.

In terms of weight loss, the Reality Diet has produced remarkably consistent results. Over the first sixteen weeks, patients I work with experience an average of 32½ pounds of weight loss. Patients with diabetes have found that the Reality Diet controls their blood sugar to the point where they have been able to reduce their medication. Those who started out on the diet with insulin resistance have reduced their blood sugar to levels where they are no longer at high risk for diabetes. Contrary to popular belief, carbohydrates and insulin are not the enemy. The enemy is obesity, and when patients get their weight under control, their underlying insulin problems decrease dramatically.

Last, but certainly not least from a cardiologist's point of view, all of my patients' lipid profiles have improved significantly on the Reality Diet. Patients have seen increases in their HDL ("good") cholesterol and reductions in their levels of total and LDL ("bad") cholesterol, triglycerides, and other risk factors for cardiovascular disease. In addition, preliminary studies are now under way in my practice, using state-of-the-art CAT-scan machines to show that the Reality Diet may actually cause arterial plaque to shrink and cardiovascular disease to regress.

Drew

One of the first people to try the Reality Diet was Drew, a talented interior decorator with a booming business whom I met when I was renovating my apartment. He was already overweight then, and over the past few years he's probably put on another thirty pounds. Drew used to be a competitive distance swimmer, but gave up exercise when he started his own business nine years ago and has put on about ten pounds a year ever since. He's an extremely sensitive person, so I was careful about talking with him about his weight in a way that wouldn't hurt his feelings. But as soon as I mentioned the Reality Diet, he seemed overcome with relief.

Drew has been a model patient—in his first sixteen weeks he lost thirty-seven pounds, 88 percent of which was fat. His body mass index (BMI) decreased from 40.3 to 34.6 and his body fat plummeted from 41.5 percent to 27.8 percent. In fact, his actual fat weight has decreased by 54.6 pounds, but he has put on nearly 15 pounds of muscle through exercise. Drew now swims for an hour a day—"me time," he calls it. The inches he sheds mean as much to him as the pounds—he's gone from a size 46 pants to a size 38. He even splurged on an expensive Prada belt with grommets all the way around so he can give himself a pat on the back every time he's able to tighten it another hole. "Even my rings are loose now—sometimes I have to take them off and put them in my pockets. A few months ago I couldn't even fit my hands in my pockets!"

When Drew met with my dietitian Shirley for the first time, he told her there was no way he could follow the Reality Diet—he absolutely never cooks; his gas is turned off and he uses his oven to store fabric samples. All of his meals are at restaurants or from prepared food he buys and eats at home. Plus, he has a major sweet tooth. So he started by simply cutting back—from four doughnuts a day to two, from two to one, and eventually to zero. At the same time, he learned how to make healthier choices and watch his portion sizes when he selected food at restaurants or stores. By the time he actually started following the Reality Diet plan, he had already shed some weight and was excited by the results. One thing he refuses to give up is his after-dinner chocolate. But he eats only a bit of it, and exercises enough so that it hasn't impeded his fat loss. Drew still has a way to go to reach his target weight, but he's motivated by the encouragement he gets from his clients and the visible changes he sees every time he looks in the mirror.

No Risk, No Reward

As twenty-first-century beings, we're accustomed to instant gratification in so many aspects of our lives—we have television stations that serve up whatever movie we want to see exactly when we want to see it, restaurants that deliver food almost as soon as we hang up the phone, catalog operators working 24/7 to take our orders and ship them to us next-day delivery, cell phones and BlackBerrys that give us instant communication. Unfortunately, our bodies are very old-fashioned and resist quick fixes.

The human body was designed to maintain the status quo—if we were to lose large amounts of weight every time we skipped a meal, the whole species would have died out long ago. Back in the hunter-gatherer days, when the food supply was unpredictable, our bodies needed to conserve weight and held on to stored energy in the form of fat so that we would have a reserve for the lean times. And in those lean times, when food was scarce, our metabolism adjusted so that we saved energy until the next woolly mammoth came our way.

So there's no getting around the fact that it's hard to lose weight. We have several million years of evolution stacked against us. Diets that promise dramatic weight loss do not make sense biologically. What you end up losing is water weight, which comes right back the minute you go off the diet. Basically, the faster you lose weight, the faster you'll put it back on. Slow, steady weight loss is the best way to ensure that you'll be able to keep the pounds off and not have to fight the same battle a year from now.

I've taken a risk here by being blatantly honest with you. If you think you're going to lose ten pounds in a week, forget it—I have to tell you that it just isn't going to happen. But you are going to lose a lot of weight on the Reality Diet, I promise you. And guess what? You're going to enjoy delicious food and feel great eating it. If you're used to eating a lot of junk food and not exercising, you'll have to make some major lifestyle changes. But it's not impossible, as you've seen from Drew's story. And the knowledge that you're not only losing fat, but also significantly benefiting your health—reducing your risk of heart disease, diabetes, and cancer; increasing your energy level; and improving your mental state—should inspire you to take the long view and put in the extra effort.

Now I invite you to take a positive risk—to risk starting a new diet, embarking on a new exercise plan, and developing a new relationship with food and with your body. Compared with the health risks of not addressing your weight concerns, this is a small risk indeed. And the potential rewards—mental as well as physical—are beyond measure. In reality, these are the things that count.

Part I

The Facts About Food and Your Body

Chapter 1

Myth Versus Reality

Fueled by reports of rampant obesity, a diet obsession has swept the land. As with anything else that requires committed personal involvement—religion, say, or politics—people become passionate on the subject. They can also become somewhat fanatical, casting their lot with a particular denomination or party, which in the realm of weight loss means a particular diet fad. Instead of red states and blue states, we have low-carb zealots, high-protein promoters, low-fat fanatics, and low-calorie devotees. What all of these diet fads have in common is that they promote an extreme change, a low or high something, which makes people feel that they are going to get extremely good results extremely quickly.

But just as in religion and politics, extremism in dieting can be a dangerous thing. Like it or not, we are at the top of our food chain, which means that our bodies were designed to survive on a varied diet that includes all types of food found in nature. Eliminating one or more can have serious health consequences—even more serious, in some cases, than being overweight. For example, as a cardiologist, I constantly remind my patients that excess pounds increase the risk of heart disease. However, eliminating foods such as potatoes and bananas—which are packed with potassium, fiber, and B vitamins—can also lay the groundwork for a major heart attack.

Many people are so driven to lose weight that they are willing to risk even their health for the chance to see the needle on the scale spin backward.

And there's no question about it: On most extreme diets, the pounds will fly off—at least in the beginning. But, for reasons I'll explain below, this is generally not real weight loss, and in most cases it is not sustainable. Let's look at some of the most common misconceptions about fad dieting to see why.

Myth: A low-carb diet is part of a healthy lifestyle.

Reality: First, let's define low carb. Glucose, a simple sugar that is created when your body metabolizes carbohydrates, is the primary energy source for the human body. When it is in short supply, many of your body's systems can adapt and get the energy they require from alternate means, such as the breakdown of fat and protein. But there are certain parts of your body, specifically red blood cells and parts of the brain, that absolutely require glucose to function. When they don't get enough, which can occur when you seriously restrict your carbohydrate intake, you can experience side effects such as lethargy, dizziness, and confusion. In extreme cases, vision problems may result.

When you take in less than 100 grams of carbohydrates a day, or about 25 percent of your total calories, your body starts breaking down fat and lean muscle to get the energy it needs. In the absence of carbohydrates, fat and protein break down incompletely to form ketone bodies, an alternate but poor fuel source, and when they start to build up in your blood, which can happen on a carb-restricted diet, we say you're in ketosis.

Although some have argued that ketosis is a benign condition, I strongly disagree and recommend that about half of your total calories come from carbohydrates to make sure you avoid it. For diabetics, pregnant or lactating women, and people with even early stages of kidney disease, ketosis can be disastrous. Because ketone bodies acidify your blood and are toxic in large quantities, your body tries to dilute and eliminate them as quickly as possible, excreting a great deal of water in the process. This puts a strain on your kidneys even if you don't have renal disease, but may be especially dangerous to the one out of eight people who have underlying renal disease and don't know it. A telling side effect of ketosis is acetone breath—bad breath that smells a bit like the main ingredient in nail polish remover.

Nevertheless, low-carb diets associated with ketosis do cause weight loss, although most of that weight is water. A potential hazard of this rapid water loss is dehydration, which leads to its own set of side effects, including constipation, fatigue, muscle cramps, sudden drops in blood pressure, electrolyte imbalances, and irregular heartbeat.

Not long ago, I saw a patient who complained of dizziness, headaches, and nearly passing out on several occasions. She was in her mid-fifties, generally healthy, and the only recent lifestyle change she'd made was starting a low-carb diet. I recommended changes in her diet to bring it in line with the Reality Diet and her symptoms resolved.

If you eat significantly below 100 grams of carbohydrates a day, your body will need to manufacture its own carbohydrates to supply your brain and red blood cells with energy. The only internal source of carbohydrates is lean muscle tissue. Now that's the last thing you want to lose if you're dieting, because muscle burns more calories than fat. By breaking down your lean muscle, you're ultimately lowering your metabolism and sabotaging the long-term success of your diet.

Myth: Losing a lot of weight in the first two weeks on a low-carb diet will help me lose more in the long run.

Reality: The reason you lose so much in the first two weeks of a low-carb diet is because you're spending a lot of time in the bathroom. The first thing that happens when you deprive yourself of carbohydrates is that your body liquidates its short-term energy reserve: glucose that is stored as glycogen in your liver and muscle tissue. When glycogen is broken down, water is released. When your glycogen reserves are used up, usually within the first twenty-four hours of low-carb dieting or within just a few hours if you're exercising, your body will begin to break down lean muscle and then fat, leading to ketosis and even more water loss.

Water loss does not equal fat loss, however, and it's as easy to put water weight back on as it is to take it off. Try weighing yourself before going for a long run or sitting in the sauna, then weighing yourself afterward. The difference is water weight, not real weight, and the minute you have a glass of water, you're back where you started.

On a low-carb diet, you may lose weight quickly, but the moment you reintroduce carbs, you'll start retaining water again. So you'll go back to restricting your carbs, lose a lot of water weight, then try again to segue into the less restrictive phase of the diet. Not only is this kind of yo-yoing bad for your immune system, it also means that the "advantage" of your quick initial weight loss will evaporate. Studies comparing people on low-carb diets with those following a balanced diet show that while low-carbers lose more weight in the first six months, after a year their total weight loss is the same as the control group.

Myth: I need to avoid all high-glycemic carbohydrates to lose weight.

Reality: A lot of fad diets rate carbohydrates as "good" or "bad" according to where they fall on something called the glycemic index. Carrots, beets, and other root vegetables are "bad," while broccoli and green leafy vegetables are "good"; bananas are "bad" and blueberries are "good." Pity the poor potato farmers who have had to take out advertising in major media to convince people that spuds are not sacrilege!

The fact of the matter is that the glycemic index is at best grossly oversimplified—and at worst downright misleading—as a determinant of the healthfulness of various foods. To show you what I mean, let's take a look at what the glycemic index is and how it's calculated.

All carbohydrates are broken down into glucose in your body. As soon as that glucose is absorbed into your bloodstream, your blood sugar level rises. The rate at which this process occurs is called the glycemic response, which is measured according to a glycemic index.

The hitch here is the standard portion size needed to measure the glycemic response. Take carrots, for instance, which have a highly unfavorable glycemic index score of 131. To test carrots, volunteers had to eat more than six times the standard half-cup portion, or more than three cups of carrots! Personally, I don't know many people who eat 1½ pounds of carrots at a sitting.

The theory behind glycemic-index-based diets is that when your blood sugar rises, your insulin level spikes, leading to increased fat storage. Then, when your insulin level drops back down, you'll experience something called relative hypoglycemia and be overcome with cravings. There are many problems with this theory, not the least of which is that these normal fluctuations in blood sugar levels have not been linked directly to obesity, insulin resistance, or hunger.

Many factors can affect the glycemic response: the amount of food eaten, the composition of the food (in terms of fat, protein, and carbohydrates), and the way a food is processed and prepared. For example, boiled red potatoes eaten cold, say in a potato salad, have a moderate glycemic index of 56, while the same potatoes eaten right out of the pot have a glycemic index of 89. Because fat slows down the absorption of glucose into the bloodstream, french fries, which are loaded with fat, have a glycemic index of 64, while a plain baked potato has a glycemic index of 77.

As a standard measure, the glycemic index is further flawed because glycemic index values vary from individual to individual, as everyone's digestive process is different. Plus, most meals include a variety of foods, not just a bowl full of carrots, and the proportion of carbohydrates, fats, and proteins in the entire meal determines your overall blood-sugar response.

The glycemic index is a simplistic and misleading way to judge the quality of food. High-fructose corn syrup, which is one of the worst things you can eat, has a low glycemic index, while certain fruits and vegetables that are packed with nutrients score high. A far better way to make healthful choices is to look for food that is high in fiber and low in saturated and trans fats.

Myth: High-protein diets are the most effective.

Reality: By definition, most low-carb diets are high in protein. After all, you have to eat something! Substituting protein for carbohydrates not only increases the likelihood of going into ketosis, with all of its attendant health problems, but also brings on a host of other even more serious ones.

Proteins are made up of amino acids, and when they are metabolized, they increase the acidity of your blood. Your body uses calcium from your bones to neutralize the acidity of your blood. Hence, high-protein diets have been associated with an increase in osteoporosis.

The calcium released into your bloodstream to neutralize the acidic byproducts of protein metabolism eventually comes out in your urine. But a high concentration of calcium in urine is a risk factor for kidney stones. In addition, increased protein in your blood puts a strain on the kidneys, making high-protein diets especially dangerous for people with renal disease.

A diet rich in red meat and shellfish can put you at increased risk for gout, a painful disease of the joints. These proteins contain a high proportion of amino acids called purines, which are broken down into uric acid. In high concentrations, uric acid forms sharp crystals that precipitate out of the blood and end up in your joints, causing them to become swollen, painful, and purplish in color.

In terms of effectiveness, high-protein diets by design are usually low in carbohydrates, putting you into a state of ketosis in which you lose a lot of water weight and burn lean muscle tissue. Because ketone bodies suppress appetite and protein is more filling than carbohydrates, high-protein diets help you lose weight because they make you want to eat less.

If you don't self-restrict on a high-protein diet, however, you can find yourself easily gaining weight. When I was in college, I was like the skinny kid on the beach in those old Charles Atlas ads—the one who gets sand kicked in his face by the mean guy with the rippling muscles. Determined to remedy the situation, I started drinking three or four protein shakes per day. At six-foot-three, I went from 140 to 160 pounds in two months. But did I look like Charles Atlas? Far from it—for the first time in my life, I was actually getting fat! The moral of the story is that protein is calorie dense, and calories, no matter where they come from, are what make you fat.

Myth: On a low-carb diet, I can eat as much protein and fat as I want and still lose weight.

Reality: A calorie is a calorie, whether it comes from carbohydrates, protein, or fat. But fat contains more than twice as many calories per gram as protein and carbohydrates—9 calories per gram versus 4 calories per gram. The reason people lose weight on diets that allow them as much protein and fat as they want is that they inadvertently begin to restrict the amount of food they eat. Patients of mine who've tried these diets say they got to the point where their stomach turned at the sight of bacon and eggs in the morning, or they simply couldn't bear the thought of another steak. With the feeling of fullness they got from eating protein and fat, and the appetite-suppressing effect of ketosis, they ended up eating a lot less than they normally would have.

The danger of these diets is that, in addition to all the risks of eating a lot of protein—osteoporosis, kidney stones and kidney disease, and gout—there are all the cardiovascular problems that can be caused by eating lots of fat, especially saturated fat, the kind found in protein-rich food such as meat and dairy products.

Research Update

As the movie *Super Size Me* graphically illustrated, a sustained diet of fatty food can do serious damage to your cardiovascular system, as well as your liver, your libido, and your mood. But how about the once-in-a-blue-moon high-fat special-occasion meal? I'm sorry to report that recent research shows that even a single high-fat meal can damage the lining of your blood vessels. A group of young, healthy volunteers ate a low-fat breakfast one day and a high-fat breakfast the next. After each meal, their blood was drawn and tested for indicators of heart health. The low-fat meal had no effect, but shortly after consuming an Egg McMuffin, sausage McMuffin, and two hash browns, there was clear evidence of damage to their arteries. Within three hours, participants experienced an 81 percent rise in triglycerides and showed evidence of damage to their blood vessels. While the volunteers were fed a breakfast of fast food, the researchers concluded that any meal high in total and saturated fats would have a similar effect.

Myth: The less fat I eat, the better.

Reality: "Fat makes you fat" was the rallying cry behind the low-fat craze of the last decade. In truth, however, all fat is not created equal, and while some fats definitely are bad for you, others can actually improve your health and your weight. People living in Mediterranean countries are slimmer and have a far lower incidence of heart disease than Americans, and much of it seems to be linked to their high consumption of fish, nuts, and olive oil. Unsaturated fats that derive from fruits, vegetables, nuts, and fatty fish actually protect your heart by lowering your cholesterol. They also fill you up, so it's easier to maintain a healthy body weight.

The fats to be careful of are saturated fats—essentially those that are solid at room temperature, such as animal fat—as well as tropical oils (palm or coconut) and dairy fat. You should also avoid trans fats, which are not found in nature but are common ingredients in processed snack foods, commercial baked goods, fast food, fried food, and certain margarines. Trans fats act like saturated fats in your body, clogging your arteries and making you susceptible to heart disease and stroke.

Following a strict low-fat diet eliminates the health risks of a diet high in saturated fats, but it also eliminates the satiety and health benefits of a diet high in polyunsaturated fats. Plus, beware—just because a food is low-fat doesn't mean it's low-calorie! I've had patients who've gained quite a bit of weight on low-fat diets because they thought they could eat as much low-fat food as they wanted. Read the labels carefully: Manufacturers often pack low-fat foods with sugar in order to give them the flavor they lose when fat is removed.

Myth: If I control my blood sugar, I can control my cravings.

Reality: A corollary to the glycemic index concept is the idea that certain foods raise your blood sugar dramatically, and when your blood sugar level drops down again, you feel ravenous and start overeating. The problem with this theory is that we are just beginning to understand what stimulates and suppresses appetite, and it seems to be primarily a factor of hormones, not blood sugar.

If you're healthy, the minute your blood glucose level rises during a meal, your pancreas secretes insulin, a hormone that escorts that glucose into your body's cells, where it can be used immediately as fuel, or into your liver or fat cells, where it can be stored for future use. When your blood glucose levels drop, if you've gone for a while without eating or are exercising heavily, your pancreas secretes another hormone, called glucagon, which releases stored glucose from your liver, ensuring that your tissues have a steady supply. Your insulin/glucagon system keeps your blood glucose level within a normal range. Only people whose insulin systems are not functioning properly—diabetics, for example—will experience appreciable blood sugar swings.

If our blood sugar is relatively stable, then what accounts for the fatigue and cravings we get, especially in the late afternoon? Fatigue can result from a number of things, the most common of which is dehydration. It's also a fact that our bodies have an internal clock, called the circadian rhythm, which was programmed millions of years ago, in sync with the rotation of the earth. Because of this rhythm, our bodies naturally undergo biochemical changes at certain times of day. One particularly noticeable one is around four P.M. At this time, our temperatures rise slightly and we naturally become sleepy. Craving a snack in the late afternoon may just be your body's way of trying to counteract that sluggishness.

Another theory is that late-afternoon cravings, especially for chocolate, are actually a symptom of caffeine withdrawal. Many of us chug a couple of cups of coffee in the morning, then lay off the caffeine for the rest of the day. Caffeine has a half-life of about six hours, so by the middle of the afternoon it is wearing off, leaving us drowsy and distracted. The British traditionally have solved that problem by taking a break for tea. Others of us reach for a Mars bar.

So while the late-afternoon slump is a reality, it's not related to carbohydrate withdrawal or plummeting blood sugar. It's a normal occurrence that can be managed with a light, healthful snack and a beverage.

Myth: Skipping breakfast and eating a light lunch help me lose weight.

Reality: While you may think you're cutting calories by skipping breakfast, research consistently shows that people who eat breakfast actually eat fewer calories per day and lose weight more successfully than those who don't. The reason is that if you skip breakfast, by lunch you're ravenous, and if you manage to keep your appetite in check at midday, by dinner you're totally out of control. By eating meals at regular intervals, you're more likely to make sane food choices and withstand temptations that, on an empty stomach, would prove irresistible.

Also, it's just not healthy to skip breakfast. Think about it—in the morning, you have been without food for around twelve hours. Having a nutrient-rich breakfast will give your body and brain the energy they need to function optimally from the get-go.

Myth: I need to avoid fruits to lose weight because they contain sugar.

Reality: Sugar is not the enemy! And fruits are definitely our friends. Fructose, the sugar contained in fruits, is easily converted to glucose, the kind of sugar our bodies need for energy. In addition, fruits are packed with essential vitamins and minerals. The fiber contained in whole fruits (in contrast to most juices) slows down absorption of the sugar and protects the heart. Plus, fruits are fat free, except for avocados and olives, which contain healthy unsaturated fats.

Contrary to popular wisdom, however, you can have too much of a good thing. Like everything else, fruit contains calories, and eating too much fruit—and especially fruit juice, which is concentrated and usually has no fiber—can pack on the pounds. A moderate amount of fruit is a crucial part of a healthy diet and should never be eliminated altogether.

Myth: On any diet, the first thing I need to cut out is alcohol.

Reality: The short response to this assumption is no, you don't need to eliminate alcohol in order to lose weight. For many people, however, stopping drinking immediately eliminates a few hundred calories a day, which can translate into a pound or more a week. Men, who tend to put on excess weight in their abdomen, may notice their "beer bellies" shrinking, but it's not because they've stopped drinking beer per se, but because they've reduced their calorie intake.

Alcohol is a complicated subject, and it's necessary to analyze the risks and benefits of drinking on a case-by-case basis. Certainly, drinking to excess is bad not only for your waistline, but for your general health and safety as well. But moderate drinking—up to one drink a day for women and two a day for men—can have health benefits, primary among which is a significantly reduced risk of cardiovascular disease.

In my practice I find out about my patients' medical, personal, and family history before advising them about alcohol use. For a young man with no risk factors for heart disease, for example, there's no reason to recommend a daily drink. For an older man with high LDL ("bad") cholesterol and low HDL ("good") cholesterol, however, there may be. Women with a family history of breast cancer should avoid alcohol altogether or take a 600 mcg folic acid supplement if they choose to drink in moderation. And anyone with a family or personal history of drug or alcohol abuse should steer clear of the bottle.

If you choose to drink, it's best to do so with food, as it maximizes alcohol's cardiovascular benefits. Also, choose a heart-healthy drink, such as red wine or a dark-colored beer, which contain beneficial antioxidants, over white wine or light-colored beer. As far as the calories are concerned, a single serving—6 ounces of dark beer, 4 ounces of wine, or 1½ ounces of spirits—contains roughly 100 calories, most of which come from alcohol, not carbohydrates as is commonly believed. To avoid weight gain, be sure to account for those extra calories by cutting back elsewhere in your daily intake or doing additional exercise to burn them off.

The bottom line is, if you've never had a drink, don't start, and if you have any personal or family history of addiction, steer clear of alcohol altogether. But if you enjoy the occasional drink to help you relax, go ahead—dieting is stressful enough and the extra calories are easily managed.

Myth: I can lose weight without exercise.

Reality: It's certainly possible to lose weight without exercising, but it's incredibly unhealthy. As a cardiologist, I'm horrified that any doctor would condone a diet that does not specifically require physical activity. The mental and physical benefits of exercise are practically innumerable, but it is especially essential for heart health: Exercise lowers blood pressure as well as both total and "bad" cholesterol levels, all independent risk factors for heart disease.

Exercise is also an essential tool for dieters. Not only does exercise promote weight loss by burning calories, but it also increases lean muscle mass, and muscle burns more calories than fat. Without exercise, an average woman would have to eat around 1,000 calories a day to lose two pounds a week—hardly enough to keep the hunger pangs at bay. By incorporating a moderate amount of exercise into her routine, that same woman can eat a filling 1,400 calories a day and lose weight just as fast. She is also building muscle mass so that when she reaches her goal weight, she can continue to eat a satisfying amount of food without putting the weight back on.

The hormones released during exercise can act as a natural appetite suppressant, making it easier to stick to your diet. Plus, the psychological benefits of exercise and the rapid changes you'll see in your body shape will give you the positive reinforcement you need to stay motivated.

Myth: Certain food combinations help you lose weight.

Reality: There are no magic food combinations that will make the pounds melt away. What combining foods does is help keep you satisfied so you eat less. For example, eating protein with starch will slow down the absorption of the starch, so you will feel fuller longer. That's why you'll find diets recommending toast with a slice of low-fat cheese rather than plain toast—the cheese will slow the digestion of the toast, making it a more satisfying breakfast.

Diets that restrict certain food combinations, such as fruit and meat, claim that our stomachs can only process one food at a time, or particular foods together. If this were the case, we never would have survived as a species. The human body has evolved to maximize nutrient absorption under all circumstances. In fact, some food combinations are highly recommended—for example, iron, which is commonly found in red meat, is absorbed best in the presence of vitamin C, which is commonly found in fruit.

Myth: I can lose belly fat first.

Reality: There is no such thing as "spot reducing." When you lose weight, you lose it wherever fat is stored in your body. You simply may notice it in your belly first, because for most of us, our waistbands are the tightest part of our clothing.

Myth: Eating before bed makes me gain weight.

Reality: As long as you stick to the amount of calories you need to lose or maintain your weight, you won't gain even if you eat them all in one huge midnight feast. The problem is that many people max out their daily calorie allotment before the end of the day, so the snack they eat at bedtime puts them over their limit and contributes to weight gain. If you're the type of person who likes to eat at night, as long as you cut back enough during the day to compensate, you shouldn't have any problem with weight gain.

Indigestion and acid reflux, two painful conditions that are exacerbated by late-night eating, can be problems for some people. If you suffer from either of these, don't eat dinner too close to bedtime, and avoid after-dinner snacks. It also helps to remain upright for a couple of hours after your last meal.

Sometimes I recommend a light snack before bedtime, especially for patients with insomnia that is not caused by indigestion or acid reflux. Foods that contain calcium, such as dairy products, and tryptophane, such as turkey, can bring on drowsiness. So next time you feel like a late-night treat, try a couple of slices of turkey breast, low-fat cheese, or a bowl of high-fiber cereal with skim milk.

Myth: I tend to put on weight because I have a slow metabolism.

Reality: For generations, people have blamed their metabolism for their weight problems. Except in cases when they have rare genetic problems, have been fasting or in a starvation situation, or have thyroid disease, however, their metabolism is not the sole culprit. More often, the reason people gain weight is because they consume more calories than they burn, pure and simple.

Our basal metabolic rate (BMR) is the amount of calories we need to support our basic bodily functions, including breathing, blood circulation, tissue maintenance and repair, and brain activity. It usually accounts for about two-thirds of our daily calorie requirement. The remaining amount is determined by our activity level.

Your BMR is primarily determined by your body size and composition: Bigger people have greater calorie requirements, and different types of tissue burn calories at different rates. Weight loss actually decreases your BMR, because there's less of you to support. That's why a 250-pound person may actually be able to lose weight on a 2,500-calorie-a-day diet, while a 150-pound person may have to cut back to 1,500 calories a day to slim down at the same rate.

Some say genetics determines up to 50 percent of your BMR—it determines your height and build, for example—and there's nothing you can do to change that. But you can influence the other 50 percent. The most significant way is by getting in shape: The resting metabolism of muscle is greater than that of fat, so the more muscle you have, the more calories your body will burn passively. Actively exercising will also increase the additional, non-BMR calories you burn, increasing your ability to lose weight without drastically cutting calories.

You can also negatively influence your BMR by eating too few calories and putting your body in starvation mode. Throughout human history, this trick helped us survive periodic famines. What it means today is that you can actually sabotage your weight loss by eating too little. One of my patients, who had been losing steadily for weeks on the Reality Diet, suddenly plateaued. When I asked him if he'd changed his diet or exercise recently, he said he had cut back on what he was eating because he was feeling really full consuming everything I told him to and thought he needed to feel hungry in order to lose weight. I told him to go back to the 1,800-calorie-a-day menu, which he did, and he began losing weight again.

Myth: If I don't eat every three hours, my body will go into starvation mode and my metabolism will shut down.

Reality: Clocks were invented long after human beings. Your body will go into starvation mode only if it's starving—that is, if it doesn't have enough calories to sustain its basic cellular functions. Just because you feel hungry, experience cravings, or have low energy doesn't mean you're starving. It just means that you've trained your body to expect food at certain intervals, so your gastric juices start pumping in expectation. The only thing you'll do by eating every three hours is ensure that you'll be hungry every three hours—the last thing you want to do if you're trying to lose weight.

Training your body not to be hungry between meals is no different than training a toddler to use the potty. By lengthening the intervals between times you eat, you eventually will lose the urge to eat so frequently. Of course, you don't want to leave such huge gaps between meals that you become ravenous and binge. Your ultimate goal should be to eat three satisfying meals a day with an occasional snack and not be distracted constantly by thoughts of food.

Myth: If I lift weights, I'll build muscle and lose weight, since muscle burns more calories than fat.

Reality: Lifting weights is not the most effective use of your gym time when you're trying to lose weight. While it's true that muscle burns more calories than fat, the difference is far less than what you'll burn in a good aerobics class. Back when I was pumping iron and slugging protein shakes, I put on plenty of muscle. I also got pretty fat. To help myself deflate, I ditched the weights and went back to playing an hour of tennis a day. As a doctor, I'm also not a huge fan of weightlifting, because it's not particularly beneficial to your heart and puts you at risk of serious injury.

Myth: Skinny people are healthier than fat people.

Reality: Don't judge a book by its cover! Skinny people who consume nothing but junk food and diet soda—or even worse, smoke cigarettes or take pills to control their appetite—may be very unhealthy on the inside. In my years as a cardiologist, I've seen heart-attack victims who were as thin as rails. I know it's hard not to envy your friend who eats nothing but Twizzlers and wears a size 2, but try to control your jealousy. It's far better to be healthy on the inside—to eat nutritious meals, keep your blood sugar and cholesterol down, and be in good cardiovascular shape—than it is to look like a fashion model who may be doing all kinds of unhealthy things to keep her weight down.

The bottom line when it comes to weight loss is that you have to eat fewer calories than you use up during the course of a day. There's no magic to the various restrictions or combinations promoted by fad diets—they're all gimmicks that, in the end, lead you to consume less. They simply make you stop and think about your food—Does this contain too many carbs? Are my carbs, proteins, and fats in perfect balance? How many points is this worth?—before you put it on your plate or in your mouth, automatically keeping you from mindless, high-calorie eating.

The danger in many of these diets is that restricting or eliminating certain food groups also can dramatically reduce your intake of beneficial vitamins, minerals, and fiber that those foods may contain. Supplements are not adequate substitutes for getting nutrition from food—many nutrients are not well absorbed or may not be as effective in supplement form as in their natural state.

Furthermore, exercise must be an essential part of any diet—whether you are actively trying to lose weight or trying to maintain. Carb-restrictive diets that cause you to feel lethargic are not conducive to maintaining the kind of activity level you need not only to slim down but also to prevent heart disease, cancer, osteoporosis, depression, and a host of other illnesses.

Losing weight in a healthy way takes work—and anyone who promises otherwise is selling snake oil. But in the long run, it's well worth the effort, because you'll shed pounds while learning healthy habits that will help you maintain your hard-won weight loss for good.

Chapter 2

Carbs: The Good, the Bad, and the Ugly

The pursuit of happiness is one of our inalienable rights, and carbs are one of life's greatest pleasures. What's summer without strawberries and corn on the cob? Sunday breakfast without waffles? Lunch-on-the-go without a sandwich and banana? A warm winter roast without carrots and potatoes? Fruits, vegetables, yogurt, bread, potatoes, pasta, rice, tortillas, cereal—the foods that grace our palates with texture, taste, and seasonal variety are also the ones that keep our bodies healthy.

Carbohydrates are a crucial element of a balanced diet and can be enjoyed as part of a successful weight-loss program as long as they are chosen wisely. In addition to the essential vitamins and minerals they provide, foods classified as carbohydrates—vegetables, fruits, dairy products, and starches—are the best sources of bone-building calcium and heart-healthy fiber. That's why on the Reality Diet, you'll get nearly half of your daily calories from delicious and nutritious carbohydrates.

Fruits and Vegetables:
Nature's Multivitamins

I was getting ready for bed one night and my beeper went off. A young woman had been brought to the emergency room with a life-threatening cardiac arrhythmia as a result of a severe potassium deficiency. If she wasn't stabilized immediately, she could suffer permanent brain damage or even death.

I threw on my clothes and raced to the hospital, where the emergency room doctors had managed to stabilize her condition with intravenous potassium. I examined the patient, then walked out to the waiting room, where her anxious family was gathered. "Tell me about your daughter," I asked the parents.

"She's twenty-eight and she's never had any health problems before," said her father, visibly stricken.

"Has anything changed in her lifestyle recently that you know about— diet, exercise, a new medication?" I continued.

"Yes," her mother interjected. "A few weeks ago she began a new diet. She was eating lots of cheese and meat, but no fruits, no bread, no rice, no potatoes. I was worried, but she was losing a lot of weight and seemed happy, so I didn't say anything."

I reassured the mother that she wasn't to blame and that her instinct to worry had been correct. Her daughter's pursuit of a low-carbohydrate diet that severely restricted fruits and vegetables had nearly cost her her life.

Fruits and vegetables contain vast amounts of vitamins and minerals that are essential to all aspects of the functioning of our bodies. Bananas and potatoes are rich sources of potassium, which is critical for the heart. The antioxidant vitamins C, E, and beta-carotene, which may play a role in fighting cancer and protecting against heart disease, are found in a diverse array of fruits and vegetables, including oranges, kiwis, strawberries, red peppers, Brussels sprouts, broccoli, spinach, kale, carrots, winter squash, sweet potatoes, and cantaloupe. Plus, there are tens of thousands of phytonutrients—compounds found in plant-derived foods—that also promote health and fight disease in ways that researchers are still discovering.

Research Update

That old saying "An apple a day keeps the doctor away" may have more than a grain of truth to it. A recent study performed at Cornell University showed that a powerful antioxidant called quercetin found in apples might help stave off both Alzheimer's and Parkinson's diseases.

Like many fruits and vegetables, apples contain phytonutrients that help them fight against bacteria, viruses, fungi, and damage caused by overexposure to sunlight. These same compounds can help us fight diseases such as cancer, heart disease, and diabetes, as well as boost our immune systems to ward off infections. What this study showed for the first time was not only that quercetin could mitigate the kind of damage to brain cells that causes these two debilitating conditions, but that it did so more effectively than vitamin C, another antioxidant.

The highest concentration of quercetin is found in the skins of red apples. Lower concentrations are also found in cranberries, blueberries, and onions.

To help you maximize your intake of vitamins, minerals, and phytonutrients, the Reality Diet includes two fruits and at least four different kinds of vegetables a day. Because most vegetables have low calorie density—they take up a lot of space on your plate and fill your stomach without containing a lot of calories—you can eat huge quantities without busting your calorie bank. One of the most frequent comments from patients on the diet has been how absolutely stuffed they feel from all these fruits and vegetables. Some even have trouble finishing the recommended amount of food!

One of the myths about fruits and certain vegetables is that they contain sugar, and since sugar causes your pancreas to produce insulin, you'll develop relative hypoglycemia and experience uncontrollable cravings after eating a handful of carrots or grapes. As I explained in Chapter 1, relative hypoglycemia is a normal response and cravings are caused by many other factors. Even though some fruits and vegetables are high in sugar, they also contain fiber, which slows the absorption of sugar into the bloodstream. That's why natural sugars, which are found in fruits and vegetables, dairy, and whole grains, are not a problem for dieters.

Added sugars, such as high-fructose corn syrup, sucrose (table sugar), and fruit juice concentrate, by contrast, are empty calories that contain no nutritive value. It's no surprise that the increase in added sugar to our diet — on average, Americans currently consume more than 150 pounds of added sweetener per capita each year — has coincided with a national epidemic of obesity. The biggest culprit is high-fructose corn syrup — ironically, a low-glycemic food — which was developed about thirty years ago and now accounts for nearly half of the added sweetener in the American diet. As far as added sugars are concerned, high-fructose corn syrup is particularly dangerous because it reduces circulating levels of the weight-loss hormone leptin that suppresses appetite and boosts metabolism.

As long as you choose whole foods with plenty of vitamins, minerals, phytonutrients, and fiber, you can enjoy all fruits and vegetables without worrying about their sugar content. Juices are another story, however. The sugars they contain are not bad for you in and of themselves, but the effect of those sugars is usually not mitigated by fiber, which is removed by the juicing process. It's also a lot easier to get carried away calorie-wise with juice than with whole fruits and vegetables. Think of how easy it is to down an eight-ounce glass of orange juice versus eating two whole oranges. They both contain 120 calories, but the effort it takes to peel and eat a whole orange slows you down and makes you conscious of what you're consuming. Plus, the fiber in the whole orange fills you up better than the juice, which may satisfy your mouth but does very little to relieve your immediate hunger or keep your appetite suppressed for any length of time. If you absolutely must have a glass of juice, look for some of the newer fiber-fortified products and cut the juice with water.

Cracking the Code

Food manufacturers are not required to distinguish between natural and added sugars on nutrition labels, so you'll only see one line marked "Sugar," with a total number of grams per serving. It takes some sleuthing to figure out whether that number includes added sugars, and if so, how much. Among the various code names for added sugars:

   High-fructose corn syrup
   Corn syrup
   Glucose syrup
   Maple syrup
   Dextrose
   Fructose
   Glucose
   Lactose
   Maltose
   Sucrose
   Cane or beet sugars
   Fruit juice concentrate
   Molasses
   Honey

   The rule of thumb is that the ingredients listed beside or below the nutrition box are in decreasing order of weight per serving, so there is most of the first ingredient and least of the last. Check the ingredient list of some of your favorite snack foods and beverages. It's quite an eye-opener to see how many added sugars are among the top items listed.

Newt and Dolores

I first met Newt and Dolores in the ICU. A colleague of mine had performed emergency triple bypass surgery on Newt after he'd had a massive heart attack on a fishing trip with his buddies down in the Keys. I was making my rounds, checking on patients, when I found him dozing in bed, with Dolores sitting anxiously by his side.

Dolores and I started talking, and I could see right away how terrified she was that Newt had had such a close call. "We've been married for forty-four years—we were childhood sweethearts back in Brooklyn. He's all I have!" she said, wringing a handkerchief in her hands. Newt was obviously the center of her universe—they had never had children—and she couldn't imagine life without him.

"My job is to make sure your husband recovers from this heart attack," I said to her. "And yours is to help prevent him from having another." Dolores looked at me questioningly. "I want you to take a break from sitting by his bedside and walk over to my office—it's right on the other side of this building," I continued. "There I want you to talk with my dietitian, Shirley DeLeon, about what kinds of food Newt should and shouldn't be eating once he leaves the hospital."

Later that day, Dolores visited with Shirley, who explained that in addition to restricting his fat and salt intake, Newt was going to have to lose a significant amount of weight. At sixty-six years old and barely five-foot-nine, he weighed 270 pounds and suffered from diabetes—a heart attack had been virtually inevitable. "You're going to have to change the way you shop and cook," Shirley explained.

"Well, actually, I don't cook," Dolores said sheepishly. Shirley looked up in surprise. "Both Newt and I have always worked such long hours—him in the garage, me at the department store—that I never had time to cook. So we just got in the habit of eating fast food. It's easy, and it's very affordable."

So Shirley began to teach Dolores about nutrition, from the ground up. She also explained the Reality Diet principles, and how she wanted Newt to begin eating from the plan as soon as he got his strength back and to come to her for weekly weigh-ins. As soon as his doctor gave the go-ahead, Newt would have to begin a regular exercise program as well.

"Shirley," Dolores interjected, "I know I'm not the patient here, but I really need to lose some weight, too." Shirley nodded—Dolores must have weighed close to 175 pounds, and couldn't have been more than five-foot-two. "Would it be all right if I went on the diet, too?"

"Of course," Shirley replied. "It would be more than all right—it would be the best thing for both of you. It's always easier to diet with a partner, and as long as you're learning to cook, you may as well enjoy the meals, too!"

Three and a half months later, I caught Dolores in the hallway on the way to her weigh-in with Shirley. "How's it going? You look great!" I greeted her.

"That's nothing, Dr. Schnur—I feel great, too! I haven't had this kind of energy since I was a teenager! Newt and I have both lost two clothing sizes, and his sugar has come down so much that Dr. Holen has reduced his medication significantly and thinks he might be able to go off it altogether in a little while. Also, we're eating the most delicious food—every time I go marketing, I try one new fruit and one new vegetable. I never realized how many different types there were!"

"Keep up the good work!" I congratulated her as she hurried off to her appointment.

Got Milk?

Since low-carb and low-fat diet fads began washing over the nation in successive waves starting in the early 1970s, milk consumption, especially among body-conscious girls and young women, has dropped precipitously. At the same time, there has been a steady rise in the incidence of osteoporosis among women as they enter middle age. Coincidence? I think not. Calcium, which is abundant in dairy products, makes up 40 percent of the weight of human bone. Inadequate intake of calcium, especially in young women, causes decreased bone density, which in turn can lead to debilitating fractures later in life.

Our bodies only build bone density until around age thirty. After that, all of us—men and women—gradually lose bone mass. While men can get osteoporosis—in fact, one in four men in the United States will have an osteoporosis-related fracture in his lifetime—80 percent of those affected are women. Why? Because men, on average, are bigger to begin with and consume more calcium in their diets than women, they build and maintain stronger bones. Plus, men have high levels of circulating testosterone, which protects them from bone loss throughout most of their lives. Women, on the other hand, who are particularly vulnerable to fad diets thanks to our culture's obsession with emaciated young models and celebrities, tend to restrict their calcium intake during the crucial years before they reach their peak bone density. So they may not reach their optimal bone mass by age thirty, giving them less of a reserve for later in life.

To exacerbate the problem, women begin to lose the protective effects of estrogen in their perimenopausal years—up to a decade *before* menopause—and lose it altogether in the years following their last period. Low estrogen accelerates bone loss, so women who don't build up enough bone to begin with can end up with a severe deficit, leading to osteoporosis. It's possible to slow the loss through exercise and calcium intake, but it is not possible to increase bone density beyond the level reached at that thirty-year-old peak. My twelve-year-old daughter, Samantha, rolls her eyes at me because I'm constantly telling her to drink her milk, but it's for a good reason. Women—especially in their teens and twenties—should be the last people to cut dairy out of their diets. And because there are so many low-fat and non-fat dairy options, there's no need to.

In addition to building and maintaining strong bones and teeth, calcium plays an important role in blood clotting, makes it possible for us to contract our muscles and transmit nerve impulses, and helps prevent hypertension, especially in conjunction with a low-sodium diet. If you don't consume enough dietary calcium to fuel these vital activities, calcium will be released from your bones to your bloodstream to make up the deficit, further jeopardizing your bone density. The recommended daily intake for calcium is 1,300 mg a day for children ages nine to eighteen, 1,000 mg a day for adults up to age fifty, and 1,200 mg a day thereafter, except for postmenopausal women who are not taking hormone supplements, who need 1,500 mg a day. If you eat much more than that or take a high dose of calcium supplements, the excess will be excreted. Because calcium supplements can put you at risk for kidney stones, it is much better to get your calcium from food, which also contains other vitamins and minerals that increase calcium absorption.

Recent studies have suggested that people who eat more calcium weigh less and have a lower percentage of body fat, indicating that calcium may

Top Calcium Sources

To help you keep track of how much calcium you're consuming, here's a list of the top food sources of calcium:

Food	Calcium Content (mg)
1 cup plain non-fat yogurt	452
3 ounces canned sardines, with bones	372
1 cup low-fat fruit-flavored yogurt	345
1 ounce Parmesan cheese	336
½ cup part-skim ricotta cheese	335
1 ounce Romano cheese	302
1 cup non-fat or low-fat milk	301
1 cup soymilk	300
1 ounce Swiss cheese	272
1 cup cooked spinach	244
1 cup oysters	226
1 cup cooked collard greens	218
1 ounce part-skim mozzarella cheese	207
1 ounce cheddar cheese	202
1 cup rice milk	200
1 cup cooked rhubarb	174
3 ounces canned salmon, with bones	167
1 ounce feta cheese	140
1 cup cooked fresh soybeans (edamame)	131
½ cup raw tofu (not silken)	128
½ cup frozen yogurt	120

There are also a number of calcium-enriched food products available, particularly cereals and breakfast snacks. Just be certain to read the rest of the nutrition label carefully to make sure these foods contain adequate fiber and are not high in fat or calories or loaded with added sugars.

play a role in healthy weight maintenance. Whether or not it promotes weight loss is still a matter of debate. Still, there are compelling reasons to include plenty of calcium in your weight-loss plan. Calcium reduces blood pressure, and hypertension—a common side effect of obesity—increases the risk of heart disease. It has also been shown that men who consume a lot of low-fat dairy in their diets have a significantly reduced risk of type 2 diabetes than men who don't eat much dairy. Furthermore, losing weight in and of itself causes bone loss, so it is especially important to include calcium-rich foods in any weight-loss plan. To make sure you get enough calcium, the Reality Diet includes a minimum of two servings of dairy each day, as well as an array of other calcium-containing foods, including tofu, dark green leafy vegetables, low-fat cheese, and canned fish with bones.

Comfort Food

There's something about the word starch—it *sounds* heavy, as if you'll gain weight just by saying it. But starches, otherwise known as complex carbohydrates, are nothing but combinations of simple sugars, the same sugars that fuel your brain and other major organs. Starches are where plants store their energy, and when we eat starchy foods, that stored energy is transferred to us. There's a reason why the Boston Marathon organizers serve 20,000 runners a spaghetti feast the night before the race. Starches can also be great sources of vitamins, minerals, phytonutrients, and fiber. Think of potatoes, corn, peas, whole grain bread, wild rice, barley, winter squash, baked beans—all starches, all good for you.

As far as starchy vegetables are concerned, pumpkin and sweet potatoes are filled with the antioxidant beta-carotene, and white potatoes pack a nutritional wallop, including vitamins B_6 and C, potassium, and even more phytonutrients. While they may be higher in natural sugar than other vegetables, starchy vegetables also contain plenty of fiber to slow the absorption of that sugar and ensure that the intestines have time to extract as many other good things from them as possible.

Whole grain products also are excellent sources of healthy starches, and in Chapter 8 you'll learn how to choose the best ones. Grains are made up of three parts: bran (the outer shell of the seed), germ (the reproductive part of the seed), and endosperm (the seed's energy reserve). Refined grains

The Scoop on Spuds

Pity the potato. Blacklisted by low-carb promoters, it has been unjustly maligned as being worse for your waistline than ice cream. I go out to eat with friends, and at the end of the meal all of their plates are empty save for sides of potatoes in various forms. Even baked potatoes have been criticized as anti-dietetic, when it's not the poor little potato's fault that people smother it with high-fat toppings like butter, bacon, cheese, and sour cream.

On their own, potatoes are one of nature's greatest inventions. Actually, that's not true. They're one of humankind's greatest inventions. You see, potatoes are one of the first and most successful examples of genetic engineering. Potatoes, which are native to South America, are part of the nightshade family, and in their original form were as poisonous as the more deadly plants in that genus. It was the Incas of Peru who, through crossbreeding experiments on terraced fields high in the Andes, developed an edible variety. To this day, if you go to a Peruvian market you will see dozens of different types of potatoes in every shade of the rainbow. After the Spanish arrived, the potato was introduced to Europe, and the rest, as they say, is history.

Potatoes in their natural state are actually one of the most healthful starches available. One medium-size potato with skin (approximately 5 ounces, or 5 inches long) is only a little more than 100 calories, yet it contains as much potassium as a banana, 20 to 25 percent of the recommended daily intake of vitamin C, and more antioxidants than any commonly eaten vegetable except broccoli. That same unassuming potato also contains 3 grams of fiber—12 percent of the recommended daily intake for women—which, in addition to its health effects, increases satiety, or the feeling of fullness between meals.

It's time we all made peace with the potato and welcomed it back onto our plates. Our tummies and our taste buds will thank us.

(basically anything made from white flour) contain only the endosperm, or the starch, which has been stripped of the fibrous and nutritious bran and the protein- and nutrient-rich germ. To make up for some of the twenty-two vitamins and minerals lost in the refining process, the federal government has required refined wheat products to be enriched with B vitamins and iron since the 1930s, and with folate, to reduce the risk of birth defects, since 1998. While it's a noble effort, enriching refined grains still deprives consumers of a host of beneficial nutrients, so whenever possible, choose whole-wheat products instead.

Switching to whole grain foods may be one of the healthiest choices you can make to lower your risk for coronary artery disease and diabetes. Whole grain foods lower triglyceride and LDL ("bad") cholesterol levels, while raising HDL ("good") cholesterol levels. They also reduce blood pressure, inflammation, and circulating homocysteine levels. The combination of vitamins, minerals, phytonutrients, and fiber in whole grains is essential to any heart-healthy diet.

Unfortunately, starchy foods can also be carriers for added sugars, saturated and trans fats, and a host of other chemical additives that are extremely bad for you. Think Twinkies, Cinnabons, Krispy Kremes, french fries, potato chips, store-bought muffins, rolls and breads that mysteriously stay fresh for months—you get the picture. The trick is to learn to distinguish between healthy starches—those that give you a nutritional bang for your buck—and unhealthy ones, which are a waste of your caloric capital.

Takeaway Tips

Carbs are an essential part of a healthy diet, providing energy for our brains and other major organs and vital nutrients to help ward off disease and keep our bodies functioning at their peak. A great way to make sure you're getting a beneficial assortment of vitamins and minerals is to select fruits and vegetables that represent a rainbow of colors. And remember to eat two servings a day of low-fat dairy (or soy) for healthy bones! Don't feel you have to skimp on the starches, either, as whole grain products are also full of nutrients and can actually help slim you down.

Chapter 3

The Pros—and Cons—of Protein

Walk over to the supplement counter at your local health food store and feast your eyes upon the vast number of protein supplements. With names like Pro Performance and Muscle Builder, they inspire visions of taut thighs and bulging biceps. You'd practically have to be a body builder just to lift those huge containers! On top of the general protein powders, there are supplements of individual amino acids that purport to bestow all kinds of magical properties—better sleep, improved mood, more beautiful hair and nails, and, of course, a slimmer body. Even at the checkout counter, you're accosted with sixteen different kinds of high-protein "energy" bars.

From the looks of it, it would appear that the American diet is woefully lacking in protein—why else would we need extra protein thrust at us from every direction? In fact, the opposite is true: The average North American diet contains far more protein than even the most enthusiastic athlete could possibly need. Supplementing or increasing consumption by following a high-protein diet only skews the balance even more, potentially leading to health problems including heart disease, kidney disease, and—yes—obesity itself!

How Protein Can Make You Fat

Back in Chapter 1, I told you about how I tried to build muscle with protein shakes in college and ended up with a spare tire instead. You'd think I'd have learned my lesson, but no! Twenty years later, I was again possessed by the urge to bulk up. This time I enlisted the help of a professional. I hired a personal trainer to train me with weights three times a week, and after each workout he would instruct me to drink a huge protein shake. Over the course of six months I went from 185 to 215 pounds. My trainer thought I looked terrific. Then one day I took a long hard look at myself in the mirror and realized I was totally bloated. I fired the trainer and hired Shirley DeLeon, a freelance dietitian, to help me lose the weight. Under her supervision, I took off twenty pounds in three months and was inspired to create the Reality Diet. Meanwhile, I offered Shirley a permanent position on my staff so that she could help my patients lose weight following the Reality Diet plan.

Protein and carbohydrates contain exactly the same amount of energy—4 calories per gram. So when fad diets advise you to cut the carbs and load up with protein, they're not saving you any calories. Adding protein supplements to your regular diet, the way I did, only increases your daily intake of calories, and unless you increase your exercise enough to burn those extra calories, you'll see the numbers on your scale begin to rise.

Your body needs a specific amount of protein to maintain its health and ability to function. Any additional protein you feed it can be metabolized in one of two ways. First, it can be broken down to provide energy if there's not enough glucose available. This occurs if you're not consuming enough carbohydrates, which are your body's preferred energy source. Second, if all your energy needs are met and you still have excess protein in your bloodstream, that protein will be converted to fat, just as excess carbs will. Unless you're on a severely carb-restricted diet or doing a lot of exercise, most of your excess protein intake will become fat.

Mom, Baseball, Apple Pie . . . and Steak

Americans are obsessed with red meat. In the popular imagination, beef conjures up images of cowboys herding cattle over the wide open plain—it's almost unpatriotic not to eat it. When we're children, we're told that red meat will make us big and strong. As we grow up, happy memories are formed around backyard barbecues of hamburgers and ribs. And when we're older and have an occasion to celebrate, it's steak and champagne for dinner. Unfortunately, we also have one of the highest incidences of cardiovascular disease in the world. Could there be a connection?

Down here in Miami, Shula's Steak House is *the* place to eat for football fans. The restaurant, now part of a nationwide chain, was founded by Don Shula, the coach who led the Miami Dolphins in their undefeated 1972 season. On the menu—which is printed on a football—is a 48-ounce porterhouse steak. If you eat the whole thing, you are inducted into the 48-Ounce Club. You receive a commemorative football personalized with your name and photo and signed by the coach, and you can have your name listed with the other 28,259 members on the restaurant's website. One proud member has met the challenge one hundred times!

Although I have failed to join the club, I can attest that eating that porterhouse is an awesome experience. It's awesome in terms of its nutritional statistics as well. One 48-ounce porterhouse has seven times the calories, nine times the fat, and nearly twelve times the cholesterol of a Big Mac! Rather than seeking fame for their richly marbled steaks, Shula's and other steakhouses should be ashamed of the damage they're doing to their customers' arteries.

It's time we break the connection between gorging on red meat and being a red-blooded American. To be as cool as a cowboy or as macho as a Miami Dolphin, you don't have to consume half a steer. Enjoy lean cuts of red meat in moderation, along with other sources of protein, and forgo the commemorative football.

How Much Protein Is Too Much?

As a general rule, protein should make up between 10 and 35 percent of your total daily caloric intake. For most people, 10 percent is plenty to fuel all of the body's protein needs. More than 35 percent can lead to the health problems associated with high-protein diets, and can also increase your risk of kidney and heart disease. Because many protein sources are also high in saturated fat—like a 48-ounce porterhouse, which contains 326 grams of protein and 262 grams of fat, 99 grams of which are saturated—eating more than the recommended amount of protein can lead to a host of cardiovascular problems, which I'll discuss in the following chapter.

On the Reality Diet, 25 percent of your daily calories will come from lean protein. In addition, you'll see that the menu plans emphasize a mix of protein sources: lean red meat, white meat, fish, eggs, low-fat dairy, and legumes, which include soy products. Vegetables, starches, nuts, and seeds also contribute to your daily protein intake. To make sure you don't go over the upper limit of your recommended protein intake, steer clear of starch products labeled "low-carb," such as breads, bagels, pasta. These are made with soy flour and often are enriched with wheat gluten, both of which increase the protein content to double that of regular starch products.

Joe

After playing tennis one Saturday morning, my buddy Joe and I decided to grab a bite of lunch. It was my treat, as I'd beaten him 6–4, 3–6, 7–5. Both of us are in good shape—we exercise regularly, try to eat healthfully, and keep our weight within the normal range. In addition to tennis, Joe pumps iron at a gym three times a week. Afterward, while he's in the sauna, he reads whatever men's health and fitness magazines are lying around.

"Steve, you're a doctor—can you explain something to me?" Joe asked as he dug into his fajita. "I read all these magazines and they talk about how important it is to eat protein if you're exercising. On top of that, there are a zillion ads for protein supplements and energy bars—what's the deal?"

I swallowed a bite of my turkey wrap before answering. "Listen, I'll tell you what I tell all my patients: Unless you have a particular medical condition that requires a specific therapy, there is no reason a normal person eating a balanced diet should ever need supplements of any kind. On top of that, most of us already eat way too much protein, so these protein powders and bars are totally overkill."

"What do you mean we eat too much protein?" Joe replied.

"Here—let's do a little math," I said, grabbing a paper napkin. "Now tell me exactly what you had to eat yesterday."

"For breakfast I had two poached eggs on an English muffin, a glass of milk, and a cup of coffee. I had a banana around ten, then lentil soup and a tuna-melt on whole-wheat for lunch."

"Big can of tuna or little can?" I interrupted.

Joe thought for a moment. "Probably a big can—it was a big sandwich."

"Okay, go on," I said, scribbling away.

"I munched a couple of handfuls of peanuts in the afternoon, and for dinner Marcy made salmon, Caesar salad, roasted potatoes, and asparagus. We had mango sorbet for dessert, plus a couple of glasses of chardonnay."

While Joe was talking, I was quickly approximating the number of calories and grams of protein in what he ate. When he had finished, I turned the napkin toward him.

"Now, this is just an estimate, but it looks as if you ate about 2,200 calories for the day, which is right on target for a guy like you. You also ate about 150 grams of protein. Protein has 4 calories per gram, which means you had about 600 calories worth of protein. Six hundred divided by 2,200 equals a little more than 27 percent. The recommended range for protein intake is between 10 and 35 percent of your total daily calories. You're right in that healthy range."

"So you're saying protein supplements are a waste?"

"A waste of money, a waste of calories. At your size, you probably need no more than 55 grams of protein a day—the rule of thumb is 0.8 grams per kilogram of body weight. You're already consuming nearly three times that amount."

"So what's happening to that extra protein?" Joe asked.

"Because of all the exercise you do, you're burning it up. In someone less active, it would turn into fat."

"In that case," Joe said, slurping up the last of his iced tea, "we'd better play two games next Saturday!"

What's the Deal with Eggs?

I can't tell you how many times a day I hear this from my patients. And it's no wonder they're confused. For years researchers told us to avoid egg yolks because they were high in cholesterol and contributed to heart disease. Then the scientists realized that the cholesterol you eat has very little to do with cholesterol levels in your blood, and eggs were redeemed. Both the Nurses' Health Study and the Health Professionals Study, two enormous long-term epidemiological studies, show that eating an egg a day is perfectly fine and doesn't increase your risk of heart disease, *except* if you're diabetic. Because insulin resistance magnifies the adverse effects of cholesterol, diabetics need to restrict their consumption of egg yolks.

For non-diabetic people, this is good news, as eggs are low in calories and are a rich source of protein, B vitamins, and, when the hens are fed flaxseed, omega-3 fatty acids. Look for organic eggs from free-range or pastured hens—they're a little more expensive but a lot more flavorful and nutritious than standard supermarket eggs. If you're diabetic, you should consult with your physician and, if you need to restrict your consumption of egg yolks, use an egg substitute or, even better, just use the whites from organic eggs.

The Pros of Protein

The human body contains somewhere between 10,000 and 50,000 different kinds of proteins, of which scientists have studied only about a thousand. Among those they've identified are proteins like collagen, which gives structure to your skin, teeth, hair, nails, and bones, and elasticity to your tendons, ligaments, and artery walls. There's also hemoglobin, which carries oxygen in your red blood cells, and the hormone insulin. Antibodies, the linchpin of the immune system, are giant protein molecules. Plus, there are innumerable enzymes made of protein that facilitate the billions of chemical reactions that are taking place in your body at any given time. In addition, protein is essential for growth and repair—and not just when you're a child or when you're injured. Day in and day out, your body is making new cells, largely of protein, replacing old ones at a steady rate. Cells in your digestive tract are replaced every three days, and skin cells are replaced once a month. Muscle cells grow larger and stronger when you exercise, and hair and nails grow without your doing anything at all.

Proteins are made up of amino acids, which are often called the "building blocks" of proteins. There are only twenty different amino acids, but they can be combined in a nearly infinite variety of ways. Our bodies can manufacture eleven of the twenty amino acids in sufficient amounts. The other nine, however, we must obtain from food. Those nine are called essential amino acids because it is essential that we consume them for our bodies to function.

The best way to acquire essential amino acids is by eating protein from a variety of high-quality sources—sources that contain all the essential amino acids in the proportions that the human body needs. High-quality proteins include those that come from animals, such as meat, fish, poultry, dairy, and eggs, as well as products made of soy protein and the "supergrains" quinoa, buckwheat, and amaranth. All other plant proteins are considered lower quality because they contain less protein on an ounce-per-ounce basis than animal sources and they do not contain a full complement of essential amino acids. That's why vegetarians, especially those who don't eat dairy or eggs, have to make sure to eat combinations of foods that together contain a full complement of essential amino acids. For you Latinos, that would mean rice and beans.

From a weight-loss point of view, it is important to include adequate protein in your diet because it helps you feel full. Numerous studies have shown that when people are fed a high-protein meal or snack, they remain hunger-free for longer periods of time than people who are given high-carbohydrate foods. They also consume fewer calories at their next meal. Why this occurs is still a mystery to scientists. What isn't a mystery is why people lose weight on high-protein diets—essentially, people who go on them end up limiting the total number of calories they eat because they simply aren't that hungry.

The Dark Side of Protein

As healthful and important as protein is, you can have too much of a good thing. As I mentioned above, excess protein can be metabolized into glucose or fat. In either case, your blood becomes more acidic. In response, your bones release calcium into your bloodstream to neutralize the acidity. This puts you at risk for both osteoporosis and kidney stones. Excreting the by-products of protein metabolism puts a strain on your kidneys and can be extremely dangerous for people with underlying renal disease or diabetes.

While I do recommend consuming red meat if you like it, as it is both a high-quality protein and an excellent source of iron and antioxidants, don't overdo it. Animal protein often comes coupled with animal fat, which tends to be saturated and therefore bad for your heart. Too much red meat, especially organ meats (liver, brains, kidneys, sweetbreads), shellfish, beans, anchovies, and gravies can also lead to the "rich man's disease," gout, which occurs when crystals of uric acid—a by-product of the metabolism of certain proteins—accumulate in the joints. Furthermore, eating a lot of meat and eggs can also raise the level of the amino acid homocysteine in your blood, a marker that is considered an independent risk factor for heart disease.

A diet high in protein inevitably will be low in something else—usually carbohydrates, because protein and fat intake are often linked. The danger here is that if you fill up on meat, poultry, fish, and eggs, you will be missing out on the enormous variety of nutrients contained in fruits, vegetables, dairy, and whole grains. Plus, animal sources of protein do not contain fiber, which is a hugely important ingredient for good health and successful weight loss.

The Joy of Soy

Not long ago, soy products were considered "hippie" food, familiar only to vegetarians and Asian food enthusiasts who dared to venture beyond spare ribs and chow mein. Now soy is everywhere, from the Tofutti Cuties in the ice cream department to the Boca Burgers in the frozen food section. Soy nut butter is replacing peanut butter in school cafeterias and boxed soy milk is available in bulk at warehouse clubs. For vegetarians and vegans (who don't eat dairy or eggs), soy is a great choice, as it provides a complete assortment of essential amino acids. It's also full of nutrients: calcium, copper, iron, magnesium, phosphorus, potassium, and zinc. Some soy foods, such as tempeh and soy flour, contain fiber as well.

Even for nonvegetarians, soy products are worth a try because they're full of phytonutrients—compounds found only in plants that may promote health and reduce risk of disease. Phytoesterols, found in full-fat soy foods and soybean oil, have been shown to reduce cholesterol levels and may also decrease the risk of colon cancer. Phytoestrogens, which include isoflavones, lignans, and coumestans, may ease peri- and menopausal symptoms such as hot flashes, mood swings, insomnia, memory lapses, and migraines, help prevent osteoporosis, and reduce the risk of uterine cancer. There's also mounting evidence that the reduced rate of breast cancer in Asian women is linked to their high consumption of soy.

While soy may seem like a wonder food, there are certain circumstances under which you should avoid soy products. Specifically, if you are a woman and suffer from heavy menstrual bleeding, fibroids, or endometriosis, steer clear of soy, as it will exacerbate your symptoms. Also, avoid soy supplements—powders or pills—as they lack the soy protein needed to activate the soy isoflavones.

Takeaway Tips

One of my mother's favorite sayings is: "Moderation in all things." Nutritionally speaking, this applies particularly well to protein. On the one hand, it's important to eat enough high-quality protein to obtain the essential amino acids your body cannot make. On the other hand, it's important not to go overboard and put yourself at risk for the often serious complications of a high-protein diet. Try to eat protein from a variety of plant and animal sources, and be sure to choose the leanest options available: strip steak over prime rib, pork tenderloin over bacon. Your heart and your kidneys will thank you.

Chapter 4

The Fats of Life

Humanity's love affair with fat is timeless. Back when we were living in caves and gnawing meat directly off the bone, fat was an important part of our diet. We weren't counting calories back then—in fact, if we had been, we would have been trying to consume as many as possible, as there was no guarantee when we might next enjoy a good meal. Because fat contains more than twice as many calories per gram as carbohydrates and protein—9 versus 4—eating it is one of the most efficient ways to obtain energy. And in those days, before cars and central heating, we needed a lot of energy just to survive. So when a big fat piece of flesh came into our hands, we went to town (or we would have, if towns had been invented).

Nowadays, we don't need to consume as many calories, and we certainly don't need as much fat as our prehistoric ancestors. And yet our brains, which were hardwired way back then, still crave the taste, smell, and texture of fat. That's why it's so hard to resist the tantalizing aromas of fast food, which generally come from cooking fat. Ditto the tub of buttered popcorn at the movies, the steaming hot dog on the street corner, and the fresh-baked cookies at the mall. More than any other nutrient, fat stimulates our sense of smell. When those olfactory nerves begin tingling, they send instant messages to the amygdala, the pleasure center of the brain, which in turn sends messages to the conscious part of our brain compelling us to eat.

So fighting the urge to gorge on fat is an uphill battle, but it's one that can be won. And the most effective strategy is not to eliminate fats altogether. Low-fat diets are notoriously difficult to maintain because fat gives food great taste and texture—or "mouth feel," as culinary professionals call it—which plays a huge role in helping us feel psychically satisfied, rather than deprived. Fat helps us feel physically satisfied as well, because it slows the breakdown of carbohydrates so we fill up quicker and can go a longer time without feeling hungry. Our bodies also need fats to help absorb and transport the fat-soluble vitamins A, D, E, and K. Furthermore, certain fats actually promote good health and should be eaten regularly as part of a balanced diet.

By far the best way to satisfy your taste buds and protect your health is to include a moderate amount of heart-healthy fats in your diet. To help you choose the right fats, let's take a look at the different kinds and how they affect your body.

The Bad Guys

Because life expectancy was low in the hunter-gatherer era, people didn't live long enough to suffer the kinds of diseases that plague modern human beings, including cardiovascular disease, which is now the number-one killer in the United States. Cardiovascular disease occurs when cholesterol deposits stick to artery walls, narrowing and stiffening them until either the blood supply to the heart is cut off and you have a heart attack, or a clot forms and travels to the brain and you have a stroke.

The primary culprit in cardiovascular disease is saturated fat, the kind found in red meat, among other foods. Since our ancestors were more afraid of dying from starvation, infected wounds, or hypothermia than from heart attacks, they could eat red meat with abandon. Unfortunately—or fortunately, depending how you look at it—times have changed.

Saturated fats are easily identifiable as fats that are solid at room temperature. They also generally come from animal products. Fatty cuts of beef and pork are high in saturated fats, as are beef tallow, lard, whole milk, cream, butter, and cheese. Other sources of saturated fats include cocoa butter, tropical oils—coconut, palm, and palm kernel oils—and products that contain them, such as candies and commercially baked cookies, cakes, pies, and doughnuts.

Saturated fats are no more fattening than other fats—all fats contain the same number of calories per gram. The reason they are so bad for you is that they raise the level of LDL ("bad") cholesterol in your body. Study after study has shown that reducing dietary intake of saturated fat lowers blood levels of LDL cholesterol and lowers the risk of heart attack.

The Good Fats

One of the best ways to cut back on bad fats is to substitute good ones. Healthful, unsaturated fats come in two forms: monounsaturated and polyunsaturated. Monounsaturated fats are the most beneficial for the heart, not only reducing LDL ("bad") cholesterol, but increasing HDL ("good") cholesterol as well. Foods that contain monounsaturated fats include olive, canola, sesame, and peanut oils, sesame seeds, peanuts and peanut butter, nuts (almonds, cashews, hazelnuts, macadamias, pecans, pine nuts, and pistachios), olives, and avocados. Olive oil is particularly good for your heart, researchers have recently discovered, because it contains a naturally occurring anti-inflammatory chemical called oleocanthal that can have effects similar to those of drugs like ibuprofen and aspirin. Extravirgin olive oil has the greatest benefit, although you don't have to buy the most expensive brand.

So right away you can begin by substituting olive or canola oil for butter or lard when you're sautéing. Rather than reach for a cream cheese–laden bagel, try a fresh avocado with a sprinkling of olive oil and balsamic vinegar. For a snack, instead of store-bought cookies, try a handful of unsalted mixed nuts.

Nuts provide a particularly healthful type of fat, as in addition to being unsaturated, they also contain an amino acid called arginine. Arginine is a precursor of nitric oxide, which relaxes the linings of your blood vessels and prevents platelets from sticking to them, thereby preventing blood clots that can lead to a heart attack or stroke. In addition, several population studies have shown that nuts protect against cardiovascular disease and reduce the risk of type 2 diabetes. Nuts also contain high amounts of magnesium, copper, folic acid, potassium, fiber, and vitamin E.

Nuts are one of nature's best snack foods. Just be careful not to overdo

The Oil of the Future?

There's a new vegetable oil on the market that may be even better for your heart and your waistline than olive or canola oil. It's called Enova oil. Already the top premium cooking oil in Japan, where it was developed, Enova oil is produced from soy and canola oils and can be used exactly the way you use regular cooking oil—in salad dressings, for baking, and for sautéing.

Unlike regular vegetable oil, which is metabolized into triglycerides that can end up stored as fat in our bodies, Enova oil cannot be converted into triglycerides. Instead, it is immediately broken down in the liver and used for energy. Studies have shown that substituting Enova oil for regular cooking oil results in a smaller increase in circulating triglycerides after eating. After twelve weeks, diabetics who used Enova oil had 39.4 percent lower triglyceride levels than diabetics who used ordinary vegetable oil. Enova oil may also help prevent fat storage—studies in both Japan and the United States showed that people who used Enova oil had lower total fat mass than people who used vegetable oil.

While researchers are still exploring other potential benefits of Enova oil, it has been generally recognized as safe by the FDA and is definitely worth a try. It's pricier than vegetable oil, but if you have elevated triglycerides, it may be a worthwhile investment.

it—nuts are highly caloric, and as the saying goes, "you can't eat just one." Once I told a patient about the benefits of nuts and suggested he incorporate them into his diet. Forty-eight hours later I got a desperate phone call from his wife. "Dr. Schnur, you've got to tell him to stop with the nuts! He's eaten two cans in the past two days. When I told him to quit, he said, 'But Dr. Schnur said they were good for me!'"

Omega-3's and Omega-6's

Polyunsaturated fats include what are known as essential fatty acids. These are molecules that our bodies cannot make and that we have to get from food. There are two types of essential fatty acids: omega-3's and omega-6's. You've probably heard a lot about omega-3's—they're the reason you're supposed to eat at least two servings of fish a week. The statistics relating fish consumption to cardiovascular health are truly astounding: In one study, women who ate fish two to four times a week were 40 percent less likely to suffer a stroke than women who ate very little fish; in another, men who consumed 7 ounces or more of fish a week had a 59 percent lower risk of having a fatal heart attack than men who consumed less than 2 ounces of fish a week. Eskimos who eat a traditional diet, which is extremely high in fat, have surprisingly low cholesterol. The reason is that the source of the fat that they're eating is mostly fish.

In addition to reducing the risk of cardiovascular disease, the anti-inflammatory properties of omega-3's may have protective effects against arthritis and diabetes. Omega-3's stabilize the cholesterol plaques that build up in your arteries, therefore preventing them from rupturing and causing major heart attacks. Some studies have also shown omega-3's to reduce symptoms of depression and bipolar disorder. In spite of popular claims, however, I can't guarantee that they'll cause your skin to be wrinkle-free or have a youthful glow.

On a recent trip to the supermarket, I was amazed at how many products are now enriched with omega-3 fatty acids—cereals, waffles, eggs. Natural sources of omega-3 fatty acids include wheat germ, cashews, flaxseed and flaxseed oil, walnuts and walnut oil, soybeans and soybean oil, and fatty fish (herring, mackerel, salmon, shad, sardines, anchovies, lake trout, bluefish, most species of whitefish, and albacore tuna). There is a difference between marine- and plant-derived omega-3's, however, and recent research suggests that men should not go out of their way to increase their consumption of omega-3's or take ALA (alpha-linolenic acid) supplements, as they may increase the risk of prostate cancer.

Omega-6 fatty acids are also good for your cardiovascular health, but because they are inflammatory agents, should not be consumed excessively. On average, Americans consume six times more omega-6's than omega-3's;

A Word of Caution

Before you raid the fish counter, do keep a couple of caveats in mind. Unfortunately, many of the rivers, lakes, and oceans where fish are caught and farmed are polluted with industrial waste. For decades, for example, General Electric dumped tons of PCBs (polychlorinated biphenyls) into the Hudson River in New York state; these chemicals formed a toxic sludge that lined the bottom of the river. PCBs, combined with various other industrial wastes, killed off the majority of the native fish, and now—around thirty years after PCBs were banned—the few fish that survive are still too contaminated for human consumption.

Similarly, years of unreserved dumping of industrial waste into the oceans has contaminated them with methylmercury. Because animals store toxins in their fat cells, large fatty fish such as shark, swordfish, king fish, tuna, and mackerel tend to have relatively high concentrations of mercury and should be eaten sparingly, especially by pregnant and nursing women. The waters where salmon are farmed may be contaminated by pesticide runoff, so try to limit your intake of farmed salmon to once or twice a month. If you have a choice between wild salmon and farmed salmon, choose the wild (canned salmon is almost always wild), as it will be lower in pesticides and other toxins.

In addition to PCBs and methylmercury, other hazardous chemicals responsible for fish contamination include chlordane, dioxins, and DDT. Be aware of news reports that mention finding any of these chemicals in your local waterways, and avoid eating locally caught fish if they do.

Because omega-3 fish oil supplements, which are available at health food stores, are made from the skins and livers of fish, they can have high concentrations of mercury and PCBs, as well as excessive amounts of vitamins A and D, which can be hazardous to your health. If you eat a healthful diet, there is no reason to take them. For patients of mine who have high triglycerides and documented coronary artery disease, I recommend the prescription omega-3 drug Omacor, which is purified and contains no toxic chemicals.

ideally, we should cut back to at most a 3-to-1 ratio in order to achieve both cardiovascular and anti-inflammatory effects. Foods that contain omega-6's include all nuts, vegetable oils, nonhydrogenated margarine, and pumpkin, sunflower, and sesame seeds. Meat, poultry, and eggs also contain omega-6 fatty acids, so by substituting a piece of broiled fish for a strip of steak, you're not only reducing your saturated fat intake, but also increasing your omega-3 to omega-6 ratio. Other ways to increase your omega-3's include consuming more flaxseeds and flaxseed oil, walnuts and walnut oil, or soybeans and soybean oil.

Cholesterol 101

I've noticed a lot of confusion among my patients about cholesterol, so I thought I'd take a moment here to explain the different types of cholesterol and how they affect your cardiovascular health. Cholesterol is simply a type of fat—or lipid—molecule with a particular shape. It is the building block for many important compounds in your body, including bile acids, sex hormones, adrenal hormones, and vitamin D (which your body makes in response to sunlight), and serves as a structural component of cell membranes. Most of the cholesterol in your body is made by your liver—*it does not come from the cholesterol you eat.* This is a popular misconception. People think that the first thing they should do when they have high cholesterol is stop eating cholesterol. In fact, saturated fats are a far greater source of high blood cholesterol than dietary cholesterol.

Dietary cholesterol is found exclusively in animal products: meat, eggs, fish, poultry, and dairy products. Vegetables, fruits, and grains are naturally cholesterol-free, which is why I always have to laugh when I see bread labeled "low cholesterol" at the supermarket. For people with extremely high cholesterol, I do recommend limiting consumption of red meat and eggs,

The Really Bad Fats: Trans Fats

The problem with cooking oils is that after a while, they react chemically with the oxygen in the air and become rancid. If you're a food manufacturer who is trying to produce and ship food that is destined to sit on supermarket shelves and in kitchen cabinets for weeks without going bad, this is a challenge. To overcome this problem, the food industry came up with a way to stabilize unsaturated fats through a process called hydrogenation. The result is what are known as trans-fatty acids. Trans fats are as bad as—if not worse than—saturated fats in terms of cardiovascular health, raising LDL cholesterol and increasing certain inflammatory markers in the blood that are independent risk factors for heart disease and diabetes.

Trans fats are most commonly found in highly processed foods, such as store-bought pastries, cookies, and doughnuts, crackers, snack chips, microwave popcorn, imitation cheese, and fast foods. They are also present in shortening, nondairy creamers, and solid margarines. Thanks to the negative publicity trans fats have received in recent years, many major food producers are curbing their use of these hazardous ingredients. Many products now announce that they are "trans fat–free" on their labels, and foods like margarine, that used to be loaded with trans fats, are now available in soft, nonhydrogenated forms. Food manufacturers are required to list the trans fat content of their products on nutrition labels. You'll notice that there is no "% daily value" amount next to trans fats. That is because you should try to avoid them altogether.

but for the general population it's fine to eat lean meat, low-fat dairy, and eggs in moderation.

The liver produces between 800 and 1,500 milligrams of cholesterol a day, far more than most people consume on a regular basis. That cholesterol is bound up with triglycerides, which are also produced by the liver, and circulating proteins to form lipoproteins (lipid plus protein). There are two main types of lipoproteins, low-density lipoproteins (LDL) and high-density lipoproteins (HDL). LDLs are considered "bad" because they hang out in the bloodstream, packed with cholesterol. This makes them more likely to clog arteries. HDL, by contrast, mops up excess cholesterol and takes it back to the liver for recycling or disposal, so it is considered "good."

Triglycerides are another form of lipid that can accumulate in your bloodstream and put you at risk of cardiovascular disease. When you eat more calories than you need, regardless of whether they come from carbohydrates, fats, or proteins, the excess nutrients are converted to triglycerides. This raises your blood levels of triglycerides, putting you at greater risk of cardiovascular disease. On the Reality Diet, patients have experienced significant drops in their triglyceride levels because they're balancing their diet and exercise so there isn't an excess of triglycerides in their bloodstream.

The best way to reduce your total cholesterol, LDL, and triglycerides is to lose weight by following the Reality Diet, which is low in saturated fat and refined carbohydrates, and by exercising. Your doctor may also prescribe cholesterol-lowering drugs, known as statins, which can reduce dangerous lipid levels dramatically. Even if you're taking cholesterol medication, however, it's still important to achieve a healthy weight through diet and exercise. Just be careful—I've seen side effects ranging from muscle aches to impaired liver function when patients for whom I've prescribed statin drugs have gone on to either take nutritional supplements or follow fad diets. Patients of mine on the Reality Diet who are also taking statin drugs have experienced no side effects.

The CRP Connection

One of the most frustrating things about being a cardiologist who's committed to preventive medicine is the number of patients I meet for the first time *after* they've had a heart attack. Their cholesterol levels are normal—in fact, half of all people stricken by heart attacks have normal cholesterol readings—so their internists had no obvious indication that they were high risk and no reason to send them to me earlier. But what many of these patients do have is a cluster of symptoms known as metabolic syndrome (also called insulin resistance, pre-diabetes, or Syndrome X), which includes mild hypertension, elevated glucose levels, high triglycerides, low levels of HDL cholesterol, and high levels of a blood marker called C-reactive protein (CRP).

CRP is a protein that is made in the liver, in the walls of coronary arteries, in abdominal fat cells, and potentially elsewhere in the body, which is released under conditions of inflammation. People with rheumatoid arthritis or gum disease, for example, have high levels of CRP. Whether CRP itself causes arteries to harden or blood clots to form, or whether it is merely a marker for other conditions that cause cardiovascular disease is still under debate. What is certain, however, is that an elevated CRP level is a risk factor for heart disease totally independent of cholesterol, and reducing CRP lowers the risk of heart attack. CRP can be lowered through lifestyle changes—weight loss, exercise, cessation of smoking—or, it has been discovered recently, through statin drugs, the same drugs that are used to control cholesterol.

So that you don't end up meeting your cardiologist for the first time in the emergency room, encourage your internist to test your blood not only for the standard lipid profile (total cholesterol, LDL, HDL, and triglycerides), but also for CRP, especially if you have risk factors for heart disease. Below is a chart showing low, borderline, and high risk levels for each of these markers (mg/dL = milligrams per deciliter; mg/L = milligrams per liter).

Blood Lipid and CRP Levels

Indicator	Low Risk	Borderline	High Risk
Total cholesterol	below 200 mg/dL	200–239 mg/dL	above 239 mg/dL
LDL cholesterol	below 130 mg/dL	130–159 mg/dL	above 159 mg/dL
HDL cholesterol	above 60 mg/dL	59–40 mg/dL	below 40 mg/dL
Triglycerides	below 150 mg/dL	150–199 mg/dL	above 199 mg/dL
CRP	below 1.0 mg/L	1.0-3.0 mg/L	above 3.0 mg/L

Joan

Joan was out to dinner with her husband at a hot new fusion restaurant, celebrating their twenty-fifth anniversary, when she suddenly groaned and slumped forward, her head hitting her plate. It was pure luck that a doctor was sitting in the booth next to hers and, realizing that she may have had a heart attack, immediately forced an aspirin down her throat and instructed the maître d' to call an ambulance. When Joan got to the hospital the emergency staff diagnosed a major heart attack—three of her arteries were completely blocked, and the other two were 50 percent blocked. She had emergency bypass surgery that very night.

The next day I met Joan and I was, frankly, surprised. She was fifty-five and no more than twenty pounds overweight. Consulting her chart, I could see that while her total and LDL cholesterol were in the normal range, her HDL was low and her triglycerides and CRP were high. I could also tell, just from the outline of the sheet over her body, that those twenty extra pounds were all in her stomach—her arms and legs were actually quite thin. Without even seeing her blood glucose level—which, when she was tested later, turned out to be elevated—I surmised that she had metabolic syndrome.

Talking to Joan's husband, Bill, I found out that they both worked hard to support three college-age children, Joan as a trade lobbyist, Bill as a pharmaceutical sales rep. Both traveled quite a bit for their jobs, so they ate out frequently and didn't have a regular exercise routine. "Well, that's exactly where you're going to be making some big changes," I informed him.

A few weeks later, when Joan was up and about, she came into my office. Before having her meet with Shirley and get educated about the Reality Diet, I performed a full blood workup and talked to her about the importance of improving her diet and committing to an exercise routine if she were to avoid another heart attack.

"Restaurant food is notoriously high in saturated fat, and that's absolutely the worst for someone with metabolic syndrome. You see how your extra pounds are in your abdominal region?" I asked her.

Joan blushed and gave a small sigh. "Yes, my waistline has always been a struggle," she confessed.

"Abdominal fat acts differently than other fat," I continued. "It produces triglycerides and C-reactive protein, both of which are bad for cardiovascular health. It also may affect how the liver deals with insulin, which may contribute to insulin resistance."

Joan looked overwhelmed—clearly I was throwing too much information at her.

"Here," I said, turning the computer monitor toward her so she could see her medical records up on the screen. "The amount of sugar circulating in your blood is high, which means that your cells are not responding normally to insulin, the hormone that's supposed to help get sugar out of your bloodstream. We call this insulin resistance—part of what's known as metabolic syndrome. People with metabolic syndrome have triple the risk of heart attack and stroke and five times the risk of developing type 2 diabetes than people who don't. The only proven cure for insulin resistance is weight loss, which is why I'm sending you to Shirley. If you don't take care of it and continue to eat poorly and not exercise, you'll end up with diabetes and, most likely, another heart attack."

I must have scared the daylights out of poor Joan, because later that afternoon Shirley cornered me in my office.

"What did you tell that woman?" she demanded. "I've never seen someone so desperate to begin the Reality Diet!"

We knew Joan was serious about changing her habits, and sure enough, the pounds started to melt away. Within three months she had lost the twenty pounds. In addition to following the menu plans at home and taking advantage of our dining-out tips when she was on the road, she committed to a serious exercise program. One or two times a week she did free-weights, which she chose because she could pack them in her suitcase easily when she traveled, and five times a week she did speedwalking, which easily fit into her peripatetic lifestyle.

More impressive than her weight loss was the change in Joan's blood profile. In only three months her total cholesterol decreased from 160 to 140, her LDL decreased from 99 to 89, and her HDL, which had been low, increased from 39 to 42, bringing her out of the high-risk category. In addition, her triglycerides decreased from 160 to 125, which is in the normal range, her CRP came down from 6.7 to 5.1, and her fasting glucose also improved, from 151 to 104.

"You're our star patient," I told Joan when she came in for her next checkup.

"You know, when you first explained my situation to me, I was petrified," Joan said. "I realized it was a life-or-death choice I had to make. Under those circumstances, it's easy to stay motivated."

Diagnosing Metabolic Syndrome

In April 2005, the International Diabetes Federation released a new definition of metabolic syndrome to increase early detection and treatment, with the hope of ultimately reducing the incidence of cardiovascular disease. The new criteria are:

Central obesity—waist equal to or more than 37 inches (94 cm) for men and 31.5 inches (80 cm) for women—together with *two or more* of the following:

- Elevated triglycerides of at least 150 milligrams per deciliter (1.7 millimoles per liter)
- HDL cholesterol less than 40 mg/dL (1.04 mmol/L) for men and less than 50 mg/dL (1.29 mmol/L) for women
- Raised blood pressure of at least 130/85 mmHg
- Fasting hyperglycemia (high blood sugar) equal to or greater than 100 mg/dL (5.6 mmol/L), or previous diagnosis of diabetes or impaired glucose tolerance

Weight loss is the only sure way to reverse metabolic syndrome, so if you have any of the above signs, talk to your doctor about starting the Reality Diet.

Takeaway Tips

The most important dietary change you can make to improve your cardiovascular health and lose weight is to cut back on saturated and trans fats. Choose lean cuts of meat over fatty ones, and vegetable and olive oils over butter, lard, or hard margarine; substitute fish for meat a couple of times a week; and snack on nuts and low-fat cheese or yogurt rather than packaged baked goods or chips.

Also, think about how you cook your food—try broiling, baking, steaming, or sautéing rather than frying your meat, chicken, or fish. Marinate your main course in olive oil and vinegar or lemon juice, perhaps with a sprinkling of herbs or spices. Store-bought marinade is often full of saturated fat and salt, and can pack a stunning amount of calories.

It goes without saying that to prevent heart disease, you should stop smoking. In addition, start exercising, both to lose weight and improve your blood profile. In Chapter 9 you'll learn more about the beneficial effects of exercise and how to choose a fitness plan that fits your lifestyle.

As Joan realized, the facts speak for themselves: If you have an unhealthy blood profile—high total cholesterol, LDL, triglycerides, or CRP, or low HDL—you simply have to take action or you'll risk ending up in the emergency room. One of the results of the Reality Diet I'm most proud of is the dramatic improvement patients have seen in their blood profiles. Long before they reach their goal weights, their lipids are coming into line and their CRP levels are dropping like stones. Even if they may have many pounds to go to feel beautiful on the outside, they look beautiful on the inside, and that counts for a lot.

Part II

The Reality Diet

Chapter 5

The 2:90 Rule

Last time I went to the supermarket, I counted 150 different types of packaged bread on the shelves, including bagels and English muffins. Many sported labels with sheaves of wheat on them to indicate their healthfulness. Others had labels promoting the numbers of grains they contained — seven, ten, twelve. Still others stated that they were made with either wheat or oat bran. They all looked delicious — dark and nubby, some even had tasty seeds stuck to their crusts — and all claimed to be nutritious. How was I ever to choose?

Fortunately, I know an easy rule. Once I applied it, I was able to pop a loaf into my shopping cart, confident that the bread I'd selected contained enough of the one nutrient that would make it worth its calories. A nutrient that can be obtained only from carbohydrate-containing foods, and one proven to reduce the risk of heart disease, gastrointestinal problems, and insulin resistance. The nutrient that is the single best predictor of success when it comes to weight loss.

Fiber.

The Skinny on Fiber

Fiber is the structural part of plants that cannot be broken down by human digestive enzymes. Among its many attributes is fiber's ability to promote satiety—in other words, it makes you feel satisfied, or full. Satiety is one of the keys to successful weight loss, because no matter how much willpower you have, if your stomach is growling and you pass a Dunkin' Donuts, you'll be hard-pressed to resist. If you're completely full, however, you'll have an easier time passing it by. The federal government recommends that adults consume a minimum of 25 grams of fiber per day. On a good day, most Americans consume 12 to 17 grams, and according to an article in the *New England Journal of Medicine,* four popular fad diets—Atkins, Ornish, Weight Watchers, and Zone, provide an average of 15 grams per day. It's not surprising, then, that so many of us find ourselves standing in line for a chocolate glazed with sprinkles.

Fiber may also help promote weight loss by preventing the absorption of calories from the small intestine. A U.S. Department of Agriculture study showed that when a man doubled his fiber intake from 18 to 36 grams a day, he absorbed 130 fewer calories daily. Similarly, when a woman doubled her fiber intake from 12 to 24 grams a day, she absorbed 90 fewer calories daily. Over a year, that could add up to nine pounds for women and more than thirteen pounds for men!

While many fad diets recommend consuming a high amount of fiber, they leave it up to the dieter to figure out how to get it. It's especially hard to get enough fiber on low-carb diets, as fruits, vegetables, and whole grains are where most fiber comes from—fats and meat contain no fiber at all, and while a few dairy and soy products contain fiber, it's in small amounts. In designing the Reality Diet, we made sure not only to talk the talk about fiber, but to walk the walk, providing a built-in mechanism to ensure adequate fiber intake.

Not only does fiber help control weight, it also prevents disease. A century ago, before our food supply was industrialized and processing became the norm, people ate an average of 28 grams of fiber per day and diabetes, heart disease, and obesity were far less common. Even today, in cultures that eat a traditional plant-based diet (sadly, there are fewer and fewer of them), diabetes, cancer, and cardiovascular disease are still rare. By contrast, the United States currently ranks lowest in fiber intake and highest in deaths from heart disease among twenty developed countries.

The 2003 European Prospective Investigation into Cancer and Nutrition, spanning ten countries and including 519,978 participants who were observed for nearly five years, found that those with the highest amounts of fiber in their diets had a 40 percent lower risk of developing colon cancer that those with the lowest fiber intake. Other recent studies have found that increasing daily fiber intake by 6 grams lowers the risk of death from heart disease by 25 percent, and that every additional 10 grams of fiber consumed on a daily basis cuts the risk of death from heart disease by 27 percent. Fiber has been proven to lower triglyceride, LDL-cholesterol, C-reactive-protein, and blood-pressure levels—all independent risk factors for heart attack and stroke. Plus, it is found in foods that are full of other health-promoting nutrients.

While you easily can increase your fiber intake through supplements, I do not recommend them. Foods that are rich in fiber are also packed with vitamins, minerals, and antioxidants, which fiber supplements cannot provide.

Slow Food Versus Fast Food

One of the problems with fast food is exactly that—that it's fast. I don't mean fast in the sense that you can pull into the drive-thru, order your meal, and be back on the road in ninety seconds or less. I mean fast in the sense that it's digested fast—it moves through your body quickly, leaving you deprived nutritionally and craving another fix.

It's far and away better to eat slow food—not necessarily food that takes a long time to prepare, but food that takes a long time to digest. Think of an apple, which is a slow food, versus apple juice, which is fast. The benefit of slow food is that it keeps you full for a long time by delaying the emptying of food from your stomach into your small intestine. Slow foods also allow for the gradual absorption of nutrients from your small intestine into your bloodstream.

So, what determines the speed of digestion? Fiber. High-fiber foods are digested much more slowly than low-fiber foods. This has significant implications for people with metabolic syndrome. With the popularization of the glycemic index theory, people with metabolic syndrome have been counseled to avoid starches and many other carbohydrate-containing foods because it is believed that these foods will lead to spikes in blood sugar and elevated insulin responses. This advice completely contradicts the latest scientific research.

A recent review article in the *Journal of Clinical Endocrinology & Metabolism* comparing popular glycemic-index-based low-carb diets to a high-fiber, high-carbohydrate diet emphasizing fresh fruits and vegetables concluded that it was the fiber content of the foods eaten, not their glycemic index, that was the best indicator of insulin sensitivity. While not a weight-loss diet, a classic Mediterranean diet, which is high-carbohydrate, high-fiber, and full of fruit, vegetables, whole grains, walnuts, and olive oil, has been shown over and over to be one of the best diets for improving metabolic syndrome. Because fiber slows the absorption of nutrients into the bloodstream, it naturally regulates blood sugar levels, eliminating insulin surges and reducing insulin resistance. It's clear that the best way to manage metabolic syndrome and decrease all of the cardiovascular risks that accompany it is by eating a diet high in complex carbohydrates, with at least 25 grams of fiber a day. And patients on the Reality Diet are proving that every day.

Carmen

In her youth, Carmen was a competitive salsa dancer. She wowed judges nationwide with her dramatic style, which was enhanced by her wide smile, sultry dark eyes, and magnificent figure. In her late twenties, Carmen settled down, married, had two children, and embarked on a second career as a homemaker. She cooked up traditional Latin delights for her family, including lots of rice and beans, plantains, fried pork, and malanga fritters. Years passed, and with her relatively sedentary lifestyle and heavy diet, she began to put on pounds. By her mid-fifties, she was a good fifty pounds more than she'd been at her salsa-dancing prime.

Carmen came in to meet with Shirley and they discussed her health, her lifestyle, and her goals.

"I know I'll never be as thin as I was in my twenties—those days are over! But I'd love to feel that kind of energy again. Now I get out of breath so easily. I take care of my two-year-old granddaughter while my daughter works, and some days I can barely carry her upstairs."

"I see you're taking medication for elevated blood sugar," Shirley noted.

Carmen nodded. "My sugar is high, my pressure is high—my doctor keeps telling me I need to do something, but it's so hard. Plus, none of the diets I've seen allow any of the foods I like to eat."

"I totally understand," replied Shirley. "I'm Cuban myself, so I've made a point of making the Reality Diet compatible with ethnic cooking. You don't need to stop eating the foods you love. You just need to change how you prepare them and eat smaller servings."

Shirley then had Carmen describe the kinds of foods she ate, and, one by one, explained how Carmen could adjust her ingredients and cooking techniques to make them compatible with the Reality Diet: less rice, more beans; less meat, more vegetables; less salty canned products, more fresh — and everything cooked with vegetable oil rather than lard. She sent her home with lists of healthful substitutions and suggested meals, and made a follow-up appointment for two weeks later.

When Carmen returned, she brought with her plastic containers of homemade red beans and bread pudding that she'd made following Shirley's guidelines. "I've had such fun these past two weeks making up new recipes. Even my granddaughter likes them!" Shirley took a taste of each and proclaimed them to be delicious.

Shirley weighed Carmen and found she'd lost eight pounds. "That's a lot for the first two weeks. About half of it is probably water weight, because you've been cutting back on the salt in your cooking," Shirley explained. "Once your body gets used to eating this way, you can expect to lose one to two pounds a week. Now let's talk about exercise."

Since Carmen hadn't been exercising at all, Shirley suggested she begin slowly. "Take your granddaughter for a stroll around the neighborhood. Walk to the playground instead of driving. Play hide and seek, Simon says — games that involve physical activity rather than ones you do sitting down."

Carmen agreed to try, and over the next four months a transformation occurred. She lost thirty-five pounds, which had been her goal, lowered her blood pressure to within the normal range, and was able to go off her blood sugar medicine completely. Most important, she was filled with energy, cooking and keeping house for her daughter, as well as chasing her granddaughter around the yard. At a recent family wedding, she even got out on the floor and did a little salsa dancing. "It's like riding a bike," she told Shirley, "once you learn, you never forget!"

Research Update

While being overweight generally increases the risk of metabolic syndrome and, eventually, of diabetes, where you carry your extra pounds may give you a clue as to how vulnerable you are in particular. The Harvard Health Professionals Follow-Up Study, which has tracked more than 27,000 men for thirteen years, recently yielded an interesting correlation between men's waist size and incidence of diabetes. Men whose waists measured 37.9 to 39.8 inches had five times as great a risk as men whose waists were between 29 and 34 inches. It appears that abdominal fat tissue is especially active, making it more risky to have a big belly, for example, than a round rear. Because there's no such thing as spot reducing, the only way to trim your tummy is to commit to a weight-loss program. In addition to promoting fat loss, the Reality Diet helps prevent metabolic syndrome by promoting adequate consumption of fiber, which regulates insulin response.

The Fiber-Calorie Connection

Study after study has shown that when people are allowed to eat as much as they want of a diet high in complex carbohydrates, they end up losing weight. Why? Because the fiber fills them up and they ultimately consume fewer calories per day. Remember, it's all about the calories! While carbohydrates and proteins have the same calories per gram, fiber-rich carbohydrates are less dense calorically, so you can eat a greater volume of them without busting your calorie bank.

But what constitutes "fiber rich"? A lot of products tout their high fiber content on their packaging, but sometimes that comes at a price: high calories. In developing the Reality Diet, I spent a lot of time reading textbooks and medical journals, doing research on the Internet, and making field trips to the supermarket trying to figure out what a healthful ratio of fiber to calories might be—one that would allow a wide variety of satisfying starches and would not require adding bran flakes to every meal or drinking those nasty-tasting fiber supplements. At last, these investigations led me to formulate the 2:90 Rule. Any starch that contains a total of at least 2 grams of fiber per 90-calorie serving is legit. It's that simple! Even if there's a bit of added sugar in the ingredient list, as long as the food meets the 2:90 Rule, you can't go wrong.

Why 2:90 as opposed to 3, 4, or 5:90? Because requiring too many grams of fiber per serving would eliminate starches such as whole-wheat pasta, waffles, and many breads that are not only important nutritionally, but also delicious, filling, and simple to prepare. Why not 1:90, or 2:150? Because requiring too few grams of fiber per serving would not ensure adequate daily intake without supplements.

To see how the 2:90 Rule works, let's compare the nutrition labels from two whole-wheat breads. The label on the right below shows less than 1 gram of fiber per 110-calorie slice; the one on the left, 3 grams of fiber per 90-calorie slice. Apparently all whole-wheat breads are not created equal! The bread indicated on the right is more highly processed than that on the left, or it contains wheat and white flour instead of being 100 percent

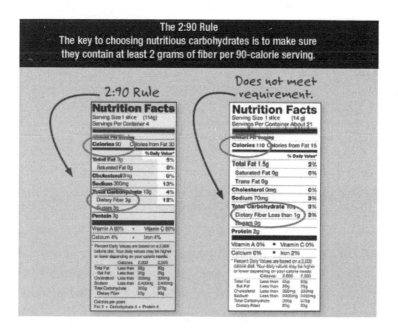

whole wheat. The bread indicated on the left meets the 2:90 Rule with 1 gram of fiber to spare and is clearly a wiser choice.

You can apply the 2:90 Rule to any starch—bread, cereal, pasta, couscous, barley, rice, frozen waffles, tortillas, prepared pizza crusts, crackers, chips, matzo, rice cakes, popcorn, bread crumbs. Once you get used to it, you'll find yourself looking for products that exceed the 2-gram requirement. In the cereal aisle, in particular, you can really have fun, as there are cereals out there with more than 10 grams of fiber per 90-calorie serving. Be careful not to buy products marked "low-carb"—most of them meet the 2:90 Rule because they are made with soy flour, which contains more fiber than wheat flour. Soy flour also contains protein, however, and can end up skewing your daily nutritional intake toward the high-protein end of the spectrum. Plus, low-carb products tend to have more fat than their ordinary counterparts. Also, be aware that some starches contain fiber additives to boost their numbers. It's much more preferable to get fiber from natural sources, such as whole grains that also contain a variety of other nutrients.

The 2:90 Rule is designed specifically to help you choose the best starches, but it really applies to virtually all carbohydrates. Most fruits and all vegetables naturally meet the 2:90 Rule (see the fruit and vegetable equivalent substitution lists, pages 383–387). Corn, peas, potatoes (with skin), carrots, squash, apples, bananas, cantaloupe, papaya—it's open season in the produce aisle! The only exceptions are grapes, watermelon, and raisins, each of which contain 1.2 grams of fiber per 90 calories. Nevertheless, I recommend that you include them in your diet as well, because they're full of other valuable nutrients. Until recently, no dairy food met the 2:90 Rule, but as I explained in Chapter 2, dairy should be consumed twice a day anyway, as it is a potent source of calcium. While it's unlikely that milk or cheese will ever be fortified with fiber, yogurt companies are now coming out with fiber-fortified yogurts that meet the 2:90 Rule. Look for them in your supermarket and use them whenever a meal or recipe calls for yogurt.

By following the 2:90 Rule and the Reality Diet menus, you'll easily meet the recommended daily intake of fiber, which is 25 grams a day for women and 38 grams a day for men. Because you'll be getting your fiber from whole foods eaten throughout the day, you'll also avoid the potentially unpleasant gastrointestinal side effects of supplements, which contain a high dose of fiber that is consumed all at once.

Takeaway Tips

The key to successful weight loss and to heart and colon health is a high-fiber diet. Once you get used to incorporating a lot of fruits and vegetables into your meals and using the 2:90 Rule to select your starches, you'll easily get enough fiber to curb your appetite and protect yourself against disease. Just remember to eat the skins of fruits and vegetables whenever possible and choose whole produce rather than juice, unless it's fiber-fortified. You can also substitute wheat germ, wheat bran, or oat bran for a starch to increase your daily intake of fiber. The 2:90 Rule automatically eliminates overly processed foods that contain lots of added sugars and promotes consumption of nutrient-dense whole grains. To ensure a comfortable transition to a high-fiber diet, make certain to drink extra water—more on that in the following chapter.

Chapter 6

The Reality Diet Plan

Now that you've learned about nutrition and the simple 2:90 Rule, you're ready to embark on the Reality Diet. Unlike any other diet you've ever been on, the Reality Diet will transform your relationship to food. One of my patients, Nadine, said that she was so satisfied by her Reality meals that, for the first time in her life, she would go for hours at a time without thinking about food. "It was a revelation to me—I'd never realized before how many of my waking hours I was spending obsessing about where my next food fix was going to come from. Now I can really focus on whatever I'm doing—work, hanging out with friends, even reading a book—without being distracted. I feel much more connected to my life now that my hunger is under control."

Many patients also report that the Reality Diet has given them a new awareness of and respect for their bodies. "After eating good, wholesome food for a while, I notice how much cleaner my body feels," one told me. "I'm honestly not tempted by the kind of junk I used to eat, because I know it will make me feel sluggish and bloated, make my skin feel greasy, and generally drag me down. It's as if I'm being good to my body, and in exchange it's giving me this gift of vibrancy and energy. I just don't want it to stop!"

First Things First

The first thing to do before starting the Reality Diet—or any new diet or exercise plan—is to visit your physician for a full checkup. If your doctor has the equipment to do a body fat analysis, have one done. If you're over forty, take a stress test and, if you're a woman, a bone densitometry scan. Also, make sure you have a complete blood workup, including thyroid hormone, lipid profile, and possibly CRP. Let your doctor know that in addition to following the diet, you will be embarking on an exercise program. If you have back or joint problems, your doctor may recommend that you avoid or pursue particular activities. Once you get the green light from your doctor, you're good to go.

On the Reality Diet you'll be eating from all of the different food groups every day, maximizing your nutritional intake through balance and variety. You also won't be restricting certain food groups, counting calories or points, or "rating" fruits and vegetables as "good" or "bad." You'll simply be eating satisfying portions of a diverse array of wholesome foods. It's that easy!

Reality Diet 101

So how does the diet work? On the most basic level, like all successful diets, it ensures you take in fewer calories than you expend. Unlike many other diets, however, that doesn't mean starving yourself or tricking your body into self-restricting by cutting out certain food groups. Rather, you'll be eating a certain number of servings from each of seven categories of healthful food. Because each meal will be filled with nutrients, healthy fats, and satisfying fiber, you'll have a continual high level of energy throughout the day without feeling hungry. Many fad diets leave you too lightheaded to exercise; the Reality Diet, by contrast, will give you plenty of energy to begin an exercise program or ramp up your existing one. Exercise isn't just for correcting dieting mistakes, but is an important component of any healthy diet—not only to burn extra calories and build muscle, which increases your basal metabolic rate, but also to protect yourself from cardiovascular disease and a host of other ailments.

The easiest way to get the hang of the Reality Diet is to follow the menus in Part IV of this book. No need to count calories, no need to worry about getting balanced nutrition or adequate fiber—Shirley has designed these meals so that you'll get everything your body needs. You'll also be eating amazing food, with recipes developed by a top food consultant, Andrew Hunter. Unless you're a professional gourmet like him, you'll find yourself being introduced to all kinds of wonderful new foods and flavor combinations. In addition to being an extraordinary chef, Andrew is also a busy dad who knows the value of quick and easy preparation. Although the dishes may sound exotic, they're all incredibly simple and tasty. I've even served them at dinner parties, to rave reviews! None of my guests could believe they were eating "diet" food.

A lot of my patients like the menu plans because they don't have to make decisions each day about what to eat, and having a set menu helps them avoid temptation in the supermarket aisles. Following the menus, even for a short time, is also a great way to teach your brain and your body the components and proportions of a well-balanced meal. In a short time you'll be able to eyeball 5 ounces of fish or ⅓ cup of cooked pasta. You'll somehow "know" at the end of the day when you've forgotten a fruit or a dairy. The habits of healthful eating will become ingrained in your subconscious, and if you break them, your body will remind you to get back on track.

For those times when you want to create your own Reality Diet menus, all you need to know are how many servings of each food group you should eat each day and what constitutes a serving. After that, it's up to you—you can distribute the food groups however you wish throughout your day; just make sure that you eat them all. The following chart indicates the daily distribution of servings, depending on whether you're a man or a woman.

As you can see, I've listed the food groups alphabetically. To remember how many servings of each I get a day, I've programmed the seven numbers into my cell phone: 422-2252. (For women, the number is 322-2141.) That way, when I'm at work or out to eat at a restaurant, I can always do a quick check to see how many servings of each food group I can have.

Reality Diet at a Glance

	Women	Men
Fats	3	4
Fruits	2	2
Milk/Yogurt	2	2
Primary Protein	2	2
Secondary Protein	1	2
Starch	4	5
Vegetables	1	2

In contrast to other diets, in which servings are defined by volume—generally, a serving of vegetables, for example, is ½ cup (enough to satisfy my two-year-old son, Dylan)—our servings are all a uniform 90 calories. So a serving of vegetables could be 1¾ cups of carrots, 3 cups of broccoli, or a whopping 18 cups of watercress! Clearly, nobody can eat 18 cups of watercress, so a serving could also be a salad composed of 1 cup of watercress, ½ cup of radicchio, 1 cup of Boston lettuce, 1 cup of tomatoes, ½ cup of cucumbers, ½ cup of mushrooms, and ½ cup of red bell peppers.

Starches should each have 2 grams of fiber per 90-calorie serving, and if you can find fiber-fortified yogurt in your local market, apply the 2:90 Rule there as well. All vegetables and most fruits naturally meet the 2:90 Rule; the only exceptions are grapes, watermelon, and raisins. As long as you're eating a variety of fruits and not exclusively those three, however, there's no reason to avoid them.

I've divided proteins into two groups because some protein sources are fattier, hence denser in calories, than others. Primary proteins are the lighter variety—chicken breast, most seafood, wild game, 95 percent fat-free turkey bacon, fat-free cheese, beans, egg whites, and deli meats or hot dogs with 1 gram of fat or less per ounce. Secondary proteins are heavier—red meat, pork, veal, dark chicken meat, fatty fish, duck, goose, rabbit, low-fat cheese, tofu, tempeh, soybeans, Canadian bacon, whole eggs, veggie burgers, and deli meats or hot dogs with between 1 and 3 grams of fat per ounce. In Part IV, you'll find lists of foods that are equivalent to one serving size from each food group.

In addition to your servings of the main food groups, you have a daily allowance of three or four "Dividends," 20-calorie portions of tasty extras you might want to use to add a little zip to your meals, for a total of 60 to 80 extra calories you can spend each day. For the price of one Dividend, you can "buy" a teaspoon of light butter for your popcorn, three tablespoons of salsa for your baked potato, or a tablespoon of steak sauce for your sirloin. You can also dress up your dessert with two tablespoons of whipped topping, a teaspoon of mini chocolate chips, or two teaspoons of marshmallow fluff—each costs only one Dividend. If you're following the menu plans, the recipes already incorporate your daily allowance of Dividends.

"Freebies" are another feature of the Reality Diet—condiments, cooking aids, drinks, and other ingredients you can enjoy liberally. You can't make a meal out of them, but they certainly can add flavor and variety to your cooking. Look for the lists of Dividends and Freebies beginning on

A Word About Salt . . .

A diet high in sodium is a significant contributor to high blood pressure, a major risk factor for cardiovascular disease. Recent research suggests sodium may also contribute to hardening of the arteries. To keep your heart as healthy as possible, it's wise to cut down on added salt. The latest federal guidelines recommend a maximum daily sodium intake of 2,300 mg (1 teaspoon of table salt) per day for healthy adults. People with hypertension, African Americans, and middle age and older folks should keep their daily intake at or below 1,500 mg.

The Reality Diet menus are carefully calibrated to be safe for all types of people. But be careful when you create your own recipes that you pay attention to the salt content of the ingredients you're using. Check the nutrition labels on canned goods, in particular, and wherever possible choose low-sodium products. On the Dividends and Freebies lists, I've indicated products that are high in sodium and should be avoided by people with hypertension. And to eliminate the temptation to add extra salt to your food, remove the saltshaker from your table.

page 395. Note that, wherever possible, I've included healthier alternatives that are often organic or caffeine- or preservative-free.

If you're following the menu plans, you'll notice that each day's recipe selection includes a Reality Reward—a delicious dessert that will make you forget you're even on a diet. One of the saddest things I see among patients who have tried other diets is how phobic they become about dessert—or, if they do indulge, how guilty they feel afterward. Life is too short! We all deserve treats now and again, and if you ask me, people making a concerted effort to live a healthier lifestyle deserve them even more. Every day you succeed on the Reality Diet—every day you eat nutritionally balanced meals and do some form of exercise—you can reward yourself with a delicious dessert made from wholesome ingredients and not feel one iota of guilt.

In addition to following the eating plan, you'll begin the Reality Diet with a new—or renewed—commitment to exercise. While you can lose weight and improve your cardiovascular health on the Reality Diet without exercising, getting active will speed up the process and confer a host of additional mental and physical benefits. Ideally, you should burn 2,000 calories a week. How you do this is up to you—you can do four supercharged 500-calorie workouts a week, or break your exercise into several small interludes each day. Everything counts, from walking up and down stairs in your house to playing in the park with your kids to gardening to housework to shooting hoops in your driveway. In Chapter 9, you'll learn exactly why from a health point of view I'm so adamant about my patients exercising. You'll also learn how to find activities you enjoy that also burn calories, how to design a sensible exercise plan, and how to work off any extra indulgences you might partake of.

Flexibility

If you choose to follow the menu plans, you'll find they're very flexible, just in case you don't like a particular food, or you find fish on sale Tuesday when it's not on the menu till Friday. Within each week, you can substitute any breakfast for any other breakfast, any lunch for any other lunch, and any dinner for any other dinner. If you like one particular breakfast, you can have it every day that week. Or if you're pressed for time, you can double a dinner recipe and eat it two nights in a row.

A Typical Day

So how does the list of servings and food groups translate into a typical day on the Reality Diet? Easily. Here's a real-life example of what one of my female patients ate on a typical day:

Breakfast

90-calorie serving 2:90 cereal	1 starch
1 cup skim milk	1 milk/yogurt
8 walnut halves	1 fat
Whole banana	1 fruit

Lunch

Sandwich:

2 slices regular 2:90 bread	2 starches
1 slice ham	½ secondary protein
1 slice low-fat cheese	½ secondary protein
Mustard and lettuce	Freebies
3 tomato slices	1 dividend
1 cup celery and ¾ cup baby carrots	½ vegetable
4 teaspoons hummus	2 dividends

Dinner

5 ounces grilled chicken breast with lemon juice	2 primary proteins, Freebie
small baked potato with olive oil	1 starch, 1 fat
1⅔ cups steamed broccoli and cauliflower	½ vegetable

Dessert/Snack

90-calorie serving 2:90 vanilla yogurt	1 milk/yogurt
½ cups raspberries	1 fruit
12 almonds	1 fat

The other way you can play around with the menus is to vary the order of the meals. As long as you eat a breakfast, lunch, dinner, and Reality Reward from the same week every day, it doesn't matter which meal you eat when. You may be out for a business lunch and find something on the menu that closely resembles one of your dinner options for that particular week. Go ahead and order it; just choose a lunch meal that night for dinner.

One of the most frequent comments Shirley and I hear from patients on the Reality Diet is that they don't normally eat breakfast and can't imagine eating everything listed on the breakfast menu first thing in the morning. My response is twofold: First, learn to eat breakfast—your mother wasn't wrong, it *is* the most important meal of the day! After twelve hours of not eating, your body and brain are starved for energy. Plus, numerous studies have shown that people who eat breakfast consume fewer calories over the course of each day than people who skip it, probably because people who skip breakfast eat high-calorie snacks mid-morning or overindulge at lunch because by that time they're ravenous.

Second, split up the breakfast if it's too much to eat at once. Eat half of it at seven, or whenever you normally wake up, and the other half at ten. Or, on a cereal and yogurt day, save the yogurt for an afternoon snack. The same thing applies to the daily Reality Reward—I've listed it after dinner, but there's no reason you can't have it in the afternoon if that's when you prefer to have something sweet. Or you may want to split it in two and have half after lunch and half after dinner—it's quite a generous serving!

Finally, because each Reality Reward is 360 calories, or four 90-calorie servings, rather than eating a single Reality Reward, you can substitute four servings of any other types of food as long as they meet the 2:90 Rule. One of my patients likes to have yogurt topped with 2:90 granola before bed, so instead of the daily Reality Reward, she has that plus an afternoon treat of 2:90 crackers and an extra piece of fruit. In addition, once a week you can splurge and use your 360 calories just for fun—a bowl of ice cream, a piece of cheesecake, a bagel and cream cheese, a couple of slices of pizza. I don't encourage doing this more than once a week, however, because the Reality Rewards are carefully designed to contain exactly the nutrients and fiber you need to complement the rest of the day's dishes. If you don't have a problem with alcohol, you can also exchange one of your weekly Reality Rewards for four alcoholic beverages, which you can spread out during the week (please, don't drink them all at once!) as long as you respect the guidelines at the end of this chapter.

Follow-up Visit

After two months on the Reality Diet, when you've lost approximately sixteen pounds, is a great time to go for a follow-up visit to your physician. Have your body fat analysis and blood profile repeated and discuss the results with your doctor. If you had high blood sugar or cholesterol at the beginning of the diet, you should already see some improvement. If you were on medication for hyperlipidemia, hypertension, or high blood sugar, you may be able to reduce your dose. The doses of many other medications are determined by body weight, so your doctor may need to change those as well. Going forward, it's a good idea to check in with your doctor at least once every three months if you're on any type of medication, or every six months if you're not, until you reach your target weight.

Snacking

As you'll see by the menus, there are no snacks built into the Reality Diet. As I explained in Chapter 1, I believe snacking is a habit that can have dangerous consequences when it comes to weight loss or weight maintenance. By snacking, or following a diet that recommends you eat at frequent intervals, you're just training your body to expect food every couple of hours. If you're not careful, you can really rack up the calories this way. I also believe that people snack because they don't eat enough nutritious, fiber-filled food at mealtimes, so they're hungry shortly afterward. Most patients on the Reality Diet tell me they're way too full to snack, even if they wanted to! It's far better to eat complete, satisfying meals three times a day and spend the rest of your time living your life, not thinking about food.

All that being said, there are legitimate reasons to snack, and healthful ways of doing so. People with certain conditions, such as diabetes or PMS, may need to eat more frequently than three times a day. People who exer-

Seven Strategies to Avoid Snacking

1. **Keep yourself busy.** When I'm in the office seeing patients one after the other, the time flies by and I don't think about food at all. Sometimes it's three in the afternoon before I get a break for lunch! As long as I'm busy, I'm not hungry, but the minute I stop, I'm starving.

2. **Avoid the kitchen.** On weekends, when I'm hanging around the house, it's really hard to withstand the magnetic pull of the refrigerator. No matter which room I'm in, but especially in the kitchen, I know in the back of my mind that the fridge is stocked with delicious food. If you live alone or with another dieter, you can empty your home of all temptations. If, like me, you don't, staying out of the kitchen and keeping yourself busy elsewhere In your home are the best ways to resist its siren song.

3. **Distract yourself.** Pick an activity, preferably a calorie-burning one, and train yourself to do it whenever you feel the urge to snack. It can be as simple as walking around the block or doing a load of laundry. Because exercise suppresses appetite, when you get moving your stomach won't feel empty and you'll forget about the urge to snack.

4. **Don't watch commercials.** Even if I've just had an enormous meal, when I sit down to watch a Miami Heat game and a commercial comes on for some fantastic-looking juicy burger, I'm instantly famished. Advertisers count on this reaction—why else would they spend billions each year on television commercials? Instead of watching commercials, take the opportunity to make a phone call, wash the dishes, or do a little straightening. Or even better, do what my daughter's P.E. teacher taught her, and do crunches during the commercials.

5. **Avoid idle hands.** If your hands are busy, you can't put food into your mouth. Hobbies such as knitting, making model air-

planes, pruning plants, and doing crosswords are all good ways to keep your hands busy and out of the candy drawer.

6. **Fool your mouth.** Substitutes for the oral gratification of smoking such as sucking on a toothpick or chewing sugar-free gum also can work when you're trying not to snack. Sometimes we eat just because we want to keep our mouths moving, and there are plenty of noncaloric ways to do so.

7. **Drink a glass of water.** If you think you're hungry between meals, first try drinking an 8-ounce glass of water. More often than not, what you interpreted as hunger was really thirst, and your "hunger" will be satisfied. Plus, you'll fulfill the urge to put something in your mouth while simultaneously hydrating your body, which is always important, but especially so when you're trying to lose fat.

cise heavily also may need to eat something after a workout. And there are people who simply prefer to eat five or six small meals a day rather than three big ones. In all of these cases, the key to snacking without putting on pounds is to keep the total daily number of calories consumed the same as if you hadn't snacked. It's also important to keep the same nutritional balance as if you'd eaten three squares.

It may sound strange, but one of the biggest challenges you may face following the Reality Diet is not resisting the temptation to snack, but the opposite—eating enough food. Fiber-rich food is extremely filling, and until your body gets used to it, you may find the quantities of vegetables, in particular, a bit overwhelming. It's tempting to eat less, because you're full anyway and—hey, if you eat less, you'll lose faster, right? Wrong. To keep up your metabolism and avoid plateauing, it's critical that you consume adequate calories. So, take a deep breath and . . . eat!

Nicholas

One of the most highly motivated patients on the Reality Diet is Nicholas, a thirty-seven-year-old recently divorced father of two. Shirley met him in a playgroup one Saturday—she was there with her daughter and he was there with his twin boys. They struck up a conversation and when Nicholas learned what Shirley did, his eyes lit up.

"I could so use a dietitian—look at me!" At five-foot-eight, he weighed around 200 pounds, according to Shirley's practiced eye. "I got so overweight during the year of our separation and divorce—my ex-wife had always done all the cooking, and without her, I relied on takeout and fast food. Now that I'm pulling my life back together, I'd love to get rid of this belly!"

Shirley and Nicholas agreed to meet, and when they did, she explained the Reality Diet and the exercise commitment that went with it. "What a great excuse to take up running again," Nicholas remarked with his usual sunny disposition. "You wouldn't know it the way I look now, but I was a high school track star twenty years ago. With my career and the kids and then the turmoil with my marriage, I haven't exercised regularly in probably a decade. This will force me to go back to it."

And did he ever—in no time flat he was running between six and seven miles a day. While he didn't take up cooking, he followed the Reality Diet guidelines when choosing his takeout meals, asking for lean meats broiled without butter, steamed vegetables, salads with dressing on the side, and sandwiches with mustard instead of mayo. The pounds melted away— sometimes up to three or four per week because of his intense exercise.

Then all of a sudden he stalled. He came in to see Shirley for his biweekly weigh-in and had only lost one pound. "Have you changed anything? Are you exercising any less?" Shirley queried him.

"No, if anything, I'm running more. I signed up for a half-marathon next month, so I've been training," Nicholas replied.

"Are you eating more?" Shirley continued to probe.

"If anything, I'm eating less," Nicholas countered. "I was feeling so stuffed eating the amount of food you recommended that I cut back a bit on the starches and fats. I guess part of me feels that to be on a diet, I have to feel a little bit hungry," he said with a grin.

"That's your problem right there," Shirley said, folding her arms across her chest. "You're not eating enough calories to support your body, especially with the amount of exercise you're doing. So you need to ensure that you're eating all of the recommended foods and add some resistance training to your workout in order to maintain your muscle mass and keep up your metabolism."

"You mean I have to eat more to start losing weight again?" Nicholas asked, incredulously.

"Absolutely." Shirley saw Nicholas's expression of disbelief and smiled. "You're going to have to trust me on this."

So Nicholas went back to eating all the food on his menus and, just as Shirley predicted, he began losing weight again. With his improved physique, he's gathered up the courage to reenter the dating game. Last time he checked in, he told Shirley about a woman he'd met through his runner's club. "And she cooks," he exclaimed and pumped his arm in the air. "Yes!"

Liquid Assets

It's just as important to drink healthfully as to eat healthfully, especially when you're dieting. Just because a beverage has no calories doesn't mean that it's good for you. And just because it's loaded with vitamins doesn't mean it's dietetic. The following guidelines for consuming beverages on the Reality Diet will help you choose anything from water to wine.

Water. If there's one thing that comes closest to melting away fat, it's water. In addition to all of the other wonderful things it does—helping to maintain body temperature, toning muscle and skin, transporting nutrients throughout the body, aiding metabolic reactions on the cellular level, relieving constipation, lubricating joints and eyes, helping to flush out waste, and preventing kidney stones—water is an appetite suppressant that helps the body break down stored fat.

If you don't have enough water in your system, your kidneys can't perform their normal function, which is removing toxins from your blood. Your liver picks up the slack, but that means it's not able to perform its normal duties, one of which is breaking down stored fat to be used for energy. If the liver can't break down stored fat, you don't lose weight.

Although it seems counterintuitive, drinking enough water is actually the key to preventing water retention. The reason is that if you're not getting enough fluids, your body perceives that you're in danger and hangs on to every last drop, which may lead to bloating and swollen feet, ankles, and hands. Diuretics offer only a temporary solution; your body still thinks it's threatened and will replace the lost water as soon as it can.

Every healthy adult should drink at least eight eight-ounce glasses of liquid a day, and at least five of those should be water. If you're overweight, you should drink an extra glass for every twenty-five pounds of extra weight to facilitate fat metabolism. You should also drink extra water in hot weather and every fifteen minutes during exercise. Don't wait until you're thirsty to drink—by then it's too late and your body is already dehydrated. Rather, drink continuously, keeping a glass of water or a water bottle on hand at all times. Filtered tap water, spring water, flat or sparkling mineral water, seltzer, and sugar-free tonic water all count as water.

Caffeinated beverages. Caffeine is a natural diuretic, so it's tempting to go on a caffeine spree and, between trips to the bathroom, watch the numbers on the scale go down. (Many diet pills contain caffeine, surprise, surprise!) This kind of reducing is illusory, however, and the risks of too much caffeine definitely outweigh the reward of temporary weight loss.

The side effects of overcaffeinating include insomnia and poor sleep quality, heartburn, headache, stomachache, nervousness, jitteriness, mood swings, and irregular heartbeat. Caffeine has mild estrogenic effects, exacerbating PMS symptoms and fibrocystic breast disease. Women who suffer from one of these ailments should avoid caffeine entirely during the week before their periods. Too much caffeine can also interfere with calcium and iron absorption, and can raise blood pressure, making it particularly dangerous for people with hypertension.

Recently a strapping young man—a personal trainer by profession—ended up in the emergency room when I was on call at ten o'clock one Sunday morning. He thought he was having a heart attack. He'd been up club-hopping all night long, and to stay awake he'd had four cans of Red Bull and several cups of coffee, with nothing but bar snacks to eat. He said he felt like his heart was jumping out of his chest. I examined him, did an EKG, and found him to be perfectly healthy. He'd just had too much caffeine.

Caffeine can also have beneficial effects. Because of its vasoconstrictive properties, it can relieve headaches when taken in conjunction with over-the-counter pain medication. Caffeine raises blood levels of epinephrine and norepinephrine, stress hormones that relax bronchial airways, thereby providing asthma relief. Caffeine protects against gallbladder disease and has antioxidant effects equal to or greater than those of vitamin C.

The trick is to consume caffeine in moderation. Whether it be in tea, coffee, or caffeinated soda, limit your caffeine consumption to two cups a day. If you're a heavy coffee drinker, you can decrease your consumption gradually by blending a little decaf with your caf, then gradually substituting more and more of the decaf. Also, try drinking an extra glass of water with each cup of coffee—you'll mitigate the diuretic effects of the coffee while increasing your water consumption. Chicory, as well as grain-based coffee substitutes such as Postum, Inca, or Kava can satisfy your taste for coffee, without the caffeine.

The reality is, many people rely on caffeine for its stimulant effects, so to them I say, drink smart. Caffeine has a half-life of six hours, so rather than have both cups first thing in the morning, have one at breakfast and the other mid-afternoon, when the effect of the first is wearing off. If you have trouble sleeping, don't drink anything caffeinated after four in the afternoon.

While drinking decaf coffee is preferable to drinking caffeinated, you should still limit yourself to two cups a day. There are other components of coffee—the terpene lipids cafestol and kahweol, which adversely affect serum cholesterol, as well as potentially carcinogenic substances created during roasting—that survive in decaf. Look for coffee labeled "naturally decaffeinated" or decaffeinated using the Swiss-water, pure-water, or mountain-water process, as these methods do not involve the toxic chemical methlylene chloride.

Tea is a great alternative to coffee—it contains far less caffeine, and the black and green varieties are full of antioxidants. Flavonoids, the phytonutrients predominant in tea, are also common in fruits and vegetables. (Herbal teas, which are naturally caffeine-free, do not have as many antioxidants as green or black tea.) Research suggests flavonoids may reduce the risk of cancer and heart disease. Tea is also rich in manganese, which is essential for bone growth, fluoride, which strengthens teeth, and potassium, which is critical for heart health. Green tea may help protect against infection with the influenza virus and also contains polyphenols that have been shown to have anti-inflammatory properties and may relieve the symptoms of arthritis and Crohn's disease. The polyphenols in green tea may also protect dental health by reducing plaque growth and absorption of cavity-causing bacteria. Just be aware that green tea has a diuretic effect, so you may not want to drink too much of it, especially before a long drive.

Research Update

Could tea be the next diet drink? In a ten-week study, mice who were fed a high-fat diet and oolong tea neither became obese nor ended up with fatty liver deposits, as would have occurred on a high-fat diet alone. Researchers surmise that the caffeine in the tea may have increased the breakdown of lipids in the mice's fat cells. At the same time, an unknown substance in oolong tea may have prevented the mice's intestines from absorbing fat from their diet. Those British may be on to something, drinking tea every afternoon! Just skip the scones and clotted cream.

Diet cola. If I ever had an addiction, it was to diet cola. But thanks to Shirley's badgering and my own nutritional research, I've gone cold turkey. Even if it's caffeine-free, cola is full of chemicals that are not what the human body was designed to consume. In the literature, I discovered that, when metabolized, caramel coloring has end products of insulin resistance and diabetes down the line. And the phosphorus contained in carbonated beverages leaches calcium out of your bones. My advice to everyone—but especially to girls and women, who are at greater risk for osteoporosis than men—is to avoid soft drinks, even the diet and caffeine-free varieties.

Fruit juice and sports drinks. As I mentioned in Chapter 2, drinking fruit juice can really pack on the pounds. Yes, it contains vitamins, but it is highly caloric and has no fiber to slow down the absorption of the natural sugars it contains. It's much preferable to eat a piece of fruit. If you can't resist fruit juice, try a fiber-fortified brand and cut it with water.

Sports drinks are another beverage to beware of. Many of them are full of sugar and calories. Some brands, like Propel Fitness Water, contain only 20 calories per 16-ounce serving and can count as a Dividend. Others, like Gatorade, contain 100 calories per 16-ounce serving and seven times the sugar of Propel. Check the nutrition label before you indulge.

As any of my tennis partners will tell you, I'm a very competitive player. While I was dieting, I restricted myself to only drinking water, even when I was working out. Now that I have reached my goal weight, I'll drink two bottles of Gatorade, each mixed with water to yield four 16-ounce servings, during the course of a two-hour match. There's no question that I'm burning off the extra calories, and the infusion of glucose definitely gives me an edge. If you're involved in very vigorous, intense exercise and have reached your target weight, you can drink glucose-based sports drinks like Gatorade more liberally.

Alcohol. Patients are always asking me whether I think it's a good idea for them to drink a glass of red wine with dinner to protect their hearts. While there's significant evidence that alcohol can protect against heart disease, and red wine in particular, because of the antioxidants it contains, I can't just say yes unconditionally. Some people have personal or family histories of alcoholism or drug abuse, in which case I absolutely do not recommend drinking. Others may be taking medications that should not be mixed with alcohol. Women who have had breast cancer should not drink, and if they do, should take a 600 mcg folic acid supplement daily.

If you don't have contraindications to alcohol and have multiple cardiovascular risk factors including high cholesterol, I do recommend a daily glass of red wine for health reasons. If you have normal cholesterol and no other problems with alcohol, it's fine to partake for pleasure. In general, women should limit themselves to one drink a day, men to two.

Just remember that, like a serving from any other food group, a single serving of alcohol equals 90 calories. That means 4 ounces of wine, 6 ounces of dark beer, or 1½ ounces of spirits. You can either substitute a serving of alcohol for a fat or play around with your Reality Reward calories to "buy" yourself a few drinks. I have a patient, Helene, who's an amateur chef and a wine enthusiast. She skips one Reality Reward a week and enjoys a glass of wine with dinner every other night.

Takeaway Tips

Think of starting the Reality Diet as embarking on an adventure in good eating. You'll be trying delicious new recipes that happen to be great for your body. To make food preparation easier, each week's menu has a corresponding shopping list that you can print from our website, www.realitydiet.com, so you won't waste time in the supermarket. Plus, check out the handy "Stock Your Pantry" list on page 115—once you've laid in a diverse array of condiments, herbs, and spices, you'll find that the recipes are super-easy to prepare. If you enjoy following the menus and haven't reached your target weight after the first eight weeks, start over again or mix and match the recipes within each week for variety.

The variety and flexibility of the Reality Diet make it easy to customize and fun to experiment with. *Bon appétit!*

Chapter 7

Setting Your Goals

One of the biggest reasons people are not successful at dieting is that they set unrealistic goals. When they inevitably fail to meet those goals, they give up in despair, feeling hopeless and oftentimes angry with themselves. They then return to their former eating habits and end up putting most or all of the weight back on—if not more. Healthy weight loss is not an overnight miracle. It requires realistic changes in eating behavior and attitudes toward food. Diet plans that promise dramatic results in a short amount of time are either exaggerating—if not just plain lying—or promoting unhealthy and sometimes even dangerous practices.

Being realistic about the time it will take to lose weight is a key factor in preventing frustration, disappointment, and failure. For example, if a diet promises that you will lose thirty pounds in thirty days, you'll feel like a failure if you lose only ten. By contrast, on the Reality Diet you can expect to lose two pounds a week. If you lose ten pounds in the first month, you'll be doing even better than expected! You'll also feel great about yourself and be motivated to stick to the plan.

Before you embark on the Reality Diet—or any weight-loss plan, for that matter—it's important to take the time for a little introspection. Why are you overweight to begin with? What exactly are you eating each day? Are you eating because you're hungry, or for other reasons? What is your motivation for losing weight? What are your goals, not just in terms of pounds, but in terms of physique, emotional well-being, and overall health? And most important, are they realistic? Until you can be honest with yourself, you'll never be able to make the kind of deep, long-term commitment and lifestyle changes that it takes to stick to a diet and to keep the weight off permanently.

The Three E's

To help you figure out the eating and behavior patterns that have led to your weight problem, buy a pocket-size notebook and begin what I call a 3-E Journal. In it you'll keep track of the three E's: Eating, Exercise, and Emotions. For at least one week before you start the Reality Diet, write down when and what you eat, when and how much you exercise, and what your emotional state is before, during, and after you eat. Try not to look at it or analyze it until a full week has gone by, as the patterns will not be clear until then. When you do go back and reread it, you'll likely see some distinct habits and associations around food.

One of my patients didn't realize it until she began keeping a 3-E Journal, but she was regularly eating two dinners a night. First she'd sit down with her young children at around five-thirty, and although she wouldn't serve herself a plate of food, she'd pick off of their plates and "clean up" whatever they didn't finish. Then she'd sit down to her "real" dinner at eight, after her husband came home and they'd put the kids to bed. Once she realized what was going on, she stopped eating with the kids, or if she did, she would have just a salad when her husband ate later in the evening.

When my patient Simone started keeping a 3-E Journal, she discovered that her binge eating was directly related to her destructive relationship with her mother-in-law, a narcissistic person who takes a sadistic pleasure in criticizing everything about Simone's life, including her weight. Every time Simone talked to her mother-in-law on the phone, she would hang up and head straight to the kitchen, either to the freezer, where she'd devour a pint of ice cream, or to the pantry, where she'd put away an entire bag of Milano cookies. Now that she's realized the pattern, she either goes to her husband for a hug after hanging up the phone or, if he's not home, calls a supportive friend for reassurance.

Another patient found, after keeping a 3-E Journal for several weeks, that he was consuming most of his excess calories on the weekends, when he would get together with friends to play poker or watch sports. They'd hang out, drink beer, eat chips, and order in pizza or fast food. "The point was never the poker or the game on TV," he told me. "The point was hanging out. When I realized that, I suggested we find something else we all liked to do that wasn't so sedentary and where we wouldn't just eat mindlessly. Now we play pick-up basketball at the town courts or, if the weather's bad, go to this great indoor sports complex a few miles away. Afterward, we grab a bite someplace that has a few healthy options on the menu."

Once you've become aware of the unconscious patterns that are leading you to overeat, make a list in your 3-E Journal of steps you can take to break them. Like Simone, try to come up with a positive alternative to eating if you are feeling upset. Negative emotions easily can cause your judgment and self-control to go out the window. If your problem is that you wait until you're ravenous and then grab high-calorie prepared food, try to plan ahead, stocking your pantry with low-cal 2:90 treats like popcorn or high-fiber cereal. Also, if you eat three healthful high-fiber meals at regular mealtimes, you shouldn't get so desperately hungry. If you discover that you're spending most of your day sitting down, budget time for exercise. It doesn't have to be a big commitment—several small intervals of activity throughout the day can be as effective as one long workout (more on this in Chapter 9).

Women and Weight Gain

Call it the latent feminist in me, but I always liked to believe that men and women were created equal, at least in terms of weight gain and loss. Calories are gender neutral, aren't they? When women patients would come in and tell me they were eating like birds but still putting on weight, I privately dismissed them as being dishonest with themselves about what they were really consuming. How could they be eating and exercising the same way they'd been for years, then suddenly begin gaining? According to the theory of calories-in, calories-out, it just didn't make sense.

Gradually I had an awakening. I began to notice that most of the women who had this complaint were in or approaching middle age. Could there be something going on hormonally that would make them gain weight? I began to do a little research and was astonished by what I discovered.

Between ages thirty-five and forty-four, more women tend to become overweight than at any other time in their adult lives. Why? Because these are what's known as the perimenopausal years—the seven to ten years *before* menopause, when women's ovaries are slowing down and producing fewer fertile eggs. When women ovulate, their ovaries produce a hormone called progesterone, which signals the hypothalamus gland in the brain to raise their core body temperature. That's why women use basal body thermometers when they're trying to get pregnant—their temperature goes up by a full degree Fahrenheit or more when they release an egg, and it remains elevated for the entire second half of their cycle.

A higher core temperature means a faster metabolism—your body needs to burn calories to produce that extra heat. All told, this adds up to 15,000 to 20,000 calories per year. When women enter perimenopause, and later in menopause when they're not ovulating at all, they can easily gain five pounds a year without changing their diet or exercise one bit.

Perimenopausal women also produce less estrogen than women in their prime childbearing years. Without estrogen, women have more free-circulating androgens, like testosterone (yes, women do produce testosterone). In addition to causing changes in women's body shape during these years, from the more feminine pear or gynoid shape to the more masculine apple or android shape, excess circulating androgens stimulate production of insulin, which stores fat.

Women with polycystic ovary disease fail to ovulate regularly, so they have lower circulating amounts of estrogen and progesterone and higher amounts of free testosterone. Not only do they struggle with their weight and other symptoms of excess androgens, but they are also at a greater risk for insulin resistance, high cholesterol, and heart disease than other women.

Recent research suggests that estrogen actually may be an appetite suppressant. In one study, rats that had their ovaries removed and therefore produced very little estrogen exhibited an increased desire to eat and drink. Their appetites went back to normal when they were given estrogen supplements. There's a chance, then, that perimenopausal women are hungrier than younger women and actually may be eating a bit more than they think.

As I'll describe in more detail in Chapter 9, all adults lose an average of half a pound of lean muscle mass each year after age thirty. Because every pound of muscle burns 50 calories per day, this can really add up over time. To make matters worse for women, after age thirty-five, a woman's rate of muscle loss doubles to one pound a year. This can cause women to gain five additional pounds a year without changing their diet or exercise at all. The combination of lean muscle and the metabolic slowdown from anovulation means that by the time a woman reaches menopause, she needs only two-thirds the calories she needed at age twenty to maintain a constant weight.

So what's a woman to do? My top recommendation is to increase exercise—not only will you burn the extra calories you're not using up through ovulation, but you'll reverse the natural loss of lean muscle mass that accompanies aging. Plus, of course, focus on nutrition. Even if you only have a small amount of weight to lose—or none at all—now is the time to start eating healthfully and following a Reality plan to make sure your weight gain doesn't get out of control during these transitional peri-menopausal years.

Research Update

As if you didn't have enough to stress you out, recent findings of the Study of Women's Health Across the Nation (SWAN) show that the stresses typical of middle age—job dissatisfaction, ill parents, teenage children, divorce—cause women to gain weight. Out of two thousand women aged forty and over, those who reported a low stress level during the year preceding the study (zero to one stressful life event) gained an average of 1.5 pounds over the subsequent four years. Those who reported a high stress level during the year preceding the study (six or more stressful life events) gained an average of eight pounds. Even after adjusting for diet, smoking, exercise, and menstrual periods—all of which can affect weight—the connection between personal issues and weight gain held, regardless of race, income, and education. The researchers theorize that the culprits are stress hormones, which for evolutionary reasons cause people to conserve fat. Unfortunately, that fat tends to be concentrated in the abdomen, which is dangerous for your cardiovascular health.

Moonlighting

Not surprisingly, a lot of people who work nights come to my office seeking help battling the bulge. Most of them are operating with a major sleep deficit, which can play havoc with the hormones that control appetite and cause cravings for high-fat and high-sugar foods (more on this in Chapter 10). In addition, because most night workers still have to take care of responsibilities during the day, they have little time to shop or cook healthfully and often rely on poor-quality convenience food.

Marco is a hospital technician who works the graveyard shift, from nine at night till seven in the morning. Starving, because he didn't eat during his shift, he used to drive straight to a diner after work and down a big breakfast of bacon, ham, sausage, eggs, and hash browns. He then went home and slept until he had to pick up his daughter from elementary school. They'd go to a fast-food joint for a snack for her and lunch for him, then home, where he would watch some television and rest for the night ahead. He'd eat dinner with his family, then grab some ice cream before heading out the door.

Fifty pounds overweight, Marco arrived in Shirley's office looking to break his pattern of unhealthy eating. Shirley explained that if he timed his meals better and didn't go all night without eating, he wouldn't crave such high-calorie food. She instructed him to eat a high-fiber breakfast when he got off his shift, a healthful lunch when he awoke from his daytime sleeping, then a sensible dinner at about eleven P.M., on his lunch break at work. At around three A.M. he has his healthy dessert.

Six months later, Marco has lost forty-two pounds. He's full of energy and feels much more alert and productive on the job. He has also found a way to combine his after-school playtime with his daughter with a workout for himself. He says he can eat this way for the rest of his life.

In our practice, we see a lot of policemen who also have a tendency to put on pounds. The ones who work the night shift are especially vulnerable, as they often snack on convenience food as they go on their rounds and are frequently given free or discounted meals at local restaurants. To stay alert, they drink way too much coffee and then crash when their shift is over and go straight to bed without eating. With erratic schedules and unexpected overtime, they rarely have time to pack meals from home. As with Marco, Shirley advises them to try to eat on a more regular schedule, and educates them to make healthful choices when they're eating on the run.

Choosing a Realistic Goal

When talking with my patients about weight loss, the conversation inevitably turns to how much weight they want to lose. Most people have a fairly specific number of pounds in mind. When I ask them how they came up with that amount, their answers vary: "It's how much I weighed in college," "It's what I read in a magazine someone my height is supposed to weigh," "It's what a friend of mine weighs and she looks fabulous." Some might even get technical: "It's what I need to lose to get my BMI below 25." To my mind, all of these rationales are completely arbitrary. None of them has to do with you as an individual. Comparing yourself with other people, whether people you know or images in a magazine, is not a psychologically healthy way to live. We all need to learn to be happy in our own skins and figure out what our optimal weight is, on an individual basis.

As a cardiologist, I can assure you that it's much more important to be healthy than skinny. I have model-thin patients with sky-high cholesterol, and patients who are definitely not bikini-ready with gorgeous lipid profiles. So the first goals I talk about with my patients are their internal figures. If they have high cholesterol, high blood pressure, or high blood sugar, those need to be brought under control. Because the best way to lower all three is through weight loss, their external figures automatically will benefit.

Next we talk about their physical size. The current vogue is to measure people's body mass index (BMI), which can give you a ballpark target for your goal weight. The formula for figuring out your BMI is to multiply your weight in pounds by 703, and divide that by your height in inches squared.* According to this equation, a person who is five-foot-eight and weighs 150 pounds has a BMI of 22.8. The standard interpretation is that a BMI of less than 18.5 is considered underweight, between 18.5 and 25 is considered normal, from 25 to 30 is considered overweight, and above 30 is considered obese. Because being underweight poses a risk for osteoporosis, however, I

---

*If you use the metric system, simply divide your weight in kilograms by your height in meters squared.

consider a healthier normal range for women of average build to be between 22 and 25.

The problem with BMI is that it doesn't take body composition into consideration. Because muscle weighs more than fat, a person who's very fit can have a high BMI, while a person who has a BMI in the normal range could still stand to lose a few pounds or get in shape. Some people simply have bigger bones and a bigger frame than others; the BMI takes none of this individual variation into account. Take me, for example—I'm six-foot-three and weigh 194 pounds. My BMI is 24.2—nearly overweight. But I'm in good shape—I play tennis at least an hour a day, and if you saw me you'd say I was pretty lean and mean. I'm simply a big guy.

A better number to be concerned with than your BMI is your percentage of body fat, as that's a far more accurate assessment of your body composition. In my office, we use a near-infrared machine that shines light through your biceps and, from the way the light scatters, extrapolates your percentage of body fat. It's totally safe and noninvasive—in fact, it's sort of like the way kids give themselves "X-rays" by shining a flashlight through their hands. Another reliable technique is dual energy X-ray absorptiometry (DEXA), the same machine used to measure bone density. Other methods commonly used are skinfold calipers and bioelectrical impedance machines, but they are more prone to error than the near-infrared or DEXA technologies.

Men and women are built differently—men have more lean muscle, while women have more subcutaneous fat. The reason for this is that, in spite of all the advances in assisted reproductive technology, nobody has yet figured out how men can carry babies. This privilege belongs exclusively to women, whose bodies are endowed with extra energy reserves to support fetuses and young children. Hence, while the normal range for men is 13 to 21 percent body fat, the normal range for women is higher—23 to 31 percent. Because all of us lose muscle mass as we age, the high end of the healthy range increases to 24 percent for men over forty and 34 percent in women over forty.

Rather than obsess and stress over numbers on a scale, it's a lot saner to set a goal based on how you feel, inside and out. When your blood profile looks good and you look good—fit, energized, able to wear what you want to wear—you've succeeded. It doesn't matter what the scale says. Remember Carmen the salsa dancer? She never got down to the size she was in her championship years—that would have been an unrealistic goal. Rather, she lost weight until she felt good about herself again and had a clean bill of health. Her ideal weight happened to be fifteen pounds heavier than she was in her youth.

One Step at a Time

I once had a personal trainer who was a terrible liar. He'd tell me I needed to do fifteen reps of a certain exercise, and when I got to fifteen, he'd say, "Just five more." Then, when I got to twenty, he'd say, "Last five!" And when I got to twenty-five, if I wasn't completely wrecked, he'd say, "Now give it your best for the final five!" I finally asked him why he kept doing this to me, and he said, "If I told you right off the bat you had to do thirty reps, you'd flat-out refuse. This way, you do fifteen, you feel good about it, and that gives you the energy to do another five, then another five, then another five."

It's the same thing with weight loss. Rather than having a single target amount that you want to lose that might be intimidating, start off with a smaller, more realistic goal—say, ten to fifteen pounds within the first two months. Then, when you've achieved that, set another incremental goal. Helene, my patient who loves good food and wine, gave herself a year to lose forty pounds so she would look good for her daughter's wedding. She met her goal in just over seven months and has figured that she's on a roll and may as well continue. Her new goal is to lose another fifteen. If she meets that, who knows? Maybe she'll give it her best for the final five!

Helene's case brings to mind another critical point about goal-setting. Be realistic about how long it takes to lose weight. While fad diets promise you'll shed large amounts of weight practically overnight, this isn't reality. As the old saying goes, slow and steady wins the race. The faster you lose weight, the faster you're likely to put it back on again. If you lose more slowly, the weight is mostly fat, not water or lean muscle mass, and it will more likely stay off in the long run. If you want to lose weight for a particular event, like a wedding or bar mitzvah or class reunion, give yourself plenty of lead time. On the Reality Diet, patients have been averaging two pounds of weight loss a week. I always advise patients to budget in a couple of extra weeks, in case they plateau or indulge a bit during holidays.

Reality Checks

Every one to two months, or whenever you meet an interim goal, I recommend you do a Reality Check. Take out your 3-E Journal, write down the date, your weight, and any other measurements you're keeping track of—waist circumference, hip size, dress size, and so on. Then spend a few minutes thinking about what's gone right since your last Reality Check and what still needs work. Are you exercising as much as you should be? Do you need to change the type of exercise you're doing or increase your activity level? Have you felt less tempted to overeat or eat unhealthful food? Are you getting better at planning ahead for meals? Are you controlling the triggers that make you want to overeat? Do you have adequate support from your friends and family? If you like, you can even make two columns on the page and label them "Achievements" and "Challenges." It's always helpful to look back over previous entries and see how many prior challenges are now under the achievement heading.

It's also motivating to see how much you've lost since your last Reality Check. While it's standard operating procedure to weigh yourself only once or twice a week when dieting, it's even more exciting to see the dramatic progress that occurs at monthly or bimonthly intervals. One of my patients takes periodic photographs of herself in an outfit she wore on the day she started the Reality Diet and pastes them into her notebook. "It's hanging off of me now, and I can't tell you how good that feels!" she exulted.

Takeaway Tips

To ensure your success on the Reality Diet, it's important that you be honest with yourself about your relationship to food and exercise. Keep a 3-E Journal for a week before starting the diet and look for self-destructive patterns you can work on breaking. It's also critical to set realistic goals. Before you begin the diet, when you visit your doctor and have a complete physical and blood workup, discuss any goals he or she might identify in terms of blood pressure, sugar, or cholesterol levels. Then think about your own goals. Are you losing weight for a particular occasion? If so, be sure to budget enough time. Is your aim to feel more attractive and energetic? Are you trying to lose inches as well as pounds? While you may have an ultimate goal in mind, set yourself an interim goal you reasonably can achieve in the next month or two. Do periodic Reality Checks in your 3-E Journal to troubleshoot your diet and exercise plan and to keep yourself motivated.

Chapter 8

Preparing Your Reality Kitchen

Now that you've learned the principles of the Reality Diet and set your goals, it's time to begin!

The purpose of the Reality Diet is not only to help you lose fat and improve your health, but also to teach you a more healthful way to eat. Unlike the days when we hunted and gathered our own meals, today most of our food is processed, packaged, and shipped hundreds if not thousands of miles before it reaches our plates. We used to know exactly what we were consuming—a bison was a bison, after all. Now there are all kinds of chemicals in our food, from pesticides, hormones, and antibiotics that increase farmers' productivity, to additives that improve flavor, color, and texture, to preservatives that help our food stay fresh when it may be days, weeks, or even months between when it's packaged and when we eat it.

If you start with healthful ingredients, you'll end up with more healthful food, pure and simple. To figure out what's what, it's important to know how to read food labels, and here I'm not just talking about the nutrition information in fine print on the back. Manufacturers claim all sorts of healthful properties on the packaging of their products, and while they're forbidden by law from making entirely false health claims, there is a gray area of misleading information that is totally unregulated. Plus, there are products tailored to all the various fad diets out there that may not be as good for you as they claim.

Once you've gotten all these delicious and nutritious ingredients home, the question becomes, what to do with them? Thanks to our recipe consultant, Andrew Hunter, you'll have a well-stocked kitchen and pantry, in addition to lots of ideas for making cooking easy and enjoyable. So what are you waiting for? Let's get started!

Know Your Labels

Nutrition labels are confusing; there's no question about it. Some of the nutrients are reported in grams, others in percentages. And what happened to the Recommended Daily Allowance (RDA)? The government keeps tinkering with labeling requirements, and if you ask me, they still have a ways to go to get it right.

Until they do, here are some basic guidelines to help you decipher the reported nutrition information:

* **Check the serving size.** For the Reality Diet, one serving equals 90 calories, which may be different from the serving size on the label.
* **Follow the 2:90 Rule on all starches.** Make sure there are at least 2 grams of fiber per 90-calorie serving.
* **Total fat should not exceed 5 grams per 90-calorie serving.** And of that total fat, as little as possible should come from saturated fat— ideally 1 gram or less. (Obviously this does not apply to oils and other foods that are from the fat group.)
* **Avoid trans fats as much as possible.** Choose spreadable margarine that is trans-fat free (hydrogenated or partially hydrogenated vegetable oil should not be on the ingredient list) and use canola oil rather than vegetable shortening.
* **Total cholesterol should not exceed 300 mg per day.**
* **Look for low-sodium products, especially if you have high blood pressure.** This means less than 140 mg of sodium per serving. Prepared foods—even "diet" ones—are often loaded with sodium, so watch out!
* **Beware of starches that have more than 4 grams of protein per 90 calories.** These foods have been pumped full of soy protein to make

them "low-carb," and as I explained in Chapter 3, there's already more than enough protein in the average American diet.

Other claims to be leery of on food labels include:

✳ **"Low-Carb" or "High-Protein."** To reduce the number of carbo-hydrates, manufacturers substitute inactive fiber or soy protein for flour when making these products. In either case, you're losing the nutrition naturally found in complex carbohydrates. These products are also often high in fat and calories, so read the labels carefully.

✳ **"Low-Fat" or "Fat-Free."** Fat adds flavor, and when you take it away, you need to add something else to make food taste good. Usually, that something else is sugar, so low-fat food is often surprisingly high in calories. Watch out.

✳ **"Low-Sugar" or "Sugar-Free."** Again, this may not mean calorie-free. Check the label.

✳ **"No Added Sugar."** There may not be any extra sugar added, but there also may have been plenty of sugar to begin with.

✳ **"Wheat," "Made with Wheat Flour," or "Made with Unbleached Wheat Flour."** Bleached or unbleached, wheat flour is not *whole* wheat flour. A product that says it's made with wheat flour could be made entirely with bleached white flour, as white flour originally comes from wheat. Look for "whole wheat" or "whole grain" on the label, and make sure it's high up in the ingredient list so you'll be getting the wheat germ and wheat bran, which contain most of the nutrients, as well as the wheat kernel. Although they are not technically whole grains, wheat and oat bran and wheat germ are also extremely healthful, as they con-tain most of the protein, fiber, and phytonutrients found in whole grains.

The Organic Question

When I tell patients that one of the main goals of the Reality Diet is to teach them to eat fresher, more nutritious food, they invariably ask, "Do you mean organic?"

That's a tricky question. For one thing, eating organic food is not a requirement of the Reality Diet, especially since it can be quite pricey. For another, the image we have of "organic" doesn't always match up with the reality. In the early days of organic food, it was produced on small farms and distributed locally. Nowadays, organic farms can be huge "factory" farms, and the food can be packed and shipped across the country. They can also be smack up next to nonorganic farms (and are often part of the same company), with all the pesticides and seeds blowing from one field to the next. Similarly, organic beef may come from a cow fed organic feed, but that doesn't mean the cow was grazing peacefully in a meadow full of clover. It could have been penned in with thousands of other cows in cramped, sunless conditions just as its nonorganic counterparts are.

While organic food is without a doubt more healthful than nonorganic food, you can do even better. Look for pasture-raised poultry (raised entirely outdoors in pens that are moved around so the birds don't eat their own droppings), or if you can't find it, free-range or cage-free. Left to their own devices, pasture-raised fowl seek out medicinal plants and don't require antibiotics. They're also more nutritious: A study sponsored by the Department of Agriculture found that pastured chickens have 21 percent less fat, 30 percent less saturated fat, 34 percent less cholesterol, 50 percent more vitamin A, and 400 percent more omega-3 fatty acids than birds raised in factory farms. Similarly, pastured or grass-fed beef contains 400 percent more vitamins A and E and more omega-3 fatty acids than grain-fed beef plus higher levels of beta-carotene and conjugated linoleic acids. Dairy products and eggs that come from pasture-fed cows and hens also have more flavor and nutrition than their conventional counterparts. Pastured eggs have up to three times the amount of omega-3 fatty acids than factory-farmed ones, and their yolks are a brilliant orange.

As far as vegetables and fruit are concerned, select seasonal, locally grown organic varieties whenever possible. It takes a lot of fertilizer and pesticides to create produce hearty enough to survive long-distance travel and still look picture-perfect on your supermarket shelves. Unfortunately, looks can be deceiving, and between the chemicals and the amount of time it has taken to get from the farm to your plate, that magnificent head of broccoli has lost up to 80 percent of its vitamin C and 95 percent of its calcium, iron, and potassium. Fruits and vegetables grown without pesticides have to fend for themselves and produce greater amounts of phenols — phytonutrients that protect plants against rot and may reduce cancer risk in humans—than their nonorganic brethren. Perhaps most important of all, fruits and vegetables that are grown without chemicals and eaten as soon as possible after being picked simply taste better than those that have been shipped and stored.

Seek out farmers' markets and roadside stands where you can buy your food as close to its source as possible. Health food stores carry a wide range of organic products, many of which come from small farms and local manufacturers. Many supermarkets also carry a good selection of organic food, although theirs tend to be mass produced at factory farms. One of the best ways to eat fresh, wholesome food and support your local farms is to join a CSA (community-supported agriculture) or cooperative farm. The way these usually work is that you pay a lump sum at the beginning of the growing season and every week receive a selection of produce. This is a great way to keep small farms afloat, and it gives you a chance to try a variety of fruits and vegetables you might not ordinarily buy.

Shopping with Shirley

Wouldn't it be nice if we could have a dietitian accompany us on all our trips to the supermarket, pointing out foods to enjoy and foods to avoid? The next best thing is to have my dietitian Shirley DeLeon's advice, which she's kindly contributed here.

First of all, shop the edges of the supermarket—the produce, meat, and dairy departments. Most of your food should come from these areas. When choosing produce, look for fresh fruits and veggies that are vibrantly colored and not wilted or bruised. If you're buying lettuce or other vegetables that have been kept moist with the supermarket's sprinklers, shake them off before you put them in the plastic produce bags, as excess water will hasten rotting. Fruits should be fragrant and yield slightly to the touch (except for apples, of course).

To save room in your refrigerator, trim the greens off the tops of carrots, turnips, and beets, leaving about half an inch of stem. You can also discard the dark green parts of leeks and scallions. If you have a little time after unpacking your groceries, you can wash and chop hard vegetables like string beans, carrots, bell peppers, leeks, scallions, broccoli, and cauliflower and store them in your fridge in individual rescalable bags or plastic containers.

Outfitting Your Kitchen

One reason chefs can whip up meals in a matter of minutes (besides the fact that they're highly trained) is that they have all the right equipment at their fingertips. They're not improvising, paring an apple with a butcher knife, or scouring hardened food off of dented old frying pans. To make it easier for you to whip up the recipes on the Reality Diet menus, it's worth investing in some quality kitchen gadgets and appliances. Think of this as a long-term investment—once you see how simple it is to cook healthful meals and how much better the food tastes than what you've been used to, you'll be a convert for life. Here's a basic list of what you'll need to Reality-ready your kitchen:

    Blender
    Electric mixer
    Food processor
    Juicer—electric or manual
    Kitchen scale

    Cast-iron skillet
    Small (8-inch) ovenproof nonstick skillet
    Large (10-inch) ovenproof nonstick skillet
    Nonstick baking sheet
    Nonstick muffin tin
    Pie plates
    Round casserole dish (5 inches in diameter)
    Small (1-quart) saucepan
    Medium (2-quart) saucepan
    Wok

    Measuring cups
    Measuring spoons
    Pepper grinder

Rolling pin
Metal spatula
Plastic spatula
Rubber spatula
Tongs
Whisk
Wooden spoons

Chef's or chopping knife
Paring knife
Serrated knife
Vegetable peeler
Zester

Small metal, glass, or plastic mixing bowl
Medium metal, glass, or plastic mixing bowl
Large metal, glass, or plastic mixing bowl
Microwaveable bowl
Colander
Salad spinner

Aluminum foil
Bamboo skewers
Plastic wrap
Resealable plastic bags—gallon and quart size
Set of containers with sealable plastic lids (e.g., Tupperware)
    for storing chopped vegetables, marinated meats, etc.

This way, when you need some for a recipe later in the week when you may not have as much time, you can just grab and go. You can also wash and dry your lettuce in advance—rolled in paper towels or a dish towel, it will stay crisp for up to a week in the refrigerator. Don't wash fresh herbs until right before you use them, however, as moisture will encourage them to rot.

Some produce keeps better and tastes better if left unrefrigerated. You don't need to refrigerate potatoes, onions, garlic, ginger, shallots, lemons, limes, or oranges. In fact, with the amount of citrus juice in the Reality recipes, you should always have a nice bowl of fresh lemons and limes on your countertop (the bottled juice just doesn't compare). Never refrigerate bananas or tomatoes, and store ripe bananas separately, as the ethylene gas that ripe bananas exude will hasten the ripening of any other fruits kept next to them. Berries are better if left out, but you may need to refrigerate them if you won't be using them for a few days. And don't wash fruits until you're ready to use them, as they will start decomposing as soon as they're wet.

When it comes to meat, poultry, and fish, be very choosy. Select the fresh-est possible—most supermarket packages have a sell-by and/or consume-by date on them. Even so, check carefully to make sure the food looks good, not watery or gray. Fish should not have a fishy smell—it should smell salty, if anything. When you're buying beef, choose Select or Choice grades of

Sweet Talk

The most popular and widely available sugar substitutes on the market are Splenda (sucralose), Equal (aspartame), Sweet'N Low (saccharine), and stevia, an herbal product. While there are health concerns with all of them, in modest quantities they have proven to be generally safe and effective weight-loss tools.

Saccharine is the great-granddaddy of all artificial sweeteners, dating back to 1879, and was popular for years until laboratory rats that were fed massive doses of saccharine started getting cancer. In human beings, saccharine is considered safe at the doses com-monly used in food preparation, but it is not recommended for pregnant or breastfeeding women. The good thing about saccha-rine is that it can be used to sweeten both hot and cold drinks and can be substituted for sugar in baking.

Aspartame, known as Equal or NutraSweet, gained a large share of the artificial sweetener market when saccharine fell out of favor. While there have been reports linking aspartame to migraines, seizures, brain tumors, and other neurological problems in human beings, it is still ubiquitous. People suffering the rare genetic condition phenlylketonuria must avoid aspartame, as it contains the amino acid phenylalanine, which they cannot metabolize. Aspartame is commonly found in diet soda and sugar-free gum, and it is best used in hot and cold beverages. It loses its flavor after being exposed to heat for a long time, though, so it is not recommended for baking.

Sucralose is derived from regular sugar, so it most closely resembles sugar in taste. It is made by adding chlorine molecules to sucrose, creating a molecule that the human body cannot digest. About 15 percent is absorbed into and can be stored by the body, however, and long-term effects have not been studied. It has been pointed out that sucralose is chemically similar to pesticides such as DDT; however, to date there have been no official reports of sucralose toxicity in either human or animal studies. The Splenda brand is a particularly useful formulation of sucralose, as it can be substituted for sugar in equal amounts and can be used for baking as well as to sweeten drinks.

Stevia is an herbal sweetener derived from a South American shrub that has been used there for centuries to sweeten beverages. The FDA has not approved stevia as a food additive because there are concerns that in high doses it may cause infertility and be carcinogenic. Stevia has been used in processed food in Japan for some time with no adverse effects, but Canada and the European Union share the reservations of the FDA. Stevia can be obtained in health food stores, where it is sold as a dietary supplement. It's expensive, but because it's about three hundred times sweeter than table sugar, a little bit goes a very long way.

Reality Diet recipes have been developed and tested using Splenda because it works well in both hot and cold foods, leaves no aftertaste, and is safe for phenylketonuriacs. If you choose to use one of the others, be aware that they are not all equally sweet, so you may have to tweak the amounts.

lean beef that have been trimmed of fat, and 90 percent lean ground beef. Also, look for cuts called "round" and "loin," as in sirloin, tenderloin (filet mignon), and top round (London broil). Lamb chops and leg or loin roast are all lean options. For pork, look for those "loin" words again—tenderloin and loin chops are both good options. Any poultry or wild fowl is fine as long as you remove the skin. Make sure your cold cuts, hot dogs, and sausages contain less than 3 grams of fat per ounce.

If you're not using your meat, poultry, or seafood in the next two to three days, freeze it as soon as you get it home. First, rinse the food in cold water and pat it dry with a paper towel. Trim off any excess fat and cut the food into serving-size portions. Either slip each portion in a separate resealable plastic bag or wrap each individually in plastic wrap before placing it in your freezer. Twenty-four hours before you plan to cook, remove however many servings you need from your freezer and place them in your refrigerator to defrost. Do not defrost on your countertop or in your sink, as bacteria are more likely to grow on moist food left at room temperature.

Whenever possible, buy organic, pastured, or free-range eggs. Many supermarkets now carry eggs marked omega-3. These have high levels of omega-3 fatty acids because the chickens are fed a diet that includes flaxseeds. They're a little more expensive, but worth it. If your doctor has recommended that you avoid egg yolks because of their cholesterol, you can use an egg substitute or, preferably, remove the yolks from organic eggs. Egg whites can be kept in the refrigerator for several days or frozen. One neat trick is to freeze individual egg whites in the compartments of an ice cube tray, then transfer the egg-white cubes to resealable plastic bags. Later on, you can simply remove the number of whites you need for a particular recipe.

When shopping for dairy, buy only non-fat or skim (0% milkfat) and low-fat (1% milkfat) milk, yogurts, and cheeses. Avoid reduced-fat (2% milkfat) and whole milk products. The same applies for soy beverages, yogurts, and cheeses. As I've mentioned before, use tub margarine rather than stick, and steer clear of anything that contains trans fats, which come from hydrogenated or partially hydrogenated vegetable oils.

Once you've shopped the perimeter of the market, you may need to delve into the aisles for a few additional items. In general, the shorter the ingredient list, the less processed and more wholesome the food. Remember to apply the 2:90 rule to any breads, crackers, and cereals and, for extra nutrition, look for "whole wheat" high up in the ingredients. Try whole-

Stock Your Pantry

In addition to the major ingredients you'll need to prepare each week's menus—which can be found on our website, www.realitydiet.com, under "Weekly Shopping Lists"—you should always have certain items on hand: herbs and spices, vinegars and extracts, nuts and seeds, stocks and sauces, condiments and garnishes. A well-stocked pantry not only makes it easier for you to follow the recipes, but also helps you liven up your own culinary creations when you branch out. Take this list along the first time you shop for the Reality Diet, and replace items as needed.

Spice Cabinet
Allspice
Basil (dried)
Black peppercorns
Cayenne pepper
Chocolate extract
Chocolate mini-morsels
Cinnamon (ground)
Cocoa powder
Coconut extract
Cream of tartar
Dry milk powder (non-fat)
Garlic powder
Ground ginger
Low-sodium soy sauce
Mustard powder
Nutmeg (ground)
Onion powder
Oregano (dried)
Paprika
Sugar substitute (Splenda is preferred)
Vanilla extract
Whole-wheat flour

Pantry
2:90 granola
2:90 light bread (45 calories per slice)
2:90 regular bread (90 calories per slice)
Balsamic vinegar
Brown sugar (light)
Cider vinegar
Cornmeal (stone-ground)
Extra-virgin olive oil
Nonstick cooking spray—both regular and olive oil
Red wine vinegar
Rice wine vinegar
Vegetable oil

Refrigerator
Basil (fresh)
Capers
Dijon mustard
Eggs (organic, cage-free)
Garlic (peeled and jarred, found in the produce section)
Margarine (light; trans-fat free)
Mayonnaise (reduced-fat and non-fat)
Nuts—whole almonds, cashews, pecan halves, walnut halves
Olives (green and Kalamata)
Peanut butter (natural)
Red peppers (roasted, packed in water)
Salad dressings (low-fat: Caesar, Italian)
Tabasco or other hot pepper sauce

Unrefrigerated Fresh Food
Ginger
Lemons
Limes
Onions

Freezer
2:90 English muffins
2:90 waffles
Whipped topping (fat-free)

wheat pasta and couscous as well—they're far more nutritious than the refined wheat variety, and once you add vegetables and sauce to them, it's
hard to tell the difference. You'll notice that some recipes in Part IV call for
"regular 2:90 bread" and sometimes they call for "light 2:90 bread." "Regular" means 90 calories per slice, or one slice per serving; "light" means 45
calories per slice, or two slices per serving.

When shopping for canned or bottled vegetables or sauces, compare the
sodium content of competing brands and choose the one with the lowest
amount per serving. Frozen vegetables and fruit are fine as long as you buy
them plain, without added sugar or sauces. And simply avoid the aisles that
contain chips, candies, cookies, or anything else you find utterly irresistible.
When it comes to checkout time, find a good tabloid or magazine and keep
your nose buried in it as you wait in line to help distract you from all those
tempting candy bars by the cash registers.

Low-Fat Cooking

The beauty of the Reality recipes is that you don't have to think about portion size or worry about sodium, fat, or cholesterol content—everything has
been figured out for you and is a hundred percent guaranteed to be nutritious and delicious. Even so, you may find yourself itching to cook up your
own recipes. Most people who create their own dishes have no problem
sticking to the recommended size and number of servings of proteins, vegetables, fruits, dairy, and starches. Where they tend to overdo it is with the
fats. Because fats contain twice as many calories as carbohydrates or proteins, small increases can have big consequences. A little extra olive oil
here, a little extra margarine there, and, before you know it, you're consuming a couple hundred extra calories a day.

The trick to avoiding this slippery slope is to use the same low-fat cooking
techniques Andrew did when he developed the Reality menus. Nonstick
cooking spray is your best friend—but only if you use it judiciously. It's
noncaloric if you spray for a third of a second, and a one-second spray contains 7 calories. Some sprays contain more than 1,000 calories in the entire
can! Lemon and lime juice are also essential companions, whether you're
flavoring a piece of fish or dressing a salad. Here are some other low-fat
cooking tips:

✳   Remove skin from all poultry and trim fat from all meat.

✳   Grill, roast, broil, bake, braise, microwave, steam, poach, and stew without adding extra fat (except nonstick cooking spray).

✳   Stir-fry with very little oil.

✳   Add low-sodium broth, tomato or citrus juice, or wine to add moisture and flavor when cooking meat, poultry, or fish.

✳   Avoid lard, vegetable shortening, and tropical oils.

✳   Remove fat from stews and soups by refrigerating them first and then skimming the fat off the top.

✳   Flavor your food with herbs, spices, interesting vinegars, and citrus juice instead of fat and salt.

✳   Don't add butter, margarine, oil, or salt to your food once it's cooked (you can take your salt shaker off the table to remove the temptation).

✳   In place of butter, put salsa on your baked potatoes.

✳   Buy only reduced-fat salad dressings.

✳   Have fresh fruit, non-fat frozen yogurt, fat-free gelatin, or sugar-free Popsicles on hand for dessert rather than chocolate, cookies, or ice cream.

Takeaway Tips

In the ideal scenario, we would all be living alone or with someone who is also on the Reality Diet. In either of these cases, you can simply purge your house of all unhealthy food. Throw away any opened packages of food and check with your local food pantry or Meals on Wheels program to see if they'll accept unopened packages.

If you're living with someone who is not on the Reality Diet and likes to have treats around that you'd rather not be tempted by, assign all those foods to a single cupboard. Then, when you're looking for, say, some balsamic vinegar to make a salad dressing, you won't run headlong into a package of fudge-stripe cookies.

To cook Reality Diet recipes for two or more, simply multiply the recipe. If you and your dining companion are different genders, you may have to add a couple more ingredients to the male portion, as men are allowed a few extra food groups. The instructions will specify if the male and female portions need to be cooked differently.

Part III

Living
with Reality

Chapter 9

Get Moving! The Importance of Exercise

People love to hear they can lose a lot of weight without exercise, and it's true, you can—either by starving or by severely restricting your carbs and losing a lot of water and muscle mass. As a medical doctor, I could never, in good conscience, promote such diets. It's much healthier for your mind, heart, and waistline to eat a balanced diet that contains enough calories to satisfy you and ensure that you're getting adequate nutrition while incorporating enough exercise into your daily routine to burn off those calories. At the same time, you'll build fat-burning lean muscle mass that will help you keep the weight off long term.

Remember, the fundamental truth about weight loss is that you have to use more calories than you consume. Just as it's entirely possible to lose weight through calorie restriction alone, it's entirely possible to lose weight through exercise alone. The difference is in the quality of the pounds lost, not the quantity. A study of overweight men who either ate 700 calories less per day and did no exercise or exercised enough to burn 700 calories a day but continued to eat as they always had showed that they lost exactly the same amount of weight. But the men in the exercise-only group lost 95 percent more fat than the calorie-only group, whose weight loss included more lean muscle mass.

Exercise is a lifelong habit you should cultivate whether or not you need to shed weight. And one of the best things about it is that it's addictive — when you give your muscles a good workout, you bathe your brain in endorphins that provide a natural high. So why not start right now, when it will help you not only lose both pounds and inches, but also gain motivation and energy?

Just in Case You Need More Convincing . . .

Regardless of your shape, size, age, or general well-being, exercise will help you live a longer and healthier life. A recent study of 936 women showed that fitness was actually a better indicator of cardiovascular health than body mass index. Why? Because by reducing blood pressure and "bad" cholesterol while increasing "good" cholesterol, as well as lowering intra-abdominal fat stores, aerobic exercise lowers your risk of heart attack and stroke. Exercise also reduces your risk of colon, breast, and other types of cancer, strengthens your immune system so you're more resistant to colds and other infectious diseases, reduces your risk of gallbladder disease, and lowers your blood sugar, helping to prevent type 2 diabetes. In women, exercise reduces premenstrual symptoms and symptoms of perimenopause, including hot flashes, mood swings, and lack of libido. Weight-bearing exercise also increases bone density and protects against osteoporosis.

Exercise benefits your mind as much as it does your body. Because exercise increases serotonin levels, it acts as a natural antidepressant. It also helps prevent insomnia and the stress associated with poor sleep quality. By lowering blood pressure and improving circulation and lung function, exercise keeps your brain oxygenated, which boosts memory and cerebral function. Recent research suggests it may even prevent Alzheimer's disease and other types of dementia. Last, but absolutely not least, exercise improves your self-image, and when you feel good about yourself, you're much more likely to take care of your body and make healthy lifestyle choices. When you're dieting, a positive mental attitude can make all the difference between success and failure.

The Reality Requirement

I've designed the Reality Diet so that you're going to lose weight. But in order to maximize and sustain your weight loss, you'll need to burn 2,000 calories a week through exercise. Did I do this just to be mean? No, I'm doing it to force you to get into the habit of exercising, because I'm concerned with your total health, not just your pants size. And I'm concerned about not just your health today, but your health a year, two years, even ten or twenty years from today.

Two thousand calories a week means an average of 300 calories a day. It's up to you how you burn those 300 calories. If you hate jogging, try biking or swimming or rowing instead. If you're snowbound all winter, don't despair—try cross-country skiing or snowshoeing. And don't forget that shoveling snow and chopping wood for your wood-burning stove can be great aerobic exercise!

I remember when my daughter, Samantha, first started tennis lessons—it was hard to get her to practice for more than ten minutes before she became bored and wanted to do something else. Now she's twelve and thinks nothing of playing for forty-five minutes to an hour. The same thing goes for other types of exercise. If you haven't exercised for a long time, start slowly. Ten minutes at a time is a worthy goal, and if you can do more than one session a day, all the better. Research shows that the beneficial effects of exercise are the same whether you do it all in one big spurt or break it up into several shorter ones.

Ideally, you'll be working your way up to an hour of exercise a day. When I tell patients that, they often look at me as if I'm from another planet. "Where do you expect me to find an hour a day?" they ask. One good way is to combine exercise with a more sedentary activity. Ride an exercise bike while you watch TV. Do leg lifts while you talk on the phone. Dr. James Levine, a nutritionist, endocrinologist, and professor of medicine at the Mayo Clinic, has substituted his desk chair for a treadmill, which he keeps at 0.7 miles per hour—fast enough to keep him moving, but slow enough that he can read and doesn't sweat.

Because the benefits of exercise are cumulative, you don't need to carve out a full uninterrupted hour. You may choose to do twenty minutes of vacuuming, twenty minutes of pulling weeds, and take a twenty-minute

Lots of Drops in the Bucket

Small lifestyle changes can add up to big calorie credits. Drs. Steven Blair and Milton Nichaman of the Cooper Institute in Dallas believe the obesity epidemic in the United States is caused primarily by our increasingly sedentary lifestyle. They analyzed twenty everyday activities and showed how they could be performed in either a sedentary or active way. Over the course of a month, a person who consistently chooses the path of least resistance will burn 8,800 fewer calories than the person who chooses the more active alternatives. This adds up to 2.5 pounds a month, or 30 pounds a year!*

Sedentary	kcal	Active	kcal
Using remote control to change TV channel	<1	Getting up and changing channel	3
Reclining for 30 minutes of phone calls	4	Standing for three 10-minute phone calls	20
Using garage-door opener	<1	Raising garage door 2 times a day	2 to 3
Hiring someone to clean and iron	0	Ironing and vacuuming, each for 30 minutes	152
Waiting 30 minutes for pizza delivery	15	Cooking for 30 minutes	25
Buying presliced veggies	0	Washing, slicing, chopping vegetables for 15 minutes	10 to 13
Using a leaf blower for 30 minutes	100	Raking leaves for 30 minutes	150
Using a lawn service	0	Gardening and mowing, each for 30 minutes a week	360
Using a car wash once a month	18	Washing and waxing car, 1 hour a month	300

The Dallas Morning News.

Sedentary	kcal	Active	kcal
Letting dog out the back door	2	Walking dog for 30 minutes	125
Driving 40 minutes and walking 5 minutes (parking)	22	Walking 15 minutes to bus stop twice a day	60
Sending e-mail to colleague, 4 minutes	2 to 3	Walking 1 minute and talking (standing) 3 minutes	6
Taking elevator up 3 flights	0.3	Walking up 3 flights	15
Parking as close as possible, 10-step walk	0.3	Parking in first spot, walking 2 minutes, 5 times a week	8
Letting cashier unload shopping cart	2	Unloading full shopping cart	6
Riding escalator 3 times in mall	2	Climbing 1 flight of stairs 3 times	15
Shopping on-line 1 hour	30	Shopping at mall, walking 1 hour	145 to 240
Sitting in car at drive-in window, 30 minutes	15	Parking and walking inside, 3 times a week, total of 30 minutes	70
Paying at the pump	0.6	Walking into gas station to pay, once a week	5
Sitting and listening to lecture, 60 minutes	30	Giving lecture	70

walk. Or you may bike a half-hour to and from work each weekday and play ultimate frisbee on the weekends. Helping your friend move into his new apartment could add up to well over an hour of exercise. I can tell you from experience, pushing your baby's stroller through the park and lifting him on and off the playground equipment, as I do with my son, Dylan, is a terrific workout.

For many people the thought of putting on sneakers and heading to the gym is a total turn-off. Fortunately, "lifestyle activity," such as scouring your tub, pruning your hedges, washing your dog, cleaning your gutters, or any other everyday task that involves at least a moderate level of exertion, has been shown to be as effective as structured exercise at improving cardiovascular fitness. Do yoga in the shower, take up the drums, have athletic sex—the possibilities are endless! Health experts actually believe that everyday integrative exercise that is woven into the fabric of people's lives, as opposed to gym exercise, may be the best way to combat the obesity epidemic. Between 2002 and 2004, the only state in the nation that did not have an increase in its percentage of obese adults was Oregon. One of the reasons, researchers surmise, is that urban planners in Oregon have made a concerted effort to design cities and suburbs to encourage outdoor activity. Portland has a system of bike paths that run throughout the city, and ten percent of the city's population bikes to work. Colorado, the state with the country's lowest rate of obesity, also promotes physical activity, and Boulder has a similar network of bike paths running through it.

If you like to walk, try wearing a pedometer, which tracks the number of steps you take each day. They're inexpensive and easy to use—just hook one to your waistband and you're off! Wear one for a few days and see how many steps you're averaging. Then set a goal to increase your number of steps by 20 percent each week until you reach 10,000 steps a day, the recommended amount for weight loss. As you become more fit, you may need to increase your daily amount to between 12,000 and 15,000 to get the same weight-loss benefit. One patient of mine started wearing a pedometer and noticed that on the first day she'd clocked more than 3,000 steps without leaving her home! On average, there are 2,000 steps in a mile, so my patient walked more than a mile and a half just tending to her regular household chores.

When you're choosing the types of activities you'd like to do, keep in mind that you should be doing a combination of aerobic and anaerobic exercise. Aerobic exercise increases your heart rate and improves your cardiovascular health. It also burns lots of calories and is the best kind of exercise for weight loss. You can tell if an activity is aerobic if it makes you breathless to the point that you can still speak but not sing. Anaerobic exercise which includes any kind of resistance training, such as calisthenics or weightlifting, gives your muscles and bones a workout. In addition, it's good to stretch for five to ten minutes before and after each workout to prevent your muscles from becoming damaged or from cramping and to improve your flexibility. And don't forget to drink water before, during, and after you exercise. By the time you feel thirsty, your body has already become dehydrated.

To keep track of your exercise program, take out your 3-E Journal and make a chart. Down the left side of the page, write the days of the week. Along the top, write "Aerobic," "Resistance Training," and "Stretching." Each day, write down the number of minutes you did of each type of exercise. Try to do at least thirty minutes of aerobic activity five to seven days a week, thirty minutes of light resistance training twice a week, and fifteen minutes of stretching two or three days a week. Consult the "Burn, Baby, Burn!" box on the following page to see how many calories you worked off and add your daily totals to your chart.

Lighten Up!

The bodybuilding era hit its zenith in the late '70s. Arnold Schwarzenegger and Lou Ferrigno were household names, and *Pumping Iron* was a box-office hit. Bodybuilding was cool, and as a teenager I idolized these giants. My friends and I spent hours in our basements or at the local gym working out with heavy weights, trying to look like Arnold.

What we didn't know back then was that musclemen of that era often seriously abused their bodies to achieve their enormous physiques. Steroids were not yet regulated, and many of these guys took them liberally. Plus, to make their muscles and veins really pop for competitions, they took diuretics and wouldn't drink water for several days before the events. In the end, many of them ended up with a multitude of health problems, including heart disease, because of how badly they treated their bodies. Even if you're not Mr. Universe, you can have a lot of muscle and actually be in very poor shape internally, because anaerobic activity such as weightlifting does very little for your cardiovascular health.

In spite of all the talk about how important it is to lift weights and build lean muscle mass that will miraculously boost your metabolism, if you want to lose fat, aerobic exercise beats anaerobic every time. Weightlifting simply doesn't burn that many calories at the level most people do it. Doing light weights a couple of times a week is a good idea to maintain your muscle mass while you're dieting, but after that your time is better spent moving your body and getting your heart rate up.

It's far better to be fit and trim than fit and bulky. During the football season, tune in to a game and check out the offensive linemen. These guys lift

Burn, Baby, Burn!

So how many calories does thirty minutes of exercise actually burn? Check this chart to find out. As you can see, heavier people burn more calories doing the same amount of exercise as people who weigh less, so as you lose weight, you'll have to put in more time exercising or increase the intensity of your workouts.*

Activity	110 lb.	125 lb.	150 lb.	175 lb.	200 lb.
Aerobics, high impact	204	234	279	327	372
Aerobics, low impact	126	142	170	198	225
Basketball, vigorous full-court	321	363	438	510	582
Bicycling, stationary	126	142	170	198	225
Bicycling, outdoor, leisurely	100	113	136	159	180
Bicycling, outdoor, 15 mph	162	183	222	258	294
Canoeing, moderate	150	168	204	237	270
Cross-country skiing, 8 mph	342	390	468	546	624
Golf (carrying your clubs)	150	168	204	237	270
Handball	258	294	351	411	468
Horseback riding (trot)	171	195	234	273	312
Lawn mowing, walking	114	128	153	178	205
Lawn mowing, riding	63	71	85	100	114
Raking	100	113	136	159	180
Rowing, vigorously	321	363	438	510	582
Running, 6 mph	243	276	333	390	444
Running, 9 mph	339	387	465	540	618

*Based on John M. Jakicic et al., "Appropriate Intervention Strategies for Weight Loss and Prevention of Weight Regain for Adults." *Medicine & Science in Sports & Exercise* (2001): 2152; and Ellie Whitney and Sharon Rady Rolfes, *Understanding Nutrition*, 10th ed. (Belmont, CA: Thomson Wadsworth, 2005), p. 258.

Activity	110 lb.	125 lb.	150 lb.	175 lb.	200 lb.
Soccer, vigorous	321	363	438	510	582
Studying	36	42	51	57	66
Swimming, 20 yds per minute	105	120	144	168	192
Swimming, 45 yds per minute	192	219	261	306	348
Table tennis (experienced)	150	168	204	237	270
Vacuuming/sweeping	63	71	85	100	114
Walking, 2.5 mph	75	85	102	119	136
Walking, 3.5 mph	117	132	156	183	210
Walking, 4.5 mph	159	180	216	252	288
Water aerobics	117	132	156	183	210
Weightlifting, light to moderate intensity	78	90	108	126	144
Weightlifting, vigorous intensity	156	180	216	252	288
Yoga	100	113	136	159	180

tremendous weight and have lots of muscle, but look at their stomachs—when they bend over to hike the ball, their bellies are almost touching the ground. If that doesn't convince you that weightlifting does not automatically bring on weight loss, nothing will.

If you choose to work out with a personal trainer, look for someone lean and trim, not someone bulked up like a bowling ball. Make sure the trainer understands your goal is fitness and weight loss, and isn't going to try to beef you up. Also, make sure the trainer is qualified—there are a lot of gym rats out there who, for want of other gainful employment, call themselves personal trainers when they've had no formal education. Look for someone who has taken courses in nutrition and exercise physiology or is certified by one or more training organizations.

Joining a gym that features a thirty-minute workout can be a great first step toward getting in the habit of exercising. But those workouts usually almost exclusively feature light weights, which are great for toning but don't burn a tremendous number of calories. Be sure to augment your

Research Update

In a fascinating study recently published in the journal *Science,* Dr. James Levine (the one with the treadmill at his desk) and his colleagues at the Mayo Clinic showed that you can actually fidget away fat. By attaching motion sensors to specially designed underwear, the scientists were able to calculate exactly how active their subjects were. What they found was that some people simply were more restless than others—they paced, they bounced their knees, they tapped their toes. And that restlessness added up to a whopping 350-calorie-a-day difference between the most active and most sedentary participants.

They also noted that the more restless people were the leanest, and the more sedentary were the heaviest. To test whether their activity level was determined by their weight—that is, whether the overweight ones were inactive because they found it more difficult to move—or vice-versa—lack of moving had caused them to be overweight—the scientists put the subjects on diets. Interestingly, the heavier participants' activity level did not increase even when they lost weight, meaning that they weren't sedentary because they were overweight—they were hardwired to be sedentary! This led the researchers to conclude that people are genetically predisposed either to fidget and burn lots of extra energy or to conserve movement and burn fewer calories. To lose weight, people in the latter group have to make an extra effort to overcome their predisposition to lounge around and consciously incorporate more movement into their lives.

thirty-minute workouts with extra aerobic exercise to maximize your weight loss and improve your cardiovascular performance.

As I say to my patients all the time, in spite of all the gadgets and gizmos and potions and lotions you'll see advertised on TV and in the back of magazines, you're not going to lose weight unless you move your body. Save your $19.95-a-month-plus-shipping-and-handling and instead spend $40 on a racquet and $2 on a ball and play racquetball with a friend. Or buy a decent pair of sneakers and go for a walk. Or hang a basket over your garage door and practice your lay-up shot.

If you have eight minutes in the morning, get on your treadmill or exercise bike—it's far more beneficial to your heart and your diet than weightlifting. Besides, if you wanted to look like the guys on the cover of *Flex* magazine, you'd have to lift weights for eight hours a day, not eight minutes. When you do lift weights, keep them light to avoid injury. Remember, your goal isn't to win the Mr. or Ms. Universe competition, it's to become healthy, inside and out.

Hank

If there ever was a couch potato, it was Hank. For years he lived on convenience food, exercising lightly once or twice a month at the most. He was a bachelor, worked from home as a freelance computer programmer, and ordered in most of his meals. Week after week, he cycled through the same menus—pizza, fried chicken, Chinese, subs—filling his refrigerator with leftovers, which he often ate for breakfast. While working at his desk, he kept a sixty-four-ounce soda at his elbow and would take a slug now and again, downing the entire bottle by the end of the day.

That was before his heart attack. When I met him in the recovery room after his emergency double bypass, he was disoriented, not only from the medication, but from having been blindsided by this health crisis. "How could this have happened to me, Doc?" he asked. "I'm only thirty-seven!"

"That may be your chronological age," I replied, "but according to your arteries, you're a heck of a lot older." I went on to explain that his unhealthy lifestyle had prematurely aged his cardiovascular system—the surgeon reported thick plaques in all his major arteries, and his blood tests showed a total cholesterol of 320, with high triglycerides, LDL, and C-reactive protein. Just looking at him, I could tell he was unhealthy. His skin was a yellowish pale, his ankles and feet were swollen, and he was probably one hundred pounds overweight.

"You were lucky this time, but you may not be the next," I warned him. "This heart attack was the canary in the coal mine. There's no reason you can't recover from this and live to a ripe old age. But you'll have to make some serious changes to your lifestyle." I explained that I wanted him to get moving as soon as possible and to make an appointment to see Shirley within the month. Eyes wide, Hank nodded obediently.

Fear can be a great motivator, and in Hank's case, it caused a total transformation. As soon as he was allowed out of bed, he began walking the halls of the cardiac unit. Once home, he started walking ten minutes a day, gradually building up to twenty minutes by the time he saw Shirley. She put him on the Reality Diet and explained that he still could order in food, but he would have to choose a less greasy array of menus and stick to the low-sodium, heart-healthy options. She also recommended that he make a weekly pilgrimage to the supermarket to stock up on produce and high-fiber breakfast cereal.

Hank followed all of Shirley's directives and lost seven pounds the first week, mostly water. During the next month, he settled into a pattern of losing two to three pounds a week. He continued to build up his walking, until he was up to an hour a day. "Now it's time to increase the intensity of your exercise," Shirley advised. "Have you ever thought about joining a gym?"

"Not really," Hank replied. "Can't I just buy some equipment and work out at home?"

"You could buy a treadmill, but after a while you'll want to vary your routine, and a gym has more equipment than you could ever fit into your apartment. Plus," Shirley added, "you need to get out and see other people each day. Sitting by yourself in front of your computer is no way to live."

Hank joined a gym and began working with one of the trainers, who showed him how to use the free weights and machines. He also introduced Hank to the cardio equipment, which he was about ready to start using, as well.

Six months later, Hank is halfway to his goal of losing one hundred pounds. He does five hours a week of cardiovascular exercise, rotating among the elliptical trainer, the Stairmaster, the treadmill, and swimming, plus three hours a week of weight training. He's now losing between 1½ and 2 pounds a week, but because of his intense exercise, it's mostly fat. His body fat has decreased from 44.7 percent to 30.3 percent, and it shows—his arms and legs are gaining definition, and he's dropped eight pants sizes. "I've never felt this good in my life!" he told me at his last appointment.

"I've got energy, I can run up the steps to my apartment, I can see my feet. You know something, Doc?"

"What?" I replied.

"In some ways, that heart attack was the best thing that ever happened to me."

I silently agreed.

Takeaway Tips

Exercise, exercise, exercise! However you can fit it in, make sure you do it, because aerobic exercise is the key to successful weight loss. Remember— couch potatoes start looking like potatoes! To maximize your chances of success at sticking to an exercise plan, choose an activity or array of activities that you enjoy. There's no "right" way to exercise, and even leisure-time occupations, household chores, and tricks such as taking the stairs instead of the elevator or parking as far away as you can from the mall count toward your daily total. Try to burn at least 300 calories a day to maximize your weight loss and to ensure that most of the weight you lose is fat, not lean muscle mass.

Chapter 10

There's No Such Thing as Cheating . . .

and Other Wise Words to Get You Through the Tough Times

Al, a fifty-year-old patient of mine, is morbidly obese and has struggled with his weight since he was six years old. He's tried numerous diets over the years, and even lost significant amounts of weight, but each time he put it all back again, and then some. He even looked into bariatric surgery, but he decided it wasn't for him. "If I get my stomach stapled, I'll feel sick when I overeat and probably lose weight because of that, but it still won't stop me from wanting to eat. My problem is willpower—I resent having to limit what I eat when all around me people are eating whatever they want and not gaining weight."

For a time, Al had some success with a food-delivery program that provided him with three diet meals a day, but he was thrown off by a family wedding and never got back on track again. His most successful experience was a doctor-supervised liquid diet, on which he lost one hundred pounds in seventeen weeks. Because he was only allowed to drink the prescribed shakes, he didn't feel tempted when he went grocery shopping or out to restaurants. "If there were a pill I could take instead of eating, I'd give up food for the rest of my life," he told me. "Alcoholics have it easy by comparison—they simply have to stop drinking. You can't stop eating or you'll die."

I was a bit taken aback when he said this, but then the truth of his words sank in. People who have dysfunctional or addictive relationships to drugs or alcohol certainly have a hard time of it, but if they can maintain total abstinence, they will succeed. People who have a dysfunctional or addictive relationship to food still have to eat, requiring them to flirt with their demons on a daily basis. For Al and others facing the same challenge, I imagined, this must be psychologically torturous.

While physically weight loss is simply a numbers game, mentally it's a complex battle between your desire and your willpower that requires an arsenal of tricks and strategies to win. While each person has his or her own personal weaknesses, I've discovered several common threads among the patients I've talked with and hope that this chapter, which is gleaned from their wisdom and experience, will provide the ammunition you need to overcome yours.

There's No Such Thing as Cheating

People are very hard on themselves. I hear it all the time from my patients: "I was bad, Dr. Schnur. It was my birthday and I ate everything I wasn't supposed to—prime rib, fries, cheesecake." "I was so good about exercising for the first two weeks, then I skipped a couple of days and never got back in the swing again. I'm such a loser."

What I tell them is, "You're not good or bad, you're human!" We may have good days, when we stick to our diet and exercise program, and bad days, when we fall off the wagon, but this doesn't make us good or bad people. Unfortunately, in our culture people tend to make assumptions about each other's character based on their appearance—people who are overweight are slapped with labels such as lazy, sloppy, and lacking in self-control, while people who are slender are hailed as smart and successful. We tend to apply these messages to ourselves, as well, which leads us to make something as simple as eating a bag of potato chips into a moral crisis.

I say relax. It's only calories. So you eat a few too many one day? Eat a few less and exercise a bit more the next. Or if you don't make up for it, you'll simply lose a little bit less this week. Keeping an eye on your long-term goal will help you put occasional blips in perspective and not let them sabotage your whole plan.

Karen, a patient who has been on the Reality Diet for close to a year, revises her short-term goal when she sees a holiday or special occasion looming on the horizon. "That week, my goal is not to gain weight, rather than to lose my usual one to two pounds. If I can hold steady, I consider it a victory. It took me twenty years to put on all this weight; if it takes me an extra month or two to lose it, it's no big deal."

Get Back in the Saddle

All too often patients tell me how they were "really good" about sticking to their diet, then ate something "bad" that "ruined" it. For many people, that's the end of their diet altogether. Others write off the rest of the week and promise themselves they'll start again "on Monday." But if you slip up on Tuesday, Monday is a long way off and you can set yourself way back by giving yourself license to eat carelessly for the next six days. Instead, forgive yourself for your lapse and consider yourself back on your diet immediately. Not the very next day—again, if you slip up at lunch, you can do a lot of damage before bedtime—but the very next meal.

By committing yourself to getting right back in the saddle again, you eliminate any possibility of negotiation. The longer you wait to return to your diet, the more chance there is for your desires to sweet-talk your willpower into letting go altogether. You also leave yourself a lot of time to wallow in self-pity and self-recrimination, both of which lead directly to the pint of Häagen-Dazs in the freezer.

Choose Real Friends

Real friends are friends who support you on the Reality Diet. Having at least one special person to cheer you on and counteract whatever negative self-talk you've been giving yourself in your head can help keep you on

Cheat Sheet

So you went a bit overboard at the office party last night, or it was Halloween and you couldn't resist "borrowing" a few pieces of candy from your kid's stash. Don't berate yourself. Rather, make sure you exercise enough the next day to counteract those extra calories. If you know how many calories your indulgence was, you can look at the chart on pages 128–129 to see how many minutes of exercise you need to do. Or check the chart below, which lists some popular temptations and the number of minutes you need to walk to burn them off.

Amount	Food	Calories	Required Walking Time (Minutes)
1	Reese's peanut butter cup miniature	42	11
1	Hershey's Kiss	26	7
1	Milky Way miniature	38	10
1	3 Musketeers miniature	24	6.3
1	Snickers miniature	42	11
1	Butter toffee candy	30	8
1	Cheez-It cracker	6	1.6
1	Wheat Thins cracker	9	2.4
1	Peanut	7	1.8
1	Peanut M&M	12	3.2
1	Plain M&M	4	1.1
1	Snackwell's reduced fat chocolate chip cookie	10	2.6
1	French fry	16	4.2

track. If you can find a friend who wants to go on the Reality Diet with you, all the better—there's no question that dieting with a friend is easier than dieting alone. In the best of all possible worlds, your Real friend will be your spouse, partner, or roommate. That way, you can eliminate tempting foods from your kitchen cabinets altogether and don't have to sit across from someone gobbling extra-cheesy pizza or deep-fried chicken wings for dinner while you're trying to eat healthfully. Newt and Dolores, who went on the Reality Diet together after Newt's heart attack, each say that it would have been much harder to stick to it if they hadn't had the other one to help them along.

Real friends can also help you fulfill your exercise commitment. Over the years I've developed a whole circle of buddies who love to exercise as much as I do. Every afternoon around three, the phone starts to ring: it's my friends calling to figure out what we're going to do that day after work. Sometimes we meet at the gym and work out, other days we hit the tennis or racquetball court. Many doctors I know are amazed that I have so much time to spend with friends—let's face it, running a large cardiology practice is not exactly a nine-to-five job. The difference is that they're going to the gym alone, if at all. I know myself well enough to know that I have to exercise every day, and by combining exercise with socializing, I can kill two birds with one stone.

As important as it is to have Real friends, it's equally important to avoid friends and situations that don't support your weight-loss effort. If you have a friend whose idea of a good time is to sit in his basement listening to Aerosmith and eating pork rinds, tell him you'll take a rain check. Instead, listen to your Aerosmith while walking on a treadmill or encourage your friend to get out of his basement and join you for a walk outside. If you have a particularly hospitable friend who would be offended if you didn't try a piece of her homemade coffee cake, meet her for a stroll in the park instead of at her house.

Be aware that there are also people out there who will try to undermine your diet for their own twisted reasons. They may like the fact that you're overweight because it makes them feel superior and they feel threatened by the fact that you're taking charge of your life. People like this may try to tempt you to stray from your diet or persuade you that you don't need to lose weight, that you can't change your body, or that you're being self-indulgent by spending so much time and energy focusing on your diet and exercise. Avoid these people like the plague, lest they sabotage your weight-loss effort through their mind games.

Embrace Your Sweet Tooth

For some people, even the delicious daily Reality Reward isn't enough to satisfy their sweet tooth. They may have a particular craving that simply isn't on the Reality Diet—Baskin-Robbins Peanut Butter 'N Chocolate ice cream, yogurt-covered pretzels, Tootsie Rolls, M&M's. My advice? Go for it—in moderation. Skip a Reality Reward once a week and use the 360 calories to satisfy your sweet tooth. You can parcel it out and have, say, thirteen M&M's or two small Tootsie Rolls a day, or a full cup of Peanut Butter 'N Chocolate ice cream once a week.

You can also do what Drew, my interior decorator, does. He simply cannot go a day without chocolate, and for him that means Godiva. So each week he visits the Godiva shop and buys a box with seven chocolates. Then he eats one every night before bed. To make up for it, he swims an extra fifteen minutes a day. He's still losing weight and has tightened his belt five holes in six months.

Three Cheers for Chocolate

While it's not exactly a diet food, chocolate could be one of the healthiest sweet treats around. Cocoa butter, while high in saturated fat, actually protects against cardiovascular disease, preventing oxidation of LDL ("bad") cholesterol, raising HDL ("good") cholesterol, reducing blood clotting, and relaxing arteries. One-third of cocoa butter's fat comes from stearic acid, which, although saturated, does not raise LDL cholesterol because the liver converts it to oleic acid, a monounsaturated fat that is good for your heart. Another third of the fat is from oleic acid itself. A study of volunteers who received most of their daily fat from either butter or chocolate found that those on the chocolate diet did not have increased LDL cholesterol, while those on the butter diet did.

Among the more than three hundred naturally occurring compounds in chocolate are phenols and flavonoids, powerful antioxidants that may protect against heart disease and cancer. One ounce of dark chocolate contains more antioxidants than a glass of red wine and more than four times the amount of black tea. The darker the chocolate, the higher the concentration of antioxidants. Chocolate also contains magnesium, phosphorus, and about one-tenth the caffeine of coffee. And, believe it or not, because of the antibacterial agents naturally present in cocoa beans, chocolate actually protects against tooth decay!

If you're going to enjoy a piece of chocolate, choose dark over light. Also, it's worth it to spend a little extra for a high-quality brand. Finer dark chocolates contain up to 70 percent cocoa butter, while commercial brands may only have 20 percent cocoa butter and lots of unhealthy tropical oils. Don't go overboard, however, as chocolate contains between 85 and 150 calories per ounce.

Women: Know Your Body

Premenstrual syndrome affects up to 80 percent of women at some point in their lives and, among its many diverse symptoms, can cause bloating and cravings. "I have two pair of jeans," one patient told Shirley, "my regular jeans and my PMS jeans, which are a size bigger." Another patient confessed that during the week before her period she eats up to six chocolate bars a day. Fortunately, the cravings and bloating disappear as soon as menstruation begins; unfortunately, the extra pounds from those chocolate bars do not.

There are several healthy ways to prevent premenstrual water retention. Start by eating lots of melons, bananas, and citrus fruit, as they all contain high levels of potassium, which balances the excess sodium that is making your body retain water. Also, munch on lots of vegetables that are natural diuretics, like celery, cucumbers, lettuce, watercress, tomatoes, onions, carrots, and bell peppers. Avoid salt, refined sugar, excess fat, caffeine, and al-

Research Update

When I was a medical resident, working thirty-six-hour shifts, I lived on junk food. There was a snack machine in the visitors' lounge and several times a night I'd pump in a bunch of change, pull the knobs, and watch the packets of Twizzlers, Dots, and Raisinets fall to the bottom of the machine. I convinced myself that I needed the extra sugar to stay awake, and that since I was on my feet for all those hours I didn't have to worry about the extra calories, either. Besides, all the other residents were doing the same thing. Here we were, learning how to restore health to other people's bodies while we abused our own.

Twenty years later, scientists have proven what any medical student could have told them—sleep deprivation makes you crave high-calorie, high-fat food. What they've also figured out is why. It turns out that sleep affects the hormones that control appetite, so you're actually hungrier when you haven't slept enough than when you have. When twelve young men were allowed to sleep only four hours a night for two nights, they showed an 18 percent reduction in leptin, a hormone that suppresses appetite, and a 28 percent increase in ghrelin, a hormone that stimulates appetite. They also chose candy, cookies, and cake over fruit, vegetables, and dairy products to assuage their hunger pangs. In a separate study, researchers looked at the sleeping patterns of 1,024 people and found that the ones who slept five hours or less a night had 15 percent less leptin and 15 percent more ghrelin than people who slept for eight hours a night. In addition, those who regularly slept less than eight hours a night also tended to have higher BMIs than those who habitually got more sleep.

While you may not exactly be able to snooze the pounds away, getting adequate sleep can help you lose weight. If you can't, at least try to limit your extracurricular eating to fruits, vegetables, and 2:90 starches.

cohol. And last but not least, drink plenty of water. Although it may seem counterintuitive, drinking water is the best way to reduce bloating from water retention.

In addition to shifts in levels of reproductive hormones, PMS is characterized by a drop in serotonin, a neurochemical that affects mood. Your brain makes serotonin from carbohydrates, so scientists believe that the typical PMS cravings for sweet and salty foods are your body's way of helping to correct this serotonin imbalance. Unfortunately, chocolate and potato chips, while high in carbohydrates, are also high in fat and calories. Far better to satisfy your cravings with complex carbohydrates and a little protein, such as low-fat turkey on 2:90 bread, or some tuna on 2:90 crackers.

One of the best things you can do to counteract both water retention and mood swings is to exercise. Keeping active will also prevent you from snacking and help burn any extra calories you do consume during this time of the month.

Keep Yourself Motivated

Whether it's buying a new belt, like Drew, or taking photos of yourself in your "fat" clothes like Helene, there are as many ways to stay motivated as there are people. Some like to keep a photo of a movie star or model or themselves at a slimmer time of life on their fridge to encourage them to withstand its temptations. Others find the opposite approach works and put up a photo of when they looked their absolute worst to scare themselves away. Ethel, a grandmother of seven, says looking at photos of her grandchildren keeps her focused on her diet because, in her words, "I want to live long enough to see every one of them graduate college."

My patient Mona always keeps an outfit two sizes too small on hand. When she is able to fit into it, she rejoices, then goes out and buys a new one two sizes smaller. Another patient, Lydia, who is striving to get down to her high school weight, made a tape of her favorite songs from back then, including Van Morrison's "Brown Eyed Girl," Simon and Garfunkel's "Cecilia," and other upbeat tunes from the late sixties. She plays the tape in her car on the way to work and whenever she needs a quick pick-me-up during the day.

Other ways to stay motivated include looking back in your 3-E Journal and seeing how much progress you've made so far or calling a Real friend and asking for a pep talk. "I find that when I'm depressed I simply can't think of ways to help myself feel better," one patient told me. "So one day when I wasn't depressed I made a list of things I could do to help me feel better right in my 3-E Journal. Now I just have to remember to look at my Journal!"

Avoid Triggers

From your 3-E Journal, you've probably identified triggers that cause you to overeat. Whether they be passing Dunkin' Donuts on the way to work or sitting in front of the TV with a box of Teddy Grahams, the best way to resist them is to avoid them. Choose a different route to work. Don't buy Teddy Grahams or, if you must because they're the only cookie your three-year-old will eat, make sure you have healthful snacks like fruits, veggies, and low-fat popcorn on hand for yourself as well. Your three-year-old may find she likes them, too!

Eat Consciously

Many of us engage in unconscious eating when we're involved in an absorbing activity like driving, reading, or watching TV. With conscious effort you can change such behavior. Institute a rule that food has to be eaten sitting down at a table in either the kitchen or the dining room. Then, when you're driving or reading or watching TV, chew sugarless gum or sip water instead of munching.

One simple way to stop yourself from finishing the whole bowl of grapes or bag of low-fat tortilla chips without thinking is to remove your allotted portion, then put the rest away. My weakness in this department is cereal—I keep pouring more and more in my bowl to sop up the excess milk. Instead, I've learned to pour exactly as much cereal as I want to eat—I actually keep a plastic measuring cup in the cereal box—then put the box back in the cabinet. If there's any extra milk, I drink it up and am done.

Weigh Yourself Regularly

Be sure to weigh yourself once or twice a week to keep track of your progress and modify your eating and exercise plan if you stall. Weighing yourself more often can be dispiriting, as you won't see significant change from day to day. Also, daily fluctuations in humidity and your salt intake can make you appear to have gained weight when it's just water retention. Weighing yourself less frequently can be a problem, too, especially if you're procrastinating because you haven't been as faithful to your diet and exercise plan as you should have.

Don't Freak Out If You Plateau

So, you're going great guns, losing a couple of pounds a week, when all of a sudden the dial on the scale appears to have gotten stuck. And it remains stuck for two or three weeks. Uh-oh, you've plateaued.

Plateauing is a common phenomenon in weight loss, and there are various explanations. One you've already heard is what happened to Nicholas, who cut back on his calories and tricked his body into starvation mode. His metabolism dropped and he stopped losing weight. He actually had to eat a little bit more to get the scale moving again.

Another reason people plateau is that after three or four weeks on a diet, their body adjusts to the reduced caloric intake and their metabolism shifts down a gear. The best way to speed it up again is to increase the duration and intensity of your exercise. Similarly, people who lose weight eating a certain number of calories a day may hit a plateau because, as they slim down, their BMR decreases and they need fewer calories to support their lighter bodies. Again, increased exercise—not necessarily reducing calories— is the preferred way to break through and begin losing weight again.

Sometimes people think they've plateaued when in reality they've been getting a little slack about their diet and exercise. To make sure you're eating and exercising as much as you should, use your 3-E Journal to keep a food and exercise log for a week. At the end, look back and assess whether you really have been sticking to the recommended amount of food and burning 2,000 calories a week through exercise. Skipping a couple of days' workouts and eating a few extra treats can make the difference between losing a pound or two a week and not.

There are medical reasons for plateaus, as well, including thyroid hormone imbalance, diabetes, and conditions requiring steroid medication. If you suspect any of these problems may be affecting your weight loss, consult your physician.

Plan Ahead

Dieting is a lot like scouting—you have to be prepared for any eventuality. If you're taking your child to a birthday party where you know the only food available will be pizza and cake, pack your own lunch. If you're going for a long car ride, pack meals and snacks so you won't be tempted by the fast-food joints along the highway. If you know your boss always brings danishes and bagels on Fridays, make sure you eat breakfast before you go to the office and avoid the company kitchen that morning. If a friend wants to meet you for lunch, choose a restaurant that has Reality-friendly entrees on the menu. If you know you'll be rushed in the morning, prepare your lunch the night before. Similarly, if you know you'll be rushed in the evening, have dinner made in advance and stored in your refrigerator or freezer so you won't be tempted to grab fast food or order in.

Planning ahead also means shopping ahead. It's all too easy to succumb to takeout if you lack the ingredients for a healthful meal. Use the shopping lists on the Reality Diet website to make sure you're prepared, and stock your pantry with the items listed on pages 115–116 so that you'll have tasty ingredients on hand for fun and hassle-free cooking.

Keep a Regular Schedule

A patient of mine named Chris says he always loses weight when he goes on vacation. This mystified me—if ever I feel tempted to overeat and slack off on exercise, it's when I'm traveling. He explained that unlike him, his wife keeps to a strict schedule, and when they go away together, he eats regular meals and doesn't snack in between. The rest of the time he works long hours at the office and rarely sees his wife from Monday to Friday.

Consequently, he eats haphazardly, grabbing food here and there and eating at odd times and places.

One of the best things you can learn from the Reality Diet is to eat three regular meals a day. As you get used to it, you gradually will lose the desire to snack in between meals. To make this schedule work, however, you have to eat your meals at reasonable intervals and not skip any of them. If you eat breakfast at seven and usually break for lunch around noon, don't wait until one or two to eat, as by that time you'll be ravenous and likely to binge. On the weekends, try to maintain the same routine you follow during the week so that you don't have to start retraining your body all over again every Monday morning.

Takeaway Tips

In addition to following the Reality Diet eating plan, it's essential to enlist support and develop strategies to keep yourself motivated. If you do stray, don't be hard on yourself—forgive yourself and go right back to the plan. Try to negate the effect of occasional indulgences with extra exercise. By planning ahead and keeping a regular schedule, you can avoid many pitfalls and temptations. And one last tip that has served me well—brush your teeth after every meal. It'll not only protect your pearly whites, but it will also help stop you from picking at leftovers or grazing your way straight through to the next meal.

Chapter 11

The Reality Diet in the Real World: Restaurants and Holidays

As long as you're motivated and organized, it's not hard to stay on a diet when you're preparing all the meals yourself. You're in control of your environment—you determine what food crosses the threshold into your home and can keep out tempting intruders. But the reality is that most Americans eat out—a lot. We're an on-the-go society, and all too often that means eating on the go—grabbing breakfast from a coffee shop, lunch from a deli or the company cafeteria, and ordering takeout or picking up prepared supermarket food for dinner because it's late and the kids are hungry and you just don't have the time or energy to cook.

We're also a multicultural society with a wide variety of ethnic cuisines available for the tasting. If you're an adventurous eater, you shouldn't have to deprive yourself of exotic flavors just because you're on a diet. Even if you're not that adventurous but just enjoy eating out—or have to eat out or travel for business—you still can lose weight on the Reality Diet. Look at

Drew—he eats out or takes in three meals a day, yet he's one of my greatest success stories.

Finally, we're human—we like to socialize and to get together with friends and family to celebrate holidays and special occasions. If you're trying to lose weight, these events may instill in you a sense of anxiety or even dread. The trick is to approach times like these with reasonable expectations, not a sense of preordained failure, and to learn some basic strategies to help keep you on track in these tempting situations.

Eat Out and Enjoy!

Just because you're on a diet doesn't mean you have to sit home every night by yourself while everyone else is out having a good time. The Reality Diet is designed to be flexible and to fit your lifestyle, even if you travel, entertain clients, or, like Drew, have nothing in your kitchen but fabric samples and a small box of Godiva chocolates.

When you dine out, just follow the guidelines of the Reality Diet as closely as possible. Avoid anything creamy, breaded, or fried. Instead, order items that approximate the kinds of food you would be eating if you were to cook for yourself—lots of veggies, lean meat, fish, chicken, or tofu, with low-fat dressings and sauces on the side. Start with a light vegetable soup or a house salad (a salad topped with chicken, fish, eggs, or cheese is a meal in itself). Avoid refined starches—this usually means skipping the breadbasket altogether—and stick to whole-grains (barley, quinoa, whole-wheat couscous), corn, baked sweet or white potato, or whole-wheat pasta. Order fish, poultry, or a lean cut of meat broiled, baked, poached, or grilled. Request that your food be prepared without butter or oil, and trim the fat off the meat and skin off the chicken when it arrives. Whenever possible, request a side of steamed vegetables without butter as well. If you have a choice between a baked potato and mashed, take the baked potato and eat it with the skin on. You can dress it with a teaspoon of olive oil, broccoli, chives, or salsa. At the salad bar, avoid high-fat toppings like bacon bits, fried noodles, high-fat cheese, or anything with mayonnaise. If you find yourself at a pizza joint, request a little cheese and a lot of veggies, and avoid pepperoni, sausage, and meatball toppings. For dessert, have fresh fruit salad. It's fine to taste a more luscious concoction—a couple of spoonfuls, max!—but avoid ordering one for yourself, or you'll be tempted to overindulge.

Speaking of dessert: Recent research has shown that we are highly susceptible to peer pressure when it comes to consuming sweets. If you're around people who eat cookies by the bagful, you will, too. If, on the other hand, you're sitting with someone who leaves half his pie unfinished, you're less likely to finish yours. I decided to do a little experiment to prove this phenomenon to myself. A few weeks ago I went out to dinner with a group of friends. Come dessert time, I took the lead and said, "We'll have one of everything, with lots of forks!" The waiter brought an assortment of desserts and everyone dug in. The next week I went back to the same restaurant with the same friends—we even happened to have the same waiter. When dessert rolled around, I let out a dramatic sigh and said, "Whew, I'm stuffed! No dessert for me." Nobody else at the table ordered dessert either.

After a lifetime of eating in restaurants, another fascinating fact finally dawned on me not too long ago: Most of the time the appetizer was just about filling me up. By the time the main course came I would eat most of it anyway, just because I had ordered it, not because I was really hungry. It turns out I'm not alone—a recent survey conducted by the American Institute of Cancer Research of more than one thousand adults showed that when eating out, 69 percent finished their entrees all or most of the time, and of those, 30 percent said they would have been satisfied with a smaller portion. So I developed five techniques to make sure I didn't overeat in restaurants:

1. I order two appetizers instead of an appetizer and a main course.
2. I order my own appetizer, but I split my main course with someone else.
3. If I'm not sharing the main course, I either order a half-portion or else immediately push half the portion to the side of my plate and, when the waiter comes to clear the meal, ask to have it wrapped to go.
4. I wait until after my appetizer to order my main course so I can see if I'm really hungry for more.
5. I stop eating when I'm no longer hungry—what a novel concept!

Once you've been following the Reality Diet for a while, you'll have developed an internal sense of what correct portion sizes are. Unfortunately,

The Reality Diet Goes Global

Ethnic restaurants can be challenging for dieters—what's in that dish anyway? Here are some general guidelines, courtesy of the American Heart Association, to help you make healthful selections when pursuing international and specialty cuisine. Remember to keep an eye on portion sizes, however—most restaurant portions will be about twice what you need.

Cajun. Avoid fried seafood and hush puppies. Blackened entrees usually are dipped in butter or oil, covered with spices, and pan-fried; ask the cook to use only a small amount of oil. Ask for all sauces and gravies on the side.

Chinese. Choose entrees with lots of vegetables—chop suey with steamed rice is an example. Substitute chicken for duck when possible. Skip the crispy fried noodles on the table. And request that the chef use no MSG.

Family Restaurants. Avoid dishes with lots of cheese, sour cream, and mayonnaise. Instead of fried oysters, fish, or chicken, choose boiled spiced shrimp, or baked, broiled, or grilled fish or chicken. Choose bread or pita pockets over croissants. Salads make great meals, but be careful of the dressing. If you must have a high-fat entree, split it with another family member. You'll save dollars—and fat!

French. Bypass the rich entrees, desserts, and sauces. Aim for simple dishes with sauces on the side. Nouvelle cuisine or Provençal tomato-and-herb-based entrees are good choices. Ask that non-hydrogenated margarine be used instead of butter for cooking—or leave it out altogether.

Greek and Middle Eastern. Ask for dishes to be prepared with less oil and for high-sodium foods like feta cheese and olives to be served on the side. Ask for salad dressing and sauces on the side, too. Phyllo pastry dishes are usually high in butter, so skip them. Most Greek desserts are high in fat and sugar. If you want to splurge, split one with a friend.

Health Food and Vegetarian. There are lots of great vegetarian sandwiches. Just avoid those with lots of cheese and oil. Ask for salad dressings on the side.

Indian. Start with salads or yogurt with chopped or shredded vegetables. Choose chicken or seafood rather than beef or lamb. Choose dishes prepared without ghee. Order one protein and one vegetable dish to cut down the fat and calories. If sodium is a concern, forgo the soups.

Italian. Enjoy pasta as an entree rather than as an appetizer, and ask if the chef can substitute whole-wheat pasta. Share foods among your dinner companions. Ask your waiter to hold the Parmesan (grated) cheese, bacon, olives, and pine nuts. If you order pizza, choose healthful ingredients like spinach, mushrooms, broccoli, and roasted peppers.

Japanese. Ask the cook to prepare your food without high-sodium marinades, sauces, and salt. And ask that sauces be served on the side. Avoid foods that are deep-fried, battered, breaded, or fried. Ask to substitute shrimp, scallops, or chicken for beef dishes.

Mexican. Ask your server not to bring fried tortilla chips to the table. And hold the sour cream and guacamole from entrees; use salsa to add flavor. Veracruz or other tomato-based sauces are better than creamy or cheesy sauces. If you order a taco salad, don't eat the fried shell.

Steakhouses. Don't order king-size cuts. About 3 ounces of a thinly sliced cut is perfect, or choose a 6-ounce steak and enjoy non-meat entrees the rest of the day. Steakhouses generally prepare your food to order, so ask to have all visible fat trimmed before cooking.

Thai. Aim for the lighter, stir-fried dishes and fresh spring rolls. Steer clear of heavy sauces and deep-fried entrees. Ask that cooking be done with vegetable oil rather than coconut oil or lard. Choose chicken over duck, but limit meat, poultry, and seafood portions. Avoid soups and soy and other sauces if you must watch your sodium intake, and ask that MSG be left out. Share portions.

Research Update

Did you know that drinking a glass of water before a meal does absolutely nothing to help you feel full? Lots of diets recommend it, but research has shown that water alone—either before or with a meal—does not contribute to satiety. But water that's *in* food does. Why? Because it decreases the energy density of the food.

Energy density is the number of calories in a particular weight of food. A 4-ounce piece of steak, for example, has a much higher energy density than 4 ounces of tomatoes. Because we naturally tend to eat the same weight of food each day, a great way to cut calories is to substitute foods with a low energy density for those with a high energy density.

Several years ago, Barbara J. Rolls, Ph.D., director of the Laboratory for the Study of Human Ingestive Behavior in the Department of Nutritional Sciences at Pennsylvania State University, University Park, performed an experiment to prove just this point. She and her colleagues fed a group of women three meals a day for two days. The volunteers were all fed the same portion sizes, but the meals had been manipulated so that they were either high, medium, or low in energy density. The women ate similar amounts of food by weight over the two days, but the ones who had been fed the lower-energy-density food consumed about 30 percent fewer calories than those who were offered the higher-energy-dense food. Nevertheless, women in the two groups reported equal levels of fullness and satisfaction. In another study that lasted a full year, Rolls and her collaborators divided their volunteers into two groups. Members of one group were advised to add two servings of low-energy-dense soup to their daily diet; members of the other group ate the same number of calories in higher-energy-dense snacks such as pretzels and crackers. After a year, the people in the soup-eating group lost significantly more weight than the people in the pretzel-eating group, proving that the soup was filling them up so they would eat fewer calories during the rest of their meals.

The Reality Diet menus are filled with large servings of vegetables and a variety of juicy fruits—all foods with low energy density that will keep you satisfied. When you're eating out, choose a big salad or clear (as opposed to cream) soup for an appetizer to satisfy your hunger and help keep you from overeating when the high-energy-dense entree arrives.

in the restaurant world—and I'm not talking just about fast-food restaurants here—everything has been super sized. Order spaghetti and you'll get half a pound of pasta, two 6-ounce meatballs, and an entire loaf of garlic bread. Arroz con pollo comes with a platter of rice and half a chicken. And don't even talk about steak—the average steakhouse dish can easily serve a family of four.

Professor Barbara J. Rolls of Pennsylvania State University, University Park, and her colleagues have shown that when offered larger portions, people simply eat more food. In one study, men and women were served 6-, 8-, 10-, and 12-inch sandwiches on different days. Each time they were offered a bigger sandwich, they ate more. When served the 12-inch sandwiches, women consumed 31 percent more calories and men consumed 56 percent more calories than when they were served the 6-inch sandwiches—yet they reported similar levels of hunger at the beginning of the meals and similar levels of fullness at the end! Basically, the more food you have in front of you, the more you tend to eat. So in restaurants that serve big portions, either share or immediately move half the entree to a separate plate.

When it comes to all-you-can-eat buffets, avoid them at all costs—the temptation to overeat is nearly irresistible, and the foods tend to be cheap and fatty. Back when I was a poor medical school student, I used to seek out these places, figuring that if I could eat $12 worth of food and pay only $3.99, I'd beat the restaurant at its own game. It turns out that from a health point of view, I was the big loser. If you simply can't avoid eating at a buffet, serve yourself half a portion of the leanest protein you can find and go back for seconds on veggies, salad, or fruit if you're still hungry.

Fortunately, many restaurants now flag heart-healthy or low-calorie items on their menus. These generally are lower in fat and salt than the rest of the selections and will be compatible with the Reality Diet. If they don't, feel free to ask how a dish is prepared so you can determine yourself whether it meets the Reality guidelines. In most cases, servers are well versed in how the various dishes are made, and if they aren't they will be happy to ask the chef for details. Don't be shy—these days, so many people have food allergies and special diets that waitstaff are used to these kinds of questions.

Have Happy *and* Healthy Holidays

Holidays can be a time of stress for anyone, but especially for dieters. For one thing, there's all that food—the groaning board laden with turkey, stuffing, and pies on Thanksgiving; roast beef, candied carrots, and mincemeat for Christmas; matzo, gefilte fish, and brisket for Passover; leg of lamb, roasted potatoes, and all those chocolate eggs for Easter. For another, there's all that family—people who, however well-meaning, may trigger in you the compulsion to overeat, either because they expect it of you or because it's a learned response when you're in their presence.

When a patient of mine named Alex went home to Indiana for Christmas last year, he not only noticed the vast quantities of heavy food his mother served, but also noticed how he felt tempted to revert to his childhood mode of eating. He practically could hear his mother telling him to clean his plate and think of all those starving children in China, to eat lots of potatoes because they'd stick to his ribs, to finish his bowl of creamed spinach "so you'll be big and strong like Popeye!" Plus, Alex's reputation as a child was that of a good eater, and he used to get lots of praise from his aunts and uncles because he had such a healthy appetite. It took a great deal of effort to break the pattern of this early imprinting and stick to his diet when he was with his family.

Holidays can also be stressful, especially if they involve getting together with family members whom you may not exactly love to be with. One of the most common ways to deal with stress is to eat, and with all that food lying around, it's all too easy to indulge in this method of escape. Try to find other outlets for your stress—sip water, chew a toothpick, play with your napkin under the table. Engage in the conversation to keep yourself focused on something other than the food. If you volunteer to serve the food

Holiday and Party Tips at a Glance

- **Arrive a little late.** You'll eat less.
- **Don't arrive hungry.** It's a bad idea to skip a meal in anticipation of all the delectable foods you'll encounter at the holiday feast. If your stomach is growling, you're more likely to lose control and overeat.
- **Limit your alcohol.** Choose wine over hard liquor and watch out for holiday drinks like eggnog and hot buttered rum—they can pack a huge number of calories. Drink them sparingly, and consider cutting the eggnog with skim milk. Try to drink a full glass of water between alcoholic beverages.
- **Don't hang out by the food table.** If possible, go to another room altogether.
- **Fill up on soup and salad.**
- **Choose a small plate and serve yourself half the usual portion of each dish.** If you are still hungry after the main meal, go back for seconds of veggies.
- **Eat only what you love.** Don't feel like you have to eat everything just because it's there. It's not as if you never will see these foods again. Choose the one food you simply cannot do without and fill the rest of your plate with vegetables, salads, and lean meats.
- **Eat slowly.** Chew every bite and enjoy every morsel.
- **Nibble on fruits instead of candies, cookies, or chocolate after the meal.**
- **Stop when you feel full.**
- **Carry a travel-size toothbrush with you.** Brush your teeth after the meal to help stop yourself from nibbling at goodies.
- **Exercise the day of the holiday or party *and* the day after.** You might even consider starting a new holiday tradition of taking a walk or bike ride, playing a little touch football or softball, or going sledding or skating after the meal.

- **If you're cooking the holiday meal, make it low-fat.** Tweak your favorite recipes and make them more healthful.
- **Send friends and family home with the leftovers.**

and help clear and clean up, you'll spend less time at the table in front of your plate and get a little exercise, too. After the meal, suggest a walk—again, you'll burn calories, but you'll also help yourself to decompress and remove yourself from the leftovers. Throughout, remind yourself that holidays only last a short time and that you'll soon be back to your own routine.

The upside of holidays is that the food can be delicious and trigger many happy memories. If you enjoy warm relations with your family, it's also a time to rejoice in each other's company. The trick is to enjoy it all—the atmosphere, the food, the company—but not get so carried away that you forget to watch what you eat. Go ahead and have a little of everything—just keep portion sizes and food groups in mind. A small bowl of matzo-ball soup or a scoop of noodle kugel can count as a starch and a fat. Green beans with fried onions count as a vegetable and a fat. Skinless turkey with a scoop of stuffing gives you a primary protein, starch, and fat. And don't forget that you have 360 calories to spend on dessert if you cash in your Reality Reward. Do your best to stick to the Reality Diet guidelines, and if you go a bit over be sure to cut back a little or do some extra exercise the next day.

Takeaway Tips

Take special care to stay focused on your diet during the holidays and other special occasions and don't feel compelled to stuff yourself just because the food is there. We're fortunate to live in a country where food is abundant. There's no need to eat everything in front of you as if there won't be any more tomorrow. When you eat out, don't be shy about asking questions and requesting that your food be prepared in a specific way. And feel free to dine out and enjoy a wide variety of ethnic restaurants—keeping your palate stimulated can help prevent you from getting bored with the diet and seeking excitement in the cookie jar.

Chapter 12

Keeping the Weight Off—for Good!

I began this book by debunking a long list of weight-loss myths. But I saved the best for last. It's a commonly held myth that permanent weight loss is impossible—eventually everyone gains the weight back. You may have experienced it yourself in prior attempts at dieting—you reached your goal, went off the diet, and within a matter of months or years were back where you started, or even heavier.

The reality is that this does not have to be the case. Maintaining weight loss—even significant weight loss—is entirely possible. One study showed that at least one in five dieters who have lost 10 percent of their body weight successfully keep the weight off for at least a year. I count myself among them—I've kept off the twenty pounds I lost with Shirley for three years now. In my own case, as well as for many of those surveyed, the increased self-confidence, better mood, and improved health we've experienced through weight loss has motivated us to keep it off long term.

So, How Do I "Stop" Dieting?

Good question. The trick is to gradually add more calories to your diet until your body finds its own equilibrium. Start by adding one extra 90-calorie serving of a fruit, vegetable, or 2:90 starch a day. Keep to this new level for a week and see whether you're still losing weight. If so, add a second. Continue to gradually add back and monitor your weight until you stop losing. Some people find that they begin to plateau naturally as they approach their goal weight. If that happens to you, your weight loss and maintenance eating plans will be exactly the same.

At the same time, don't stop exercising! If you slack off, you'll see the numbers on the scale going up immediately. Plus, you'll begin losing the hard-won lean muscle mass you've built up, which will help keep you fit and trim into the future.

As soon as you notice weight creeping back on, do an intervention. Return to your 3-E Journal and do a diet and exercise inventory for up to a week. Then look back and see where you may be letting yourself slide. If it's in the exercise department, commit to a more regular and rigorous routine. If it's in the food department, pay closer attention to your portion sizes and the distribution of your food groups. Also, address the regained weight immediately by returning to the weight-loss plan until you get back to where you want to be. The longer you let those pounds hang around, the harder it will be to get rid of them.

Rebecca

About a year and a half ago, a colleague referred a patient to me because he thought she could benefit from the Reality Diet. Rebecca was forty and divorced, with two school-age girls. She also was about sixty pounds overweight. She worked from home editing textbooks and told me that apart from doing errands and taking her children to their after-school activities, she spent most of her time in her house.

Rebecca had been overweight since she was a child—she brought in photos of herself when she was her own children's age to show Shirley and me, and she definitely was chunky. She told us she had been teased all the way through grade school, and as a consequence she had become shy and withdrawn. In high school she lost a lot of weight on the Scarsdale Diet, which was popular at the time, and for a brief period she enjoyed a more normal social life, going to parties and wearing fashionable clothes. But as college loomed, she became anxious about the prospect of leaving home and began to gain the weight back. By the end of college, she was heavier than ever. She moved home, floundered around for a couple of years, then made a conscious effort to take charge of her life. She went on a liquid diet, lost fifty pounds, got a job at a women's magazine, and moved to her own apartment. Once again, she entered the social scene, attracting many friends and admirers. After a few years, she met a man and got married, but it became apparent quickly that they weren't a good match. Stressed out by her situation, Rebecca quit her job and gained back all the weight she had lost. In a desperate attempt to save her marriage she agreed to have children, but the marriage continued to deteriorate, and shortly after her second daughter was born she and her husband decided to separate.

"So what's motivating you to try to lose weight again this time?" Shirley asked.

"Looking back at my life, I realize that I've been hiding behind my weight," Rebecca replied. "When I was a normal size, I was more engaged with the world around me. Since the divorce I've basically been holed up in my home. It's not healthy for me, and it's even worse for my daughters. What kind of a role model am I? This time I'm determined to succeed, not just for me, but for them, too."

Satisfied that Rebecca was serious about her commitment to a more healthful lifestyle, Shirley got her started on the Reality Diet. It was challenging for her to resist temptation, especially with young children in the house, but she remained focused. At first she exercised on a stationary bike at home, but after she dropped the first twenty pounds she felt confident enough to join a gym, where she became a regular in a morning aerobics class. When she was within ten pounds of her goal she plateaued for a couple of weeks, so Shirley advised her to increase her exercise. Rebecca decided to try the spinning class at her gym. "I feel like I'm going to die—sixty minutes of nonstop pedaling—but it's such a rush that now I'm totally addicted."

It took nine months for Rebecca to lose the sixty pounds. Toward the end, Shirley noticed her becoming anxious about the prospect of tapering off her weight loss. "In some ways, dieting has been like a security blanket for me these past nine months," Rebecca explained. "The thought of going off the diet terrifies me!"

"But you're not 'going off' the diet," Shirley explained. "The Reality Diet is as much about learning the habits of healthful eating and exercise as it is about losing weight. Those are habits you should keep up for the rest of your life. You'll be doing exactly what you're doing now, eating exactly the same kinds of foods, just maybe a little bit more.

"The problem a lot of people have with 'going off' diets," Shirley continued, "is that they see it as a license to go back to the unhealthy eating patterns that got them into trouble in the first place. To be successful at maintaining your weight loss, you need to realize those days are gone for good. And why would you want to go back to them? Not only were you overweight back then, but you didn't have the energy or the self-confidence to leave your home. Look at you now—you're at the gym every day, you're more involved at your daughters' school—"

"And I've just gotten a job as an in-house copywriter for this hot new ad agency!" Rebecca chimed in. "I wanted to wait till it was for sure before telling you the news."

"Congratulations!" Shirley cried. "With all these great things going on in your life, you should be totally motivated to keep the weight off."

So Rebecca transitioned into maintenance. The first week she added an extra serving of fruit a day, but she still lost a pound. The second week, she added an extra serving of 2:90 starch in addition to the fruit. She seemed to level off, but after two weeks she noticed that she'd lost another pound. One more serving of vegetables a day did the trick—she stopped losing and didn't gain, either.

Even though Rebecca was no longer actively dieting, Shirley kept tabs on her and invited her to come in every three months or so for a chat. "You've lost more weight, haven't you?" she accused Rebecca at her most recent visit.

"No, I promise!" Rebecca replied, holding up her right hand. "Scout's honor!"

"You look thinner to me," Shirley said, still suspicious.

"I weighed myself just this morning and can assure you I'm exactly the same," Rebecca replied.

"It must be all that spinning—you may not have lost more pounds, but you've definitely continued to lose inches."

"Maybe a bit," Rebecca admitted. "Going to the gym is one of the high points of my day—when I skip a class, my daughters complain that I'm the Wicked Witch of the West. I took my girls to Disney World for a long weekend, and I didn't exercise for four days—it was torture! Plus, all that restaurant food. When we got back, I weighed myself and had gained three pounds. I put myself back on the diet and took the weight off in less than two weeks. I was so afraid that if I didn't get it off right away, I'd 'learn to live with it' and that would be the beginning of the end. In general, I find that if I weigh myself and notice I've gained a pound, I'm very careful what I eat for the next couple of days until I lose it. That scale really keeps me in line!"

"You should be very proud of yourself," Shirley said.

"I don't feel proud, exactly," Rebecca replied thoughtfully. "I feel like I've finally got it all together—as if I've finished one of those thousand-piece puzzles and can now see the picture clearly. I also feel like I'm in control of my life in a way that I didn't before. When I was overweight, everything seemed overwhelming to me; now, I'm excited by new challenges and have the energy and self-confidence to meet them head-on. But most of all, I feel grateful that I had the opportunity to turn my life around and show my girls that by setting a goal and working hard, anything is possible."

Proven Maintenance Strategies

Rebecca is just one of many patients of mine who have successfully maintained their weight loss. So how do these people do it? Thanks to the National Weight Control Registry (NWCR), an organization founded in 1994 by Rena R. Wing, Ph.D., of Brown University, and James Hill, Ph.D., of the University of Colorado, we have some very good ideas. The NWCR is a self-selected group of people over age eighteen who have lost a minimum of thirty pounds and have kept the weight off for at least one year. In general, registry participants have done much better than that, however—the average participant has lost 72.6 pounds and has kept it off for more than five and a half years, going from a BMI of 36.6 to 25.1! More than four thousand people are currently enrolled in the NWCR, and they respond to periodic surveys in order to help researchers distill the essential qualities that make for successful weight maintenance. Here are the most important lessons they have taught us so far:

✳ **Exercise, Exercise, Exercise.** Eighty-nine percent of the participants
    lost their weight through a combination of diet and exercise, and 91
    percent exercise regularly to maintain their weight loss. And by exer-
    cise, I don't mean just ten minutes on the stationary bike a couple of
    times a week—these people really work! Most perform moderate to in-
    tense exercise for sixty to ninety minutes a day, every day. Walking is
    the most frequently cited activity, and participants who walk exclu-
    sively take an average of 11,000 to 12,000 steps a day, covering 5 to 6
    miles. So don't stop exercising once you reach your goal—if anything,
    make a renewed commitment, as there's no better way to maintain
    your hard-won weight loss.

✳ **Continue to Watch Your Diet.** When surveyed about their food intake,
    NWCR participants reported that they all continue to watch their calo-
    rie intake. They also follow a low-fat (less than 30 percent of total calo-
    ries), high-carbohydrate (more than 50 percent of total calories) diet,
    with less than 20 percent of their calories coming from protein. This is
    nearly identical to the proportion of calories you've been getting from
    fat, protein, and carbohydrates on the Reality Diet! So just continue
    the healthful eating habits you've established and you'll help your
    body resist regaining the weight.

✳ **Don't Believe You're Genetically Doomed.** When patients tell me
    they've tried other diets and invariably gained the weight back, I tweak
    the line my stockbroker always tells me and reply, "Past performance is
    no indication of future failure." Just because you've never succeeded at
    maintaining your weight loss before, have been overweight your whole
    life, or have a family history of obesity doesn't mean you're doomed to
    a lifetime of yo-yo dieting. Ninety percent of the NWCR participants
    had tried to lose weight before and failed to keep it off. About one half
    were overweight as children, and nearly three-quarters have at least
    one obese parent. The difference between their past failures and their
    current successes is that they now consider watching their diet and ex-
    ercising a lifelong commitment.

✳ **Eat Breakfast Every Day.** If you're ever tempted to skip breakfast,
    don't—78 percent of NWCR participants eat breakfast every single
    day, typically cereal and fruit. While the jury is still out on exactly why
    eating breakfast makes such a difference in weight-loss maintenance, it

may be because breakfast eaters have more energy for exercise, or because they are less likely to overeat later in the day.

* **Weigh Yourself Often.** Three-quarters of the NWCR participants weigh themselves at least once a week, and of those, two-thirds weigh themselves at least once a day. Because your weight can vary from day to day due to water retention and other factors, I recommend weighing yourself once or twice a week. This kind of vigilance will help you to catch small weight gains and correct your behavior before things get out of control. Remember, always weigh yourself at the same time of day so that you're comparing apples to apples.

* **Be Consistent.** More than half of the NWCR participants report that they eat the same way seven days a week, and nearly half maintain their eating routine during holidays and vacations as well. This consistency is directly related to their success. When followed for two years, those who reported a consistent diet were 1½ times more likely to maintain their weight than those who were strict on weekdays and let loose on weekends. Similarly, those who relaxed their standards on holidays and vacations also had a greater risk of weight gain.

* **Limit Restaurant Visits.** This goes along with the importance of consistency—it's hard to maintain a regular eating pattern if you're not in control of how your food is prepared and if you're constantly putting yourself in situations where you're tempted by a variety of high-fat dishes. On average, NWCR participants eat out two to three times a week at restaurants and less than once a week at fast-food joints.

* **Remember, It Gets Easier with Time!** Just as it took you a little while to get used to following the Reality Diet plan, it may take a few weeks to get in the swing of maintaining. Continue to be vigilant, and you'll succeed. As time goes on and you keep the weight off, you'll be less tempted to revert to your pre-Reality days and more motivated to stick to your healthful diet and exercise routine. A study of NWCR participants showed that people who kept their weight off for two years reduced their risk of subsequent weight gain by 50 percent, and the longer people had kept weight off, the more likely they were to continue to do so. Plus, nearly half volunteered that it was easier to maintain than it was to lose!

Conclusion

When everything is said and done, there's only one simple way to ensure successful maintenance: making healthful living your top priority. And that's the same commitment you've had to make in order to lose weight on the Reality Diet in the first place. So you've already proven that you're perfectly capable of keeping the weight off as long as you keep up the habits you've learned: Exercise regularly and eat nutritious food in moderation.

In my own experience, I don't see myself as being on a diet—I'm simply living a healthy lifestyle, eating great food, and participating in all the athletic activities I love. I weigh myself twice a week, and if I've gained a pound or two I don't get all bent out of shape. I just make it a point to exercise a little extra and cut back on dessert for the next few days. But in general I eat lots of vegetables, fruit, lean meat, and whole-wheat 2:90 carbs; I have an occasional drink; and when I'm out to eat, I always taste dessert. On my daughter's birthday, I have cake and ice cream and savor every bite of it. Then I challenge her to an hour of tennis.

The reality is, if you're good to your body, your body will be good to you. It will shed weight, it will stay healthy, and it will treat you to a longer and more enjoyable life. In the end, that's what the Reality Diet is all about.

Part IV

Meal Plans and Recipes

Week 1

Day 1   Monday Menu

Breakfast
Caramelized Banana and Peanut Butter Toast
1 cup skim milk or one container 2:90 strawberry yogurt
with fiber (providing up to 90 calories)
MEN: Add 1 serving 2:90 calcium-fortified dry or hot cereal
(providing up to 90 calories)
Morning Dividend*

Lunch
California Veggie Burger with Garlic-Basil Aïoli
Ten 2:90 potato chips (low-fat gourmet baked potato chips,
such as Kettle Krisps)
or 8 Garden of Eatin' Black Bean tortilla chips
MEN: Add 1 mozzarella string cheese (with no more than
4 grams of total fat per string); 4 tablespoons chopped
avocado

Dinner
Tandoori Chicken
Garlic Spinach and Tomatoes

Reality Reward
Mango Lassi
12 cashews
1 dessert starch of your choice (see Equivalents Lists,
page 381)

---

*Morning Dividend—Choose one sweetener OR one creamer from the following:
1 teaspoon honey, 1 teaspoon white granulated sugar, or 1 teaspoon brown
sugar OR 2 tablespoons 2% milk, 1 tablespoon half-and-half, 1 tablespoon
soymilk creamer, 1 tablespoon nondairy liquid creamer, 2 teaspoons nondairy
powdered creamer

Recipe items are in boldface.

Day 2   Tuesday Menu

Breakfast
1 serving 2:90 calcium-fortified dry or hot cereal (providing up to 90 calories)
1 cup skim milk or one container 2:90 peach yogurt with fiber (providing up to 90 calories)
8 walnut halves
1 large orange
MEN: Add ⅓ cup fruit muesli
Morning Dividend

Lunch
Pepper Steak Pita
Ten 2:90 potato chips (low-fat gourmet baked potato chips, such as Kettle Krisps)
or 8 Garden of Eatin' Black Bean tortilla chips
MEN: Add 12 cashews and ⅓ cup carrot sticks

Dinner
Thai Chicken Satay with Crunchy Vegetable Salad

Reality Reward
Banana-Chocolate Crêpes

Day 3   Wednesday Menu

Breakfast

Raspberry Breakfast Smoothie

1 slice toasted regular 2:90 bread with 2 tablespoons light
margarine

MEN: Add 1 slice toasted regular 2:90 bread

Morning Dividend

Lunch

Turkey Caesar Wrap

Ten 2:90 potato chips (low-fat gourmet baked potato chips,
such as Kettle Krisps)

or 8 Garden of Eatin' Black Bean tortilla chips

MEN: Add 1 mozzarella string cheese (with no more than
4 grams total fat per string); 4 tablespoons chopped
avocado

Dinner

Cornmeal-Crusted Sole
Tomato and Basil Salad

Reality Reward

Strawberry Shortcake Napoleon

1 cup ice-cold skim milk

Day 4   Thursday Menu

Breakfast   1 serving 2:90 oatmeal (providing up to 90 calories)

3 tablespoons raisins

8 pecan halves

1 cup skim milk or one container 2:90 apple yogurt with fiber (providing up to 90 calories)

MEN: Add ¼ cup 2:90 granola

Morning Dividend

Lunch   **Tofu Stir-fry**

MEN: Add 20 peanuts; ¼ cup jicama sticks

Dinner   **Blackened Red Snapper
with Baby Spinach Salad**

Reality Reward   **Gingered Pear Crumble**

1 cup ice-cold skim milk

Day 5   Friday Menu

Breakfast

1 2:90 multigrain waffle

1⅛ cups blueberries

8 pecan halves

1 cup skim milk or one container 2:90 strawberry yogurt
with fiber (providing up to 90 calories)

MEN: Add 1 2:90 multigrain waffle

Morning Dividend

Lunch

Vegetarian Gyro Sandwich

Ten 2:90 potato chips (low-fat gourmet baked potato chips,
such as Kettle Krisps)

or 8 Garden of Eatin' Black Bean tortilla chips

MEN: Add 8 walnut halves

Dinner

Maryland Crab Cake Salad

Steamed Artichoke with Lemon and Herbs

MEN: Add ½ cup carrot sticks and ¼ cup cucumber slices

Reality Reward

Gingered Pear Crumble

1 cup ice-cold skim milk

Day 6   Saturday Menu

Breakfast	1 serving 2:90 calcium-fortified dry or hot cereal (providing up to 90 calories) 1 cup skim milk or 1 container 2:90 peach yogurt with fiber (providing up to 90 calories) 12 almonds 1 large nectarine MEN: Add ⅓ cup fruit muesli *Morning Dividend*
Lunch	**BLTB Sandwich** **(Bacon, Lettuce, Tomato, and Basil Sandwich)** MEN: Add 1 mozzarella string cheese (with no more than 4 grams of total fat per string); 4 tablespoons chopped avocado
Dinner	**Garlic-Glazed Chicken and Vegetables**
Reality Reward	**Maple Peach Cobbler**

Day 7   Sunday Menu

Breakfast

2:90 Swedish Pancakes

MEN: Add ¼ cup 2:90 granola

Morning Dividend

Lunch

Canadian-Bacon-and-Mushroom-Stuffed Baked Potato

MEN: Add 1 cup celery sticks; ½ cup broccoli florets; and 12 almonds; 1 mozzarella string cheese (with no more than 4 grams of fat per string)

Dinner

Seared Peppercorn Ahi Tuna

MEN: Add ¾ cup celery sticks

Sautéed Green Beans with Leeks and Dill

Reality Reward   **Apple Streusel**

Monday

Caramelized Banana and Peanut Butter Toast

Turn simple bananas and peanut butter into a delicious gourmet breakfast with just a few extra minutes of cooking.

Nonstick cooking spray
1 banana, cut in half lengthwise
1 slice 2:90 whole-wheat bread
1 tablespoon natural peanut butter
Pinch of ground cinnamon
Pinch of ground nutmeg

Heat an 8-inch nonstick skillet over medium heat. Spray with nonstick cooking spray. Place the halved bananas, cut-side down, in the skillet and cook for 2 minutes. Turn the bananas over and cook for another 2 minutes, or until soft and golden-brown.

While the bananas are caramelizing, toast the bread, spread with the peanut butter, and sprinkle with the cinnamon and nutmeg. Cut the caramelized bananas in half crosswise and arrange side by side on the peanut butter.

Serves 1

CALORIES 280; FIBER 6g; FAT 9g; PROTEIN 9g; CARB 42g; SODIUM 160mg

California Veggie Burger with Garlic-Basil Aïoli

This burger makes a great lunch for either home or the office. If you're taking it to work, bring the tomato salad in a small container and add it to the sandwich just before eating. This will keep the bun from getting soggy.

Nonstick cooking spray
1 veggie burger patty

½ cup chopped tomatoes   MEN: 2 cups

½ cup alfalfa sprouts   MEN: 1 cup

1 tablespoon non-fat mayonnaise

1 teaspoon chopped fresh basil   MEN: 2 teaspoons

¼ teaspoon minced fresh garlic

¼ teaspoon sherry vinegar

One 2:90 hamburger bun

1 teaspoon Dijon mustard

Freshly ground black pepper

Heat an 8-inch skillet over medium heat. Spray with nonstick cooking spray. Cook the veggie burger patty for 3 to 4 minutes on each side, or until heated through.

In a small bowl, combine the tomatoes, sprouts, mayonnaise, basil, garlic, and vinegar. Toss well to coat the tomatoes and sprouts with the mayonnaise dressing.

Spread both sides of the bun with mustard. Place the cooked patty on the bottom bun, top with the tomato salad, and season with black pepper to taste.

MEN: *Make a side salad with the extra chopped tomatoes and alfalfa sprouts that don't fit on your burger. Top the salad with the cheese and avocado from the menu list, and dress with sherry vinegar or lemon juice and freshly ground black pepper.*

Serves 1

WOMEN: CALORIES 220; FIBER 7g; FAT 5g; PROTEIN 16g; CARB 31g; SODIUM 820mg

MEN: CALORIES 260; FIBER 9g; FAT 6g; PROTEIN 16g; CARB 40g; SODIUM 840mg

Tandoori Chicken

A tandoor is an Indian clay oven that cooks with very intense heat. This dish is spicy—for a milder flavor, eliminate the cayenne pepper.

1 tablespoon nondairy creamer

2 teaspoons canola oil

1 teaspoon fresh lemon juice

1 teaspoon minced fresh garlic

1 teaspoon minced fresh ginger

½ teaspoon paprika

½ teaspoon ground turmeric

½ teaspoon curry powder

¼ teaspoon ground coriander

¼ teaspoon ground cumin

⅛ teaspoon cayenne pepper

6 ounces boneless, skinless chicken breast, cut into 1-inch-wide strips
    (will yield 5 ounces cooked)

Place all of the ingredients, including the chicken, in a large resealable plastic bag. Press the air out of the bag and seal tightly. Turn the bag to distribute the marinade. Refrigerate for 30 minutes, turning occasionally.

Set a rack at the highest level of the oven and preheat to broil. Remove the chicken from the marinade and place on a nonstick baking sheet. Discard the remaining marinade. Place the chicken under the broiler for 3 minutes. Turn and broil for another 3 minutes, or until the chicken is no longer pink inside and the juices run clear.

Serves 1

CALORIES 270; FIBER 2g; FAT 12g; PROTEIN 34g; CARB 6g; SODIUM 95mg

Garlic Spinach and Tomatoes

This is a fast and clever way to cook several different vegetables in a single skillet. The beans, which need liquid to cook, will blanch in the juices from the tomatoes.

Nonstick cooking spray

½ cup chopped tomatoes   MEN: 1 cup

¼ cup chopped onions   MEN: ½ cup

⅓ cup chopped green beans   MEN: ⅔ cup

1 teaspoon minced fresh garlic   MEN: 2 teaspoons

1 cup fresh spinach leaves   MEN: 2 cups

Fresh lemon juice
Freshly ground black pepper

Heat a nonstick skillet over medium heat. Spray with nonstick cooking spray. Add the tomatoes and cook for 3 minutes, stirring occasionally. When the tomatoes are soft and juicy, add the onions, green beans, and garlic. Cook for another 4 to 5 minutes, until the vegetables have softened. Add the spinach and cook until wilted, about 30 seconds. Season with lemon juice and black pepper to taste.

Serves 1

WOMEN: CALORIES 60; FIBER 4g; FAT 0g; PROTEIN 2g; CARB 14g; SODIUM 50mg

MEN: CALORIES 100; FIBER 8g; FAT .5g; PROTEIN 4g; CARB 23g; SODIUM 95mg

Mango Lassi

Lassi is a cool and refreshing yogurt drink that helps temper spicy Indian food. A ripe mango will taste and blend the best. Select a mango that is heavy for its size and gives slightly when pressed by your thumb. A potato peeler works well to remove the mango skin.

One container 2:90 vanilla yogurt with fiber
    (providing up to 90 calories)
¾ cup peeled and diced ripe mango
1 teaspoon sugar substitute
½ teaspoon fresh lemon juice
5 to 6 ice cubes

Combine the yogurt, mango, sugar substitute, and lemon juice in the jar of a blender. Cover and blend until smooth and frothy, about 30 seconds. Add the ice cubes and blend on high speed for another 60 seconds.

Serves 1

CALORIES 170; FIBER 4g; FAT 0g; PROTEIN 7g; CARB 38g; SODIUM 95mg

Tuesday

Pepper Steak Pita

This pita sandwich is a clever way to bring a stir-fry to work or the park for lunch. The smell of garlic and ginger will perfume your kitchen.

Nonstick cooking spray

2 ounces beef round, cut into bite-size strips (will yield 1½ ounces cooked)

    MEN: 4 ounces (will yield 3 ounces cooked)

½ cup diced red bell pepper   MEN: 1 cup

¼ cup diced green bell pepper   MEN: ½ cup

¼ cup diced yellow onion   MEN: ½ cup

1 teaspoon minced fresh garlic   MEN: 2 teaspoons

1 teaspoon minced fresh ginger   MEN: 2 teaspoons

1 tablespoon bottled teriyaki sauce

Freshly ground black pepper

One 2:90 whole-wheat pita, toasted and cut in half

½ cup fresh spinach leaves

Heat an 8-inch nonstick skillet over high heat. Spray with nonstick cooking spray. Add the beef, stirring constantly, and cook until browned and caramelized, about 3 minutes. Spoon the cooked meat into a small bowl and set aside.

With the heat still on high, spray the skillet with more nonstick cooking spray. Add the bell pepper, onions, garlic, ginger, and teriyaki sauce, and cook until tender-crisp, about 3 minutes. Season with black pepper to taste.

Open the toasted pita bread and stuff half the spinach in each pocket. Spoon in the vegetables and steak and serve.

If you are bringing the sandwich to work, allow the pepper steak to cool and place in an airtight container and store in the refrigerator. When ready to serve, reheat the steak in the microwave and spoon the mixture into the pita as described above.

MEN: *There is more stir-fry than will fit in the pita, so either stuff the pita and eat the stir-fry that falls out with chopsticks, or place the stir-fry on a plate and cut the pita into triangles to eat like crackers.*

Serves 1

WOMEN: CALORIES 230; FIBER 5g; FAT 4g; PROTEIN 18g; CARB 32g; SODIUM 430mg

MEN: CALORIES 330; FIBER 11g; FAT 7g; PROTEIN 32g; CARB 41g; SODIUM 460mg

Thai Chicken Satay with Crunchy Vegetable Salad

You'll feel like you're sitting in your neighborhood Thai restaurant. But since you're cooking at home, you won't spend the fat grams or the tip money.

6 ounces boneless, skinless, chicken breast, cut into 1-inch-wide strips
   (will yield 5 ounces cooked)
Nonstick cooking spray
1 teaspoon garlic powder
½ teaspoon freshly ground black pepper
½ cup thinly sliced cucumber   MEN: 1 cup
1 cup shredded romaine lettuce   MEN: 2 cups
¼ cup grated carrot   MEN: ½ cup
¼ cup thinly sliced red bell pepper   MEN: ¾ cup
1 tablespoon fresh lime juice   MEN: 2 tablespoons
Peanut Sauce (recipe follows)

Soak 3 bamboo skewers in water for 10 minutes to prevent charring when broiling.

Set a rack at the highest level of the oven and preheat to broil. Thread the chicken strips onto the skewers and place on a baking sheet. Spray the chicken skewers with nonstick cooking spray and sprinkle evenly with the garlic powder and black pepper.

In a medium bowl, combine the cucumbers, lettuce, carrot, red bell pepper, and lime juice. Toss to coat and mound in the center of a dinner plate.

Place the chicken under the broiler for 3 minutes. Turn and broil for another 3 minutes, or until the chicken is no longer pink inside and the juices run clear.

While the chicken is broiling, make the Peanut Sauce. To serve, lean the chicken skewers against the mounded salad and drizzle with Peanut Sauce.

Serves 1

WOMEN: CALORIES 230; FIBER 3g; FAT 4g; PROTEIN 41g; CARB 8g; SODIUM 135mg

MEN: CALORIES 280; FIBER 7g; FAT 4.5g; PROTEIN 43g; CARB 18g; SODIUM 160mg

Peanut Sauce

Make this peanut sauce ahead of time and store it in the refrigerator in an airtight container for up to two weeks. You can also multiply the ingredients to make larger batches. Bring to room temperature before serving.

    1 tablespoon natural peanut butter
    1 teaspoon sugar substitute
    1 teaspoon fresh lime juice
    ½ tablespoon naturally brewed reduced-sodium soy sauce
    ½ tablespoon Worcestershire sauce
    2 teaspoons rice vinegar
    Dash of hot pepper sauce, or to taste

In a small bowl, whisk together all of the ingredients until well combined.

Serves 1

CALORIES 110; FIBER 0g; FAT 8g; PROTEIN 4g; CARB 5g; SODIUM 310mg

Banana Chocolate Crêpes

The joy of dessert is alive and well this evening. The crêpes are sweet and decadent, but the fruit and whole-wheat flour make them healthful.

    ⅓ cup non-fat dry milk powder
    3½ tablespoons whole-wheat flour

1 teaspoon sugar substitute

¼ teaspoon ground cinnamon

¼ teaspoon baking powder

½ cup water

1 teaspoon canola oil

1 teaspoon vanilla extract

¼ teaspoon coconut extract

Nonstick cooking spray

½ banana, sliced

2 pitted dates, chopped

4 toasted pecan halves, chopped

1 teaspoon semisweet chocolate mini-morsels

In a small bowl, combine the dry milk, flour, sugar substitute, cinnamon, and baking powder. Whisk in the water, oil, vanilla, and coconut extract until the batter is smooth. A few lumps in the batter are okay.

Heat an 8-inch nonstick skillet over medium heat. Spray with nonstick cooking spray. Remove the skillet from the heat and pour in half of the batter. Lift and tilt the skillet to spread the batter across the bottom. Return the skillet to the heat and cook for 30 seconds. Carefully turn over the crêpe with a spatula, and cook the second side for another 30 seconds. Slide the cooked crêpe onto a plate and repeat the cooking process with the remaining batter.

Arrange half of the banana slices, dates, pecans, and chocolate morsels across the lower third of each crêpe. Lift the bottom edge of each crêpe and roll it up to serve.

Serves 1

CALORIES 370; FIBER 6g; FAT 12g; PROTEIN 14g; CARB 56g; SODIUM 135mg

FOR BLACKBERRY CRÊPES

Substitute 1⅛ cups blackberries for the banana, dates, pecan halves, and chocolate morsels. Sprinkle the crêpes with 1 teaspoon of powdered sugar.

CALORIES 370; FIBER 6g; FAT 12g; PROTEIN 14g; CARB 56g; SODIUM 135mg

Wednesday

Raspberry Breakfast Smoothie

Keep a couple of tall beer glasses in the freezer to add a frosty touch to your breakfast drink. Strain the smoothie through a fine-mesh strainer if the raspberry seeds bother you.

   1 cup skim milk (or plain non-fat yogurt for a creamier texture)
   1½ cups fresh or frozen raspberries
   ½ teaspoon sugar substitute
   1 teaspoon vanilla extract
   ⅛ teaspoon ground nutmeg
   4 or 5 ice cubes (if you're using fresh raspberries)

Combine the milk, raspberries, sugar substitute, and vanilla in the jar of a blender. Cover and blend until smooth and frothy, about 30 seconds. Add the ice cubes if you're using fresh raspberries and blend an additional 30 seconds.

Pour into a tall glass, sprinkle with the nutmeg, and serve.

Serves 1

CALORIES 170; FIBER 5g; FAT 0g; PROTEIN 11g; CARB 31g; SODIUM 135mg

Turkey Caesar Wrap

Caesar salad was invented in Mexico by an Italian, which explains why both countries try to lay claim to this venerable dish. Wrapping the Italian flavors in a Mexican tortilla acknowledges contributions from each.

   1½ ounces turkey deli meat (with more than 1 but no more than 3 grams of
      fat per ounce), sliced into bite-size pieces
   1 cup chopped celery   MEN: 2 cups
   ½ cup shredded romaine lettuce   MEN: 1 cup

½ cup chopped tomatoes or halved cherry tomatoes

¼ cup thinly sliced red onion   MEN: ½ cup

1 tablespoon fat-free Caesar dressing

One 2:90 wrap (serving size: 35 grams) or tortilla

Freshly ground black pepper

In a medium bowl, toss the turkey, 1 cup celery, ½ cup lettuce, ½ cup tomatoes, and ¼ cup red onions with the Caesar dressing. Microwave the wrap for 10 to 15 seconds to soften it. Mound the dressed salad in a line across the center of the wrap. Sprinkle with black pepper to taste, wrap, and serve.

MEN: *Make a side salad with the extra celery, lettuce, cherry tomatoes, red onions, and avocado. Dress the salad with fresh lemon juice and basil if you prefer Italian flavors, or with fresh lime, cilantro and hot sauce if Mexican is more your style.*

Serves 1

WOMEN: CALORIES 200; FIBER 11g; FAT 3.5g; PROTEIN 15g; CARB 28g; SODIUM 750mg

MEN: CALORIES 230; FIBER 14g; FAT 4g; PROTEIN 16g; CARB 36g; SODIUM 850mg

Cornmeal-Crusted Sole

Stone-ground cornmeal, which is available in natural food stores, will add texture and flavor to this simple fish dish.

2 teaspoons cornmeal, preferably stone-ground

¼ teaspoon freshly ground black pepper

¼ teaspoon paprika

⅛ teaspoon ground cumin

One 6-ounce sole fillet (will yield 5 ounces cooked)

Nonstick cooking spray

Juice of ½ lemon

In a small bowl, combine the cornmeal, black pepper, paprika, and cumin. Spray the top of the sole fillet with nonstick cooking spray and sprinkle with the cornmeal mixture. Gently pat the cornmeal mixture to help it stick.

Heat an 8-inch nonstick skillet over medium heat. Spray the skillet with the nonstick cooking spray. Carefully place the sole, cornmeal side down, in the hot skillet. Cook for 3 minutes and turn over. Cook another minute, or until fish flakes to the touch, then sprinkle with lemon juice, and serve.

Serves 1

CALORIES 180; FIBER 0g; FAT 3.5g; PROTEIN 32g; CARB 4g; SODIUM 140mg

Tomato and Basil Salad

Ruby-red tomato slices contrast beautifully with rich green basil leaves for a taste of the garden. Serve with any fish dish.

    2 small tomatoes, sliced   MEN: 4 small tomatoes, sliced
    10 to 12 fresh basil leaves   MEN: ½ cup
    2 teaspoons olive oil
    Aged balsamic vinegar
    Freshly ground black pepper

Place the spinach on a plate and arrange alternating slices of the tomatoes and the basil leaves over the spinach. Drizzle with the vinegar and season with black pepper to taste.

Serves 1

WOMEN: CALORIES 120; FIBER 2g; FAT 10g; PROTEIN 2g; CARB 8g; SODIUM 15mg
MEN: CALORIES 160; FIBER 4g; FAT 11g; PROTEIN 4g; CARB 17g; SODIUM 45mg

Strawberry Shortcake Napoleon

This napoleon will look like a leaning tower when you've finished building it. A fork and knife will be your best tools to eat it with. Serve it on a large plate to accommodate its collapse.

    1¾ cups sliced fresh strawberries
    1 teaspoon sugar substitute
    8 pecan halves

One 2:90 waffle

2 tablespoons light or non-fat whipped topping

Preheat the oven to 375°F. Sprinkle the sliced strawberries with the sugar substitute and set aside. Crumble the pecans into small pieces and toast in the oven for 3 to 5 minutes, or until golden brown. Remove from the oven and let cool.

Toast the waffle and cut it in half. Spoon some of the sweetened strawberries on a large plate, place a half waffle on top, and top with another heaping spoonful of berries. Repeat the process with the remaining waffle and berries. Finish with the whipped topping and toasted pecans.

Serves 1

CALORIES 270; FIBER 9g; FAT 12g; PROTEIN 6g; CARB 40g; SODIUM 220mg

Thursday

Tofu Stir-fry

The natural juices from the chard mingle with the marinade to create a light but flavorful sauce. If you like heat, add as many chili flakes as you can stand. To save time, marinate the tofu overnight. This lunch is easy to reheat at work—simply spoon the stir-fry over the rice in a plastic container with a tight-fitting lid and bring it along in your briefcase.

3 ounces diced organic firm plain tofu   MEN: 6 ounces

1 tablespoon naturally brewed reduced-sodium soy sauce

¼ cup vegetable broth

1 tablespoon minced fresh ginger   MEN: 2 tablespoons

2 teaspoons minced fresh garlic   MEN: 4 teaspoons

⅛ teaspoon crushed chili flakes

Nonstick cooking spray

¼ cup sliced yellow onion   MEN: ½ cup

¼ cup sliced carrot

½ cup chopped asparagus   MEN: 1 cup

½ cup green chard

⅔ cup steamed 2:90 blend of wild and brown rice

In a small bowl, combine the tofu, soy sauce, vegetable broth, ginger, garlic, and chili flakes. Stir to coat the tofu in the marinade, and marinate 30 minutes.

Heat a nonstick skillet or wok over medium-high heat. Spray with nonstick cooking spray. Add the onion, carrot, and asparagus, and stir-fry for 3 to 4 minutes. Add the marinated tofu with the marinade and cook for another minute. Add the chard and cook until wilted, about another minute. Serve with the steamed 2:90 rice.

MEN: *Garnish the stir-fry with the peanuts.*

Serves 1

WOMEN: CALORIES 280; FIBER 6.5g; FAT 5g; PROTEIN 14g; CARB 49g; SODIUM 690mg

MEN: CALORIES 360; FIBER 7.5g; FAT 8g; PROTEIN 22g; CARB 57g; SODIUM 700mg

Blackened Red Snapper with Baby Spinach Salad

It's best to make your own Cajun seasoning, as store bought versions are usually filled with salt and sugar. Turn on your exhaust fan before blackening the fish.

One 6-ounce red snapper fillet (will yield 5 ounces cooked)

Nonstick cooking spray

1 tablespoon Cajun seasoning (recipe follows)

Juice of ½ lemon, plus more to taste

½ cup baby spinach leaves   MEN: 1 cup

¼ cup sliced red onion   MEN: ½ cup

½ cup sliced red bell pepper   MEN: 1 cup

¼ cup sliced green bell pepper   MEN: ½ cup

2 teaspoons canola oil

1 tablespoon fat-free salad dressing, your choice

1 tablespoon chopped fresh flat-leaf parsley

Spray the fish with nonstick cooking spray and sprinkle both sides with the Cajun seasoning to evenly coat.

Heat a heavy skillet, preferably cast iron, over high heat. When the skillet is very hot, place the fish in the skillet and cook for 3 to 5 minutes or until the rub starts to blacken. Turn the fish and sprinkle the cooked side with lemon juice to keep it moist. Cook for another 3 to 5 minutes, until the second side starts to blacken.

While the fish is cooking, mound the spinach, red onions, and bell peppers in the center of a large plate. Drizzle with the oil and salad dressing. Remove the fish from the skillet and place on the vegetables. The hot fish will wilt the spinach. Garnish with chopped parsley and sprinkle with lemon juice to taste.

Serves 1

WOMEN: CALORIES 300; FIBER 6g; FAT 13g; PROTEIN 37g; CARB 10g; SODIUM 150mg

MEN: CALORIES 340; FIBER 8g; FAT 14g; PROTEIN 38g; CARB 18g; SODIUM 170mg

Cajun Seasoning

This seasoning blend is a starting point for many great meals. Don't be afraid to experiment with different quantities and kinds of spices to make your own signature flavor.

    1 teaspoon ground black pepper
    1 teaspoon ground white pepper
    1 teaspoon onion powder
    1 teaspoon crushed dried thyme leaves
    1 teaspoon garlic powder
    ½ teaspoon celery seeds
    ½ teaspoon cayenne pepper

In a small bowl, combine the spices. Mix together with a fork until well combined. Store in a plastic bag or an airtight container until ready to use; the mixture will keep for 6 months.

Makes just under 2 tablespoons

CALORIES 35; FIBER 2g; FAT 0g; PROTEIN 0g; CARB 0g; SODIUM 0mg

Gingered Pear Crumble

The baking time will vary a little depending on how ripe the pears are. If the pears you're using are very green or unripe, allow for a little extra cooking time. This recipe makes 2 servings, so save half for Day 5.

½ cup 2:90 granola
2 teaspoons brown sugar
2 teaspoons sugar substitute
2 teaspoons minced fresh ginger
½ teaspoon ground cinnamon
4 tablespoons light margarine, melted
2 teaspoons vanilla extract
2 large sliced fresh ripe pears
Nonstick cooking spray

Preheat the oven to 375°F. In a medium bowl, stir together the granola, brown sugar, sugar substitute, ginger, cinnamon, margarine, and vanilla until the mixture is moist and crumbly. Add the sliced pear, tossing to coat.

Spray a small round (5 inches in diameter) baking dish with nonstick cooking spray and spoon the mixture into the dish. Cover with foil and bake for 30 minutes. Uncover and bake another 15 minutes or until browned and bubbly.

Serves 2

CALORIES 300; FIBER 6g; FAT 14g; PROTEIN 4g; CARB 46g; SODIUM 200mg per single serving

Friday

Vegetarian Gyro Sandwich

Gyros are classic street food. While you won't be able to buy this version on a street corner, you can certainly walk down the street to eat today's lunch on a park bench. Bring a couple of napkins, though, because it gets messy.

1 ounce reduced-fat feta cheese (with no more than 4 grams
    of total fat per ounce)   MEN: 2 ounces
½ cup shredded romaine lettuce   MEN: 1 cup
½ cup chopped cucumber   MEN: 1 cup
½ cup diced tomato   MEN: 1 cup
½ cup thinly sliced red bell pepper   MEN: 1 cup
2 tablespoons chopped flat-leaf parsley
3 chopped peperoncini
1 tablespoon red wine vinegar
⅛ teaspoon dried oregano
⅛ teaspoon dried thyme
Freshly ground black pepper
One 2:90 whole-wheat pita, toasted and cut in half

In a medium bowl, toss together the feta, ½ cup lettuce, ½ cup cucumber, ½ cup tomato, ½ cup bell pepper, the parsley, peperoncini, vinegar, oregano, thyme, and black pepper to taste. Open the toasted pita and stuff half the gyro mixture into each pocket.

MEN: *Make a side salad with the extra lettuce, cucumbers, tomato, and bell pepper. Dress the salad with red wine vinegar and dried oregano.*

Serves 1
WOMEN: CALORIES 170; FIBER 6g; FAT 3.5g; PROTEIN 11g; CARB 28g; SODIUM 490mg
MEN: CALORIES 270; FIBER 8g; FAT 7g; PROTEIN 20g; CARB 40g; SODIUM 880mg

Maryland Crab Cake Salad

Maryland is known for crab cakes that rely on the fresh flavor of the crab without using lots of breading. Because there isn't lots of fat and breading in this recipe, you'll need to pack each cake tightly so it holds together in the skillet.

    5 ounces crabmeat, fresh or canned
    2 tablespoons reduced-fat mayonnaise
    2 tablespoons chopped fresh flat-leaf parsley
    1 teaspoon Dijon mustard
    1 teaspoon minced fresh garlic
    Nonstick cooking spray
    ½ cup mixed baby lettuce leaves
    ½ cup thinly sliced radishes
    Juice of ½ lemon
    2 teaspoons balsamic vinegar

In a small bowl, gently blend the crab, mayonnaise, parsley, mustard, and garlic together. Shape the mixture into 8 to 10 small, tightly packed crab cakes, about 1 tablespoon each, place on a plate, cover, and refrigerate for 30 minutes. Heat an 8-inch nonstick skillet over medium heat. Spray with nonstick cooking spray. Cook the crab cakes for 3 minutes on each side, or until golden brown.

While the crab cakes are cooking, toss together the lettuce, radishes, lemon juice, and vinegar. Mound on a large plate and place the cooked crab cakes around the salad like little constellations.

Serves 1

CALORIES 220; FIBER 1.5g; FAT 8g; PROTEIN 27g; CARB 9g; SODIUM 600mg

Steamed Artichoke with Lemon and Herbs

In its purest form, the artichoke is a regal vegetable. When simply steamed, the grand choke is on a pedestal. Be sure to eat the tender heart, as it's the best part, but scrape away any prickly center.

1 small artichoke   MEN: 1 medium artichoke

Several sprigs of fresh tarragon or parsley

1 teaspoon fresh lemon juice   MEN: 2 teaspoons

Peel away the tough outer leaves of the artichoke and discard. Place the artichoke on its side and trim off the top ½ inch.

Place the artichoke, bottom up, in a pot filled with 1 inch of water, along with the sprigs of fresh herbs, cover, and steam for 30 to 35 minutes, or until the base can be pierced with a sharp knife. Sprinkle with the lemon juice.

Serves 1

WOMEN: CALORIES 60; FIBER 7g; FAT 0g; PROTEIN 4g; CARB 13g; SODIUM 120mg

MEN: CALORIES 80; FIBER 9g; FAT 0g; PROTEIN 5g; CARB 17g; SODIUM 150mg

Saturday

BLTB Sandwich
(Bacon, Lettuce, Tomato, and Basil Sandwich)

Get ready for a really delicious sandwich that's short on preparation time and long on enjoyment.

4 slices Canadian bacon

1 tablespoon non-fat mayonnaise

2 slices regular 2:90 whole-wheat bread, toasted

½ cup sliced tomatoes   MEN: 1 cup

½ cup shredded romaine lettuce   MEN: 1 cup

½ cup sliced cucumber   MEN: 1 cup

4 fresh basil leaves

Freshly ground black pepper

Heat an 8-inch nonstick skillet over medium-high heat. Arrange the bacon slices side by side in the hot skillet. Cook for 3 to 4 minutes on each side, or until the bacon is crisp.

Spread the mayonnaise evenly over both slices of the toasted bread. Layer the ½ cup tomato slices, ½ cup lettuce, ½ cup cucumber, the basil, and cooked Canadian bacon over the bread. Top with the second slice of bread. Close the sandwich and cut in half diagonally.

MEN: *Make a small side salad with the extra tomatoes, lettuce, and cucumber.*

Serves 1

WOMEN: CALORIES 350; FIBER 8g; FAT 15g; PROTEIN 17g; CARB 42g; SODIUM 890mg

MEN: CALORIES 380; FIBER 9g; FAT 15g; PROTEIN 19g; CARB 47g; SODIUM 900mg

Garlic-Glazed Chicken and Vegetables

The most delicious dinners are often the most simple. This one-pan meal is comforting, filling, and tasty. While a tablespoon might seem like a lot of garlic, it will mellow while it cooks.

Nonstick cooking spray

One 6-ounce boneless, skinless chicken breast, cut into strips (5 ounces cooked)

2 tablespoons light margarine

1 tablespoon minced fresh garlic   MEN: 4 teaspoons

⅔ cup cauliflower florets   MEN: 1⅓ cups

½ cup broccoli florets   MEN: 1 cup

¼ cup carrots thinly sliced into coins   MEN: ½ cup

¼ cup diced yellow onions   MEN: ½ cup

¼ cup sliced leeks   MEN: ½ cup

¼ teaspoon fresh thyme   MEN: ½ teaspoon

1 teaspoon brown sugar

2 tablespoons vegetable broth

Heat an 8-inch nonstick skillet over medium-high heat. Spray with nonstick cooking spray and add the chicken strips. Sear the chicken for 2 minutes on each side, or until golden-brown.

Add the margarine to the skillet and stir until melted. Add the garlic, cauliflower, broccoli, carrots, onions, and leeks. Cook until the vegetables begin to soften, about 4 minutes. Add the thyme, brown sugar, and vegetable broth. Cook for another 2 to 3 minutes, stirring often, until the broth is bubbling and the vegetables are fork-tender.

Serves 1

WOMEN: CALORIES 340; FIBER 5g; FAT 14g; PROTEIN 36g; CARB 20g; SODIUM 360mg

MEN: CALORIES 410; FIBER 9g; FAT 14g; PROTEIN 40g; CARB 35g; SODIUM 420mg

Maple Peach Cobbler

As a time-saving tip, pat the prepared dough flat instead of forming it into a ball. This will make it easier to roll out when you remove it from the refrigerator.

3½ tablespoons whole-wheat flour

2 tablespoons light margarine, chilled and cut into pieces

1 teaspoon cold water

Nonstick cooking spray

1 large fresh ripe peach, peeled, pitted, and sliced

1 teaspoon fresh lemon juice

1 teaspoon sugar substitute

½ teaspoon ground cinnamon

⅛ teaspoon ground nutmeg

2 tablespoons sugar-free maple-flavored syrup

One container 2:90 vanilla yogurt with fiber (providing up to 90 calories)

In a medium bowl, combine the flour and margarine. Using a pastry cutter or 2 knives, cut the margarine into the flour until the mixture resembles coarse meal. Add the cold water, stirring it in with a fork, and form the dough into a ball. Pat the dough ball flat, wrap it in plastic wrap, and refrigerate it for at least 1 hour.

Preheat the oven to 375°F. Spray a small round (5-inch-diameter) baking dish with nonstick cooking spray and set it aside.

In a small bowl, gently toss the peach slices with the lemon juice, sugar substitute, cinnamon, nutmeg, and maple syrup. Place the peach mixture into the prepared baking dish. When the dough has chilled, gently roll it to the approximate size of the baking dish to form the top crust. Place the crust over the peach filling and cut several steam vents in the crust.

Bake the cobbler for 30 to 45 minutes, or until the crust is golden brown and the filling is bubbling. Transfer to a wire rack to cool slightly. Top with the yogurt and serve.

Serves 1

CALORIES 340; FIBER 5g; FAT 12g; PROTEIN 11g; CARB 50g; SODIUM 300mg

FOR BLUEBERRY COBBLER

Substitute 1⅛ cup blueberries for peaches. Reduce sugar-free maple-flavored syrup to 1 teaspoon.

CALORIES 370; FIBER 9g; FAT 13g; PROTEIN 11g; CARB 58g; SODIUM 300mg

Sunday

2:90 Swedish Pancakes

Layer the pancakes with raspberries for a "tall stack." Make sure to leave enough berries to crown the stack with a colorful cap.

3½ tablespoons whole-wheat flour
1 teaspoon sugar substitute
½ teaspoon baking powder
⅓ cup non-fat dry milk powder
About ¼ cup water
Nonstick cooking spray
1½ cups raspberries
2 tablespoons sugar-free maple-flavored syrup
8 pecan halves, chopped and toasted

In a medium bowl, sift together the flour, sugar substitute, and baking powder. Stir in the dry milk and slowly stir in enough water to form a batter.

Heat a nonstick griddle over medium-high heat. Spray with nonstick cooking spray. Pour the batter into 3 or 4 small pancake shapes and cook until the batter begins to bubble. Flip the pancakes and brown the other side.

On a large platter, stack the pancakes, with raspberries between the layers, finishing with the raspberries. Drizzle the syrup and pecans over the top.

Serves 1

CALORIES 350; FIBER 16g; FAT 11g; PROTEIN 15g; CARB 55g; SODIUM 125mg

Canadian-Bacon-and-Mushroom-Stuffed Baked Potato

This hearty meal can be eaten straight from the skillet or reheated later in a microwave.

One small russet potato
Nonstick cooking spray
4 slices Canadian bacon, cut into bite-size pieces
1 cup chopped celery
½ cup sliced mushrooms   MEN: 1 cup
2 teaspoons minced fresh garlic
½ cup broccoli florets
¾ cup chopped tomatoes   MEN: 1½ cups
1 cup chopped chard
Freshly ground black pepper

Preheat the oven to 375°F. Scrub the potato under cold running water with a stiff brush. Poke holes in the potato with a fork and place it on the middle rack of the oven. Bake for 45 minutes to 1 hour, or until the potato is tender when pierced with a knife.

About 15 minutes before the potato is done, heat an 8-inch nonstick skillet over medium-high heat. Spray with nonstick cooking spray. Add the bacon, celery, ½ cup mushrooms, and the garlic and sauté until softened, about 3 minutes.

While there is still liquid remaining in the skillet from the mushrooms, add the broccoli and ¾ cup tomatoes, and cook for another 3 to 5 minutes, or until the broccoli has softened. Add the chard and cook until wilted, about 2 minutes.

Take a lengthwise slice off the top of the baked potato and squeeze the ends toward one another to open it. Stuff the potato with the bacon mixture, allowing it to spill over the sides. Season with black pepper to taste.

MEN: *Make a side salad with the extra mushrooms and tomatoes. Drizzle the veggies with aged balsamic vinegar and chopped fresh basil, if you have some on hand.*

Serves 1

WOMEN: CALORIES 260; FIBER 9g; FAT 4g; PROTEIN 17g; CARB 44g; SODIUM 700mg

MEN: CALORIES 300; FIBER 9g; FAT 4.5g; PROTEIN 20g; CARB 51g; SODIUM 710mg

Seared Peppercorn Ahi Tuna

Tuna is one of the easiest fish to cook because you can actually watch the color go from deep red to golden-brown in the skillet. If you like it rare, allow a band of red to remain in the middle.

Nonstick cooking spray
One 6-ounce fresh ahi tuna steak, about ½ inch thick
    (will yield 5 ounces cooked)
1 teaspoon freshly ground black pepper
1 tablespoon chopped fresh flat-leaf parsley
1 teaspoon chopped fresh dill

Heat an 8-inch nonstick skillet over medium-high heat. Spray with non-stick cooking spray. Season both sides of the tuna with the black pepper. Place the tuna in the hot skillet and cook for about 2 minutes on each side, depending on the thickness of the steak and how well you like it cooked. Remove the tuna from the skillet and top with the fresh herbs.

Serves 1

CALORIES 190; FIBER 0g; FAT 3g; PROTEIN 31g; CARB 0g; SODIUM 65mg

Sautéed Green Beans with Leeks and Dill

Blanching is a technique fancy restaurants use to make perfectly cooked vegetables every time. What it is is simply plunging vegetables into boiling water to partially cook them, and then transferring them to iced water to stop the cooking.

½ cup fresh green beans, trimmed   MEN: 1 cup

2 teaspoons olive oil

1 tablespoon thinly sliced shallots   MEN: 2 tablespoons

1 teaspoon minced fresh garlic   MEN: 2 teaspoons

2 tablespoons thinly sliced leeks   MEN: ¼ cup

2 tablespoons chopped fresh dill   MEN: 3 tablespoons

MEN: ¾ cup chopped red bell peppers

Fill an 8-inch nonstick skillet with water. Bring the water to a boil over high heat. Add the green beans and blanch them until crisp-tender, about 3 minutes. Drain and plunge them into a bowl filled with ice water. Drain again.

Dry the skillet and heat the olive oil over medium-high heat. Add the shallots, garlic, and leeks, and sauté until soft and aromatic, about 2 minutes. Add the blanched beans and fresh dill. Stir to combine.

Serves 1

WOMEN: CALORIES 110; FIBER 2g; FAT 9g; PROTEIN 1g; CARB 7g; SODIUM 5mg

MEN: CALORIES 160; FIBER 6.5g; FAT 10g; PROTEIN 4g; CARB 19g; SODIUM 15mg

Apple Streusel

Streusels, along with cobblers and crisps, are American classics. But like most things American, streusel has its roots in another country, in this case Germany—and *Streusel* is a German word meaning "sprinkling."

¼ cup 2:90 granola

1 teaspoon brown sugar

1 teaspoon sugar substitute

¼ teaspoon ground cinnamon

2 tablespoons light margarine, chilled and cut into pieces

Nonstick cooking spray

1 large unpeeled apple, cored and sliced

One container 2:90 vanilla yogurt with fiber (providing up to 90 calories)

Preheat the oven to 375°F. In a large bowl, mix together the granola, brown sugar, sugar substitute, and cinnamon. Using a pastry cutter or 2 knives, cut the margarine into the granola until the mixture resembles coarse meal.

Spray a small, round (5-inch-diameter) baking dish with nonstick cooking spray. Evenly arrange the apple slices in the prepared baking dish. Sprinkle with the streusel topping and bake for 45 to 60 minutes, or until bubbling. Remove from the oven and place on a wire rack to cool slightly. Serve from the baking dish topped with the yogurt.

Serves 1

CALORIES 360; FIBER 6g; FAT 14g; PROTEIN 9g; CARB 53g; SODIUM 300mg

Week 2

Day 1　Monday Menu

Breakfast

1 serving 2:90 calcium-fortified dry or hot cereal (providing up to 90 calories)

1 cup skim milk or one container 2:90 strawberry yogurt with fiber (providing up to 90 calories)

8 pecan halves

1¾ cups fresh strawberries

MEN: Add 1 serving 2:90 calcium-fortified dry or hot cereal (providing up to 90 calories)

Morning Dividend*

Lunch

Mozzarella, Tomato, and Basil Pita

MEN: Add 1 mozzarella string cheese (with no more than 4 grams of total fat per string)

Dinner

Lemon-Herb Shrimp Salad

Reality Reward

Summer Berry "Tart"

---

*Morning Dividend—Choose one sweetener OR one creamer from the following: 1 teaspoon honey, 1 teaspoon white granulated sugar, or 1 teaspoon brown sugar OR 2 tablespoons 2% milk, 1 tablespoon half-and-half, 1 tablespoon soymilk creamer, 1 tablespoon nondairy liquid creamer, 2 teaspoons nondairy powdered creamer

Recipe items are in boldface.

Day 2   Tuesday Menu

Breakfast   **Caramelized Banana and Peanut Butter Toast**
                 1 cup skim milk or one container of 2:90 strawberry yogurt
                 with fiber (providing up to 90 calories)
                 MEN: Add 1 serving 2:90 calcium-fortified dry or hot cereal
                 Morning Dividend

Lunch   **Herbed Tuna Salad Sandwich**
                 ¼ cup carrot sticks
                 MEN: Add 1 mozzarella string cheese (with no more than
                 4 grams of total fat per string) and 4 tablespoons chopped
                 avocado

Dinner   **Santa Maria Chicken**
                 Arugula and Cherry Tomato Salad
                 with Aged Balsamic Vinegar

Reality Reward   **Summer Berry "Tart"**

Day 3   Wednesday Menu

Breakfast

1 serving 2:90 calcium-fortified dry or hot cereal (providing up to 90 calories)

1 cup skim milk or one container 2:90 apple yogurt with fiber (providing up to 90 calories)

12 cashews

6 fresh apricots

MEN: Add 1 serving 2:90 calcium-fortified dry or hot cereal (providing up to 90 calories)

Morning Dividend

Lunch

Mediterranean Couscous and Feta Salad

MEN: Add 8 walnut halves

Dinner

Seared Sea Scallops over Baby Greens

Reality Reward

Blackberry Crêpes (see pages 180–181)

Day 4   Thursday Menu

Breakfast   1 serving 2:90 calcium-fortified dry or hot cereal (providing up to 90 calories)

1 cup skim milk or one container 2:90 peach yogurt with fiber (providing 90 calories)

¼ cup unsalted pistachios (with shells)

4 pitted dates

MEN: Add 1 serving 2:90 calcium-fortified dry or hot cereal (providing up to 90 calories)

Morning Dividend

Lunch   **French Cheese Sandwich**

½ cup celery sticks

MEN: Add 4 tablespoons chopped avocado and ½ cup celery sticks

Dinner   **Kung Pao Stir-fry**

Reality Reward   **Piña Colada Slush**

1 dessert starch of your choice (see Equivalents Lists, page 381)

12 cashews

Day 5   Friday Menu

Breakfast	**Blackberry Granola Parfait**
	MEN: Add ¼ cup 2:90 granola
	Morning Dividend
Lunch	**BLTB Sandwich**
	(Bacon, Lettuce, Tomato and Basil Sandwich)
	MEN: Add 1 mozzarella string cheese (with no more than 4 grams of total fat per string) and 4 tablespoons chopped avocado
Dinner	**Tarragon Halibut Steak**
	Field Greens Salad
Reality Reward	**Banana Split**

Day 6   Saturday Menu

Breakfast   1 serving 2:90 calcium-fortified dry or hot cereal (providing
up to 90 calories)
1 cup skim milk or one container 2:90 strawberry yogurt
with fiber (providing 90 calories)
8 walnut halves
1½ cups honeydew melon slices
MEN: Add 1 serving 2:90 calcium-fortified dry or hot cereal
(providing up to 90 calories)
Morning Dividend

Lunch   **Chicago-Style Hot Dog**
Ten 2:90 chips (low-fat gourmet baked potato chips, such
as Kettle Krisps) or 8 Garden of Eatin' Black Bean tortilla
chips
MEN: Add 1 mozzarella string cheese (with no more than
4 grams of total fat per string) and 20 peanuts

Dinner   **Chipotle BBQ Chicken**
Avocado-Cilantro Slaw
Steamed Artichoke with Lemon

Reality Reward **Blueberry Cobbler** (see pages 193–194)

Day 7   Sunday Menu

Breakfast	1 serving 2:90 calcium-fortified dry or hot cereal (providing up to 90 calories)
	1 cup skim milk or one container 2:90 peach yogurt with fiber (providing up to 90 calories)
	12 almonds
	1 medium Asian pear
	MEN: Add 1 serving 2:90 calcium-fortified dry or hot cereal (providing up to 90 calories)
	Morning Dividend
Lunch	**Penne with Melted Cherry Tomato Ragoût**
	MEN: Add 12 almonds
Dinner	**Sole Meunière**
	Spring Mixed-Lettuce Salad
Reality Reward	**Strawberry Custard Cups**

Monday

Mozzarella, Tomato, and Basil Pita

Thanks to the wonders of an international fresh market, you can enjoy a summer salad year-round.

One 2:90 whole-wheat pita
1 mozzarella string cheese (with no more than 4 grams of total fat per
    string), thinly sliced
1 cup chopped tomato   MEN: 2 cups
½ cup baby spinach leaves   MEN: 1 cup
¼ cup chopped scallions   MEN: ½ cup
4 or 5 chopped fresh basil leaves
1 teaspoon extra-virgin olive oil   MEN: 2 teaspoons
1 teaspoon balsamic vinegar
Freshly ground black pepper

Cut the pita in half and toast it. Set aside.

In a medium bowl, combine the mozzarella, 1 cup tomato, ½ cup spinach, ¼ cup scallions, and the basil. Drizzle with the olive oil and vinegar, and season with black pepper to taste. Spoon the mixture into the toasted pita pockets and serve.

MEN: *Make a side salad with the extra tomato, spinach, and scallions. Dress the salad with balsamic vinegar, and your extra 2 teaspoons olive oil.*

Serves 1

WOMEN: CALORIES 260; FIBER 6g; FAT 8g; PROTEIN 14g; CARB 36g; SODIUM 490mg
MEN: CALORIES 350; FIBER 8g; FAT 13g; PROTEIN 16g; CARB 46g; SODIUM 520mg

Lemon-Herb Shrimp Salad

Chefs order shrimp by the "count per pound." Large 21–25 count shrimp are the most popular, but they are also expensive. To save a few bucks, ask for 31–35 count shrimp. The fishmonger will be impressed with your knowledge and you will get a shrimp in every bite.

6 ounces shrimp, shelled and deveined (will yield 5 ounces cooked)

Juice of ½ lemon

2 teaspoons olive oil

1 teaspoon dried or 1 tablespoon fresh rosemary

⅛ teaspoon freshly ground black pepper, or more to taste

1 cup baby greens   MEN: 2 cups

¼ cup fresh flat-leaf parsley leaves

3 or 4 fresh basil leaves   MEN: 6 to 8

½ cup halved cherry tomatoes   MEN: 1 cup

½ cup blanched chopped asparagus   MEN: 1 cup

1 tablespoon chopped capers (high sodium)

Set a rack at the highest level of the oven and preheat to broil. In a small bowl, toss the shrimp together with the lemon juice, olive oil, rosemary, and black pepper. Arrange the shrimp on a nonstick baking sheet and broil for 1 to 2 minutes, depending on the size of the shrimp. Turn the shrimp over and broil another 1 to 2 minutes, or until bright pink.

In a medium bowl, toss together the baby greens, parsley, basil, cherry tomatoes, asparagus, and capers. Mound the salad in the center of the plate and arrange the shrimp on top of the salad. Pour any of the remaining juice from the baking sheet over the salad. The heat of the shrimp will wilt the greens slightly and their juices will dress the salad.

Serves 1

WOMEN: CALORIES 300; FIBER 2.5g; FAT 13g; PROTEIN 37g; CARB 9g; SODIUM 520mg

MEN: CALORIES 330; FIBER 5g; FAT 13g; PROTEIN 40g; CARB 15g; SODIUM 540mg

Summer Berry "Tart"

A tart is an open-faced pie. In this case the granola doubles as the crust and the crunch. Save a little bit of the yogurt to dab on top of the berries if you like. This recipe makes two servings, so save half to eat on Day 2.

½ cup 2:90 granola
Two containers any berry-flavored 2:90 yogurt with fiber
    (providing up to 90 calories)
1 cup sliced strawberries
1 cup raspberries
⅔ cup blueberries
1 teaspoon lemon juice
2 teaspoons sugar substitute
4 tablespoons toasted walnuts, crumbled
4 teaspoons powdered sugar

Line the bottom of a dessert bowl with the granola. Spoon the yogurt onto the granola.

In a medium bowl, toss the berries together with the lemon juice and sugar substitute. Top the yogurt with the berries and walnuts, and dust with the powdered sugar. Keep refrigerated until ready to serve.

Serves 2

CALORIES 390; FIBER 12g; FAT 11g; PROTEIN 13g; CARB 64g; SODIUM 100mg per single serving

Tuesday

Herbed Tuna Salad Sandwich

Since tuna comes from the sea, this salad is seasoned with lemon to bring out its natural flavor. You won't miss the gooey version you used to buy at the corner deli.

1½ ounces canned tuna in oil

½ cup halved cherry tomatoes   MEN: 1 cup

½ cup shredded iceberg lettuce   MEN: 1 cup

¼ cup chopped yellow onion   MEN: ½ cup

1 tablespoon chopped fresh dill   MEN: 2 tablespoons

1 tablespoon chopped flat-leaf parsley   MEN: 2 tablespoons

1 tablespoon non-fat mayonnaise

1 teaspoon fresh lemon juice   MEN: 1 teaspoon, plus more to taste

Freshly ground black pepper

2 slices regular 2:90 bread

In a small bowl, combine the tuna, cherry tomatoes, lettuce, onions, dill, parsley, and mayonnaise. Mix with a fork to combine. Season with fresh lemon juice and black pepper to taste. Spoon the salad onto one slice of the bread. Top with the second slice of bread. Close the sandwich and cut in half diagonally.

MEN: *Make a side salad with the extra veggies, plus the avocado from the menu list, seasoned with lots of extra fresh dill, parsley, and fresh lemon juice.*

Serves 1

WOMEN: CALORIES 310; FIBER 8g; FAT 6g; PROTEIN 21g; CARB 46g; SODIUM 680mg

MEN: CALORIES 340; FIBER 9g; FAT 6g; PROTEIN 22g; CARB 54g; SODIUM 690mg

Santa Maria Chicken

You will feel like a ranch hand at the table this evening, especially if you grill the chicken over an open fire. After cooking, allow the chicken breast to rest before slicing—the resting time will make the meat juicier.

6 ounces boneless, skinless chicken breast,
    cut into 1-inch-wide strips (will yield 5 ounces cooked)

Nonstick cooking spray

1 teaspoon Santa Maria dry rub (recipe follows)

Set a rack at the highest level of the oven and preheat to broil. Place the chicken breast on a broiling pan and spray both sides of the chicken with nonstick cooking spray. Sprinkle half of the dry rub on one side of the chicken. Pat the breast lightly to make the dry rub stick. Turn the chicken over and sprinkle the remaining seasoning on the other side.

Place the chicken under the broiler for 3 minutes. Turn the chicken over and broil for another 3 minutes, or until golden-brown.

Remove the chicken from the broiler and let it rest for 3 to 5 minutes before serving.

Serves 1

CALORIES 210; FIBER 0g; FAT 4g; PROTEIN 40g; CARB 2g; SODIUM 110mg

Santa Maria Dry Rub

This dry-rub is a great make-ahead recipe. You can multiply the recipe as many times as you want. It will stay fresh in an airtight container for several weeks. Use as a seasoning for meat, vegetables, and even scrambled egg whites.

3 tablespoons garlic powder

2 teaspoons dry mustard

2 teaspoons paprika

1 teaspoon ground black pepper

¼ teaspoon cayenne pepper

In a small bowl, combine the spices. Mix together with a fork until well combined. Store in a plastic bag or an airtight container until ready to use.

Makes 14 teaspoons

CALORIES 10; FIBER 0g; FAT 0g; PROTEIN 0g; CARB 2g; SODIUM 0mg

Arugula and Cherry Tomato Salad with Aged Balsamic Vinegar

Balsamic vinegar is like fine wine—the flavor and aroma get better with age. A little bit of the good stuff goes a long way.

½ cup green beans   MEN: 1 cup
¼ cup sliced yellow onion   MEN: ½ cup
¾ cup fresh arugula leaves   MEN: 1½ cups
½ cup chopped tomatoes   MEN: 1 cup
2 teaspoons olive oil
2 teaspoons aged balsamic vinegar
Freshly ground black pepper

Fill an 8-inch nonstick skillet with water. Boil the water over high heat. Add the green beans and blanch them until crisp-tender, about 3 minutes. Add the onions and blanch another 15 seconds. Drain and plunge them into a bowl filled with ice water. Drain again.

In a medium bowl, toss together the arugula, tomatoes, olive oil, and vinegar. Add the blanched green beans and onions and toss. Season with black pepper to taste.

Serves 1

WOMEN: CALORIES 150; FIBER 4g; FAT 10g; PROTEIN 3g; CARB 14g; SODIUM 15mg
MEN: CALORIES 200; FIBER 8g; FAT 10g; PROTEIN 4g; CARB 24g; SODIUM 25mg

Wednesday

Mediterranean Couscous and Feta Salad

Whole-wheat couscous adds both flavor and texture to this classic Mediterranean salad. It will fill you up and the whole grain will give you energy for hours to come.

⅔ cup cooked whole-wheat 2:90 couscous, cooled

½ cup mixed salad greens   MEN: 1 cup

½ cup halved cherry tomatoes   MEN: 1 cup

½ cup sliced red bell pepper   MEN: 1 cup

¼ cup sliced red onion   MEN: ½ cup

1 ounce reduced-fat feta cheese (with no more than 4 grams of total fat per
   ounce), crumbled   MEN: 2 ounces

2 tablespoons chopped fresh flat-leaf parsley

2 tablespoons chopped fresh basil

2 teaspoons balsamic vinegar

In a medium bowl, toss together the couscous with remaining ingredients.

Serves 1

WOMEN: CALORIES 310; FIBER 11g; FAT 4.5g; PROTEIN 16g; CARB 58g; SODIUM 380mg

MEN: CALORIES 410; FIBER 14g; FAT 8g; PROTEIN 24g; CARB 72g; SODIUM 770mg

Seared Sea Scallops over Baby Greens

This entree is both elegant and easy to prepare. The heat from the seared
sea scallops will slightly wilt the salad greens, creating a wonderful contrast
of flavor, texture, and aroma. The orange zest is a functional garnish, which
means it adds both beauty and flavor to the dish.

½ cup mixed salad greens   MEN: 1 cup

½ cup sliced cucumber   MEN: 1 cup

½ cup halved cherry tomatoes   MEN: 1 cup

¼ cup sliced carrots   MEN: ½ cup

4 or 5 fresh basil leaves

2 teaspoons olive oil

6 ounces sea scallops (will yield 5 ounces cooked)

Balsamic vinegar

Freshly grated orange zest

Freshly squeezed orange juice, to taste

In a medium bowl, toss together the salad greens, cucumber, cherry tomatoes, carrots, and basil. Mound the salad in the center of a large plate.

Heat an 8-inch nonstick skillet over medium-high heat. Add 1 teaspoon of the olive oil and carefully place the scallops in the hot pan. Cook for 2 minutes, or until golden brown. Turn the scallops over and cook for another minute. Add the vinegar and swirl it around the scallops to coat. Cook for another minute.

Place the cooked scallops onto and around the salad. Drizzle with the remaining teaspoon olive oil and sprinkle the orange zest over the top of the salad. Cut the orange in half and squeeze the juice onto the scallops.

Serves 1

WOMEN: CALORIES 310; FIBER 3g; FAT 11g; PROTEIN 35g; CARB 16g; SODIUM 380mg

MEN: CALORIES 350; FIBER 5g; FAT 12g; PROTEIN 37g; CARB 24g; SODIUM 400mg

Thursday

French Cheese Sandwich

The peppery arugula is softened by the sweet blend of dried herbs, creating a balance that only the French could imagine.

    1 teaspoon Dijon mustard
    2 slices regular 2:90 bread
    1½ ounces any cheese (with more than 1 but no more than 3 grams of fat
        per ounce) MEN: 3 ounces any cheese (with more than 1 but no more
        than 3 grams of fat per ounce)
    1 teaspoon French Seasoning Mix (recipe follows)
    Freshly ground black pepper
    1 cup arugula leaves MEN: 2 cups
    1 cup chopped tomato MEN: 2 cups

Spread the mustard over both slices of bread. Place the cheese on one slice of bread. Sprinkle with the French seasoning mix and black pepper to taste. Top with 1 cup arugula and 1 cup tomato. Top with the second slice of bread. Close the sandwich and cut it in half diagonally.

MEN: *Season the extra tomato and arugula leaves with an extra pinch of the French seasoning mix, and toss the salad with white wine vinegar from the pantry.*

Serves 1
WOMEN: CALORIES 330; FIBER 8g; FAT 7g; PROTEIN 24g; CARB 48g; SODIUM 680mg
MEN: CALORIES 470; FIBER 11g; FAT 12g; PROTEIN 40g; CARB 58g; SODIUM 880mg

French Seasoning Mix

Tarragon, chives, parsley, and marjoram are members of an elite group called fines herbs. French chefs use these herbs for seasoning delicate sauces and fish.

½ teaspoon dried tarragon

½ teaspoon dried chives

½ teaspoon dried parsley

½ teaspoon dried marjoram

½ teaspoon dry mustard

½ teaspoon garlic powder

½ teaspoon onion powder

¼ teaspoon ground white pepper

¼ teaspoon cayenne pepper

In a small bowl, combine the spices. Mix together with a fork until well combined. Store in a plastic bag or an airtight container until ready to use.

Makes 4 teaspoons
CALORIES 5; FIBER 0g; FAT 0g; PROTEIN 0g; CARB 1g; SODIUM 0mg

Kung Pao Stir-fry

This spicy Szechuan dish is great with chicken, shrimp, or tofu. You can adjust the spiciness to your taste by adding more or less of the garlic, ginger, and chilies.

1 tablespoon teriyaki sauce (reduced sodium)

1 tablespoon rice vinegar

1 tablespoon water

1 tablespoon sugar substitute

½ cup broccoli florets   MEN: 1 cup

¼ cup snow peas   MEN: ½ cup

¼ cup chopped red onion   MEN: ½ cup

2 teaspoons minced fresh garlic   MEN: 1 tablespoon

1 teaspoon minced fresh ginger   MEN: 2 teaspoons

1 or 2 small dried red chilies, or to taste

20 unsalted peanuts, chopped

Nonstick cooking spray

6 ounces boneless, skinless chicken breast, cut into ½-inch cubes
   (will yield 5 ounces cooked)

1 cup chopped chard   MEN: 2 cups

¼ cup chopped fresh cilantro leaves

In a small bowl, whisk together the teriyaki sauce, vinegar, water, and sugar substitute. In another small bowl, combine the broccoli, snow peas, and red onion. In a third bowl, combine the garlic, ginger, chilies, and peanuts.

Heat a wok or nonstick skillet over high heat and spray with nonstick cooking spray. Add the chicken and cook for 2 to 3 minutes, stirring constantly. Remove the chicken from the wok and set aside. Add the vegetable mixture and cook for another 2 to 3 minutes, or until the vegetables begin to color. Add the garlic mixture and cook for another 30 seconds.

Add the chicken back to the wok, along with the chard and the soy mixture. Bring to a boil and cook for 30 seconds, or until the chard is wilted. Stir in the cilantro.

Serves 1

WOMEN: CALORIES 350; FIBER 4g; FAT 12g; PROTEIN 47g; CARB 15g; SODIUM 520mg

MEN: CALORIES 410; FIBER 7g; FAT 14g; PROTEIN 50g; CARB 24g; SODIUM 610mg

Piña Colada Slush

A favorite of tropical drink lovers, a piña colada is a cool and refreshing drink to finish the day with. Serve it in a frosted glass for an even cooler experience.

1 ⅛ cups diced fresh or canned pineapple

One container 2:90 vanilla yogurt with fiber (providing up to 90 calories)

2 teaspoons marshmallow fluff

2 teaspoons sugar substitute

1 teaspoon coconut extract

6 to 8 ice cubes

Combine all of the ingredients in the jar of a blender. Cover and blend until smooth and frothy, about 30 seconds. Add a little water to thin the consistency if necessary.

Pour into a tall glass and serve with a straw.

Serves 1

CALORIES 190; FIBER 4g; FAT 0g; PROTEIN 7g; CARB 42g; SODIUM 100mg

Friday

Blackberry Granola Parfait

The fancier the glass, the fancier the presentation. Shop around at flea markets for a tall, fluted glass of unknown vintage for this fruity breakfast.

One container of any 2:90 vanilla yogurt with fiber (providing 90 calories)

¼ cup 2:90 granola

1 ⅛ cups blackberries

8 toasted pecan halves, crumbled

2 or 3 fresh mint leaves

Fill a tall glass with alternating layers of the yogurt, granola, and black-berries. Finish with either the berries or a sprinkling of granola. Garnish with the pecans and fresh mint.

Serves 1

CALORIES 350; FIBER 5g; FAT 10g; PROTEIN 13g; CARB 56g; SODIUM 100mg

FOR CHERRY-ALMOND GRANOLA PARFAIT

Subsitute 18 fresh, pitted and sliced cherries and 12 chopped and toasted almonds for the blackberries and pecans.

CALORIES 360; FIBER 9g; FAT 10g; PROTEIN 13g; CARB 59g; SODIUM 95mg

Tarragon Halibut Steak

Tarragon is the most sophisticated of the French herbs. Its sweet aniselike flavor tastes best when used alone or with a little lemon juice.

One 6-ounce halibut steak (will yield 5 ounces when cooked)

2 tablespoons fresh lemon juice

2 teaspoons olive oil

1 tablespoon chopped fresh flat-leaf parsley

1 teaspoon chopped fresh tarragon

Preheat the oven to 400°F. Place the halibut steak in an ovenproof dish and sprinkle with the lemon juice and olive oil. Bake for 4 to 6 minutes, or un-til the fish feels firm. Add the parsley and tarragon and bake another minute, or until the herbs are aromatic.

Serves 1

CALORIES 270; FIBER 0g; FAT 13g; PROTEIN 35g; CARB 0g; SODIUM 90mg

Field Greens Salad

Simple greens dressed in citrus and sea salt can brighten up any meal.

1 cup field greens   MEN: 2 cups
1 cup radicchio
½ cup chopped cucumber   MEN: 1 cup
½ cup broccoli florets   MEN: 1 cup
½ cup cauliflower florets   MEN: 1 cup
Fresh lemon juice

In a large bowl, toss all the vegetables together and season with lemon juice and salt to taste.

Serves 1

WOMEN: CALORIES 50; FIBER 4g; FAT 0g; PROTEIN 4g; CARB 10g; SODIUM 55mg
MEN: CALORIES 90; FIBER 9g; FAT .5g; PROTEIN 7g; CARB 19g; SODIUM 100mg

Banana Split

Reminiscent of an old-time ice cream parlor treat, without all the calories, this banana split will satisfy your craving for something indulgent.

One container 2:90 vanilla yogurt with fiber (providing up to 90 calories)
1 ripe banana
1 tablespoon low-sugar raspberry or strawberry jam
20 unsalted peanuts, crushed
⅓ cup muesli

Empty the yogurt into a shallow metal bowl and place it in the freezer. Freeze for 40 minutes, stirring every 10 minutes, until the yogurt feels like ice cream. Peel the banana, slice it in half lengthwise, and arrange it on opposite sides of an oval dish. Scoop the frozen yogurt into two scoops between the banana halves. Top each scoop with a little jam, crushed peanuts, and muesli.

Serves 1

CALORIES 390; FIBER 8g; FAT 10g; PROTEIN 14g; CARB 69g; SODIUM 170mg

Saturday

Chicago-Style Hot Dog

These high-piled hot dogs are a Chicago tradition, and the celery salt is the Windy City's signature flavor. There are so many goodies, in fact, that you'll probably want to eat this hot dog with a fork and knife.

Nonstick cooking spray

One 1-ounce hot dog (with between 1 and 3 grams of fat per ounce)

One 2:90 whole-wheat or multigrain hot dog bun

1 teaspoon yellow mustard

¾ ounce Jack cheese (with more than 1 gram but no more than 3 grams of fat per ounce)

½ cup chopped tomato   MEN: 1 cup

¼ cup chopped yellow onion   MEN: ½ cup

1 teaspoon chopped peperoncini

½ large dill pickle

⅛ teaspoon celery salt

    MEN: 1 cup sliced cucumber

    MEN: ¾ cup sliced fennel

    MEN: ¼ cup shredded carrot

    MEN: Lemon juice, to taste

    MEN: Freshly ground black pepper, to taste

Heat an 8-inch nonstick skillet over medium-high heat. Spray with nonstick cooking spray. Place the hot dog in the skillet and cook until browned, about 3 minutes, turning once.

Split the bun open and spray it with nonstick cooking spray. Place cut-side down on the skillet for 30 seconds, or until toasted. Spread mustard on both sides of the bun; put in the hot dog and cheese. Top with tomato, onion, peperoncini, and pickle. Sprinkle with celery salt.

MEN: *Make a side salad with the cucumbers, fennel, and carrots. Season to taste with lemon juice and black pepper.*

Serves 1

WOMEN: CALORIES 220; FIBER 5g; FAT 6g; PROTEIN 19g; CARB 29g; SODIUM 580mg

MEN: CALORIES 340; FIBER 11g; FAT 7g; PROTEIN 22g; CARB 54g; SODIUM 700mg

Chipotle BBQ Chicken

Chipotle chilies are smoked jalapeños. They're typically sold in small cans with a spicy red sauce called adobo. Puree the contents of a whole can in your food processor—the pureed peppers will stay fresh in the refrigerator for a couple of weeks.

    2 teaspoons pureed chipotles in adobo sauce
    1 tablespoon fresh lime juice
    1 teaspoon sugar substitute
    6 ounces boneless, skinless chicken breast, cut into 1-inch-wide strips
        (will yield 5 ounces cooked)
    Nonstick cooking spray

In a small bowl, combine the chipotles, lime juice, and sugar substitute. Mix until smooth.

Place the chicken strips in a resealable plastic bag, add the chipotle BBQ marinade, shake to coat, and refrigerate until ready to cook.

Heat an 8-inch nonstick skillet over high heat. Spray with nonstick cooking spray. Remove the chicken pieces from the marinade, shaking gently to allow any excess to drip off. Discard the remaining marinade. Arrange the pieces in a single layer in the skillet and cook for six minutes, turning once.

Serves 1

CALORIES 200; FIBER 0g; FAT 3.5g; PROTEIN 39g; CARB 0g; SODIUM 110mg

Avocado-Cilantro Slaw

This cool, crisp salad is the perfect accompaniment to a spicy dish like Chipotle BBQ Chicken. Instead of chopping the cilantro, pluck the leaves from the stems and toss them into the salad. The cilantro flavor will pop in your mouth.

½ cup shredded green cabbage   MEN: 1 cup

¼ cup thinly sliced red bell pepper   MEN: ½ cup

¼ cup grated carrot   MEN: ½ cup

¼ cup chopped avocado

2 tablespoons fresh cilantro leaves   MEN: 3 tablespoons

Juice of 1 lime, or more to taste

⅛ teaspoon chili powder   MEN: ¼ teaspoon

Hot sauce

In a small bowl, combine the cabbage, bell pepper, carrot, avocado, and cilantro. Drizzle with the lime juice, salt, and chili powder. Toss again to combine and season with hot sauce to taste. Refrigerate until ready to serve.

Serves 1

WOMEN: CALORIES 130; FIBER 6g; FAT 9g; PROTEIN 2g; CARB 12g; SODIUM 30mg

MEN: CALORIES 150; FIBER 8g; FAT 9g; PROTEIN 3g; CARB 19g; SODIUM 55mg

Steamed Artichoke with Lemon

The outer leaves of an artichoke are tough and often have prickly little spikes sticking out. The spikes will be cut away, though, when you trim off the top ½ inch of the choke.

1 small artichoke

Several sprigs of fresh tarragon or parsley

1 teaspoon fresh lemon juice, plus more to taste

Peel away the tough outer leaves of the artichoke and discard. Place the artichoke on its side and trim off the top ½ inch.

Place the artichoke, bottom up, in a pot filled with 1 inch of water, along with the sprigs of fresh herbs, cover, and steam for 30 to 35 minutes, or until the base can be pierced with a sharp knife. Sprinkle with fresh lemon juice.

Serves 1

CALORIES 60; FIBER 7g; FAT 0g; PROTEIN 4g; CARB 13g; SODIUM 120mg

Sunday

Penne with Melted Cherry Tomato Ragoût

Melted is a fun way to describe tomatoes that have been cooked until they begin to lose their shape and share their juices with the other vegetables in the pan. A quick note on leeks: Wash them very well, as they can harbor sand between their layers.

⅔ cup cooked 2:90 whole-wheat penne pasta

2 tablespoons light margarine

¼ cup chopped yellow onion   MEN: ½ cup

¼ cup chopped carrot   MEN: ½ cup

¼ cup chopped leek   MEN: ½ cup

½ cup halved cherry tomatoes   MEN: 1 cup

1 teaspoon garlic powder   MEN: 2 teaspoons

½ teaspoon red pepper flakes

1 tablespoon chopped fresh flat-leaf parsley   MEN: 2 tablespoons

1 tablespoon chopped fresh basil   MEN: 2 tablespoons

3½ tablespoons grated Parmesan cheese   MEN: 7 tablespoons

Heat an 8-inch nonstick skillet over medium heat. Add the margarine to the skillet and continue to heat for another 15 seconds. Add the onions, carrots, and leeks, and cook for 5 minutes, stirring often. Add the tomatoes and cook for another 5 minutes. Add the garlic powder, red pepper flakes, parsley, basil, and Parmesan, stir to combine, and cook until the cheese is melted, about 30 seconds.

Serves 1

CALORIES 330; FIBER 7g; FAT 6g; PROTEIN 16g; CARB 54g; SODIUM 490mg

MEN: CALORIES 460; FIBER 10g; FAT 12g; PROTEIN 24g; CARB 68g; SODIUM 790mg

Sole Meunière

This classic French preparation will make you feel like you've traveled to a Parisian bistro for dinner. Sole is extremely delicate, especially when cooked, so make sure to slide your spatula under the whole fillet before lifting it out of the skillet.

2 tablespoons non-fat margarine
1 tablespoon finely chopped fresh flat-leaf parsley
One 6-ounce sole fillet (will yield 5 ounces cooked)
2 teaspoons fresh lemon juice
Nonstick cooking spray

Heat an 8-inch nonstick skillet over medium-high heat. Add the margarine and let it melt. Add the parsley and carefully place the sole over the parsley. Cook for 2 minutes, then turn the sole over and cook for another minute. Add the lemon juice and swirl it around the sole to coat. Cook for another minute, or until the fish begins to flake. Carefully lift the fillet onto a plate and pour the lemon sauce over the top.

Serves 1

CALORIES 170; FIBER 0g; FAT 3.5g; PROTEIN 32g; CARB 0g; SODIUM 320mg

Spring Mixed-Lettuce Salad

This mixed green salad is a classic accompaniment to a simple dinner. The fresh lemon juice gives it a bright and tart taste.

1 tablespoon fresh lemon juice

2 teaspoons extra-virgin olive oil

Freshly ground black pepper

1 cup prepackaged mixed salad greens (or a combination of romaine, Bibb,
    escarole, arugula and/or radicchio)   MEN: 2 cups

¾ cup chopped tomato   MEN: 1½ cups

½ cup broccoli sprouts   MEN: 1 cup

Combine the lemon juice, olive oil, and black pepper to taste in a medium
bowl. Add the salad greens, tomato, and broccoli sprouts. Toss well to coat
with dressing.

Serves 1

WOMEN: CALORIES 160; FIBER 7g; FAT 10g; PROTEIN 2g; CARB 8g; SODIUM 25mg

MEN: CALORIES 230; FIBER 13g; FAT 10g; PROTEIN 4g; CARB 16g; SODIUM 50mg

Strawberry Custard Cups

If you have a minute to spare, you have time to prepare this dessert. It's
quick and easy, and tasty too.

1¾ cups whole strawberries, sliced

One container 2:90 strawberry yogurt with fiber (providing up to 90 calories)

⅓ cup 2:90 fruit muesli

1 teaspoon semisweet chocolate mini-morsels

8 pecan halves, crumbled

In a small bowl, combine the strawberries and yogurt. Spoon the fruit
muesli into the bottom of a dessert cup and top with the strawberry-yogurt
mixture. Top with the chocolate chips and crumbled pecans.

Serves 1

CALORIES 380; FIBER 11g; FAT 12g; PROTEIN 12g; CARB 65g; SODIUM 160mg

Week 3

Day 1 Monday Menu

Breakfast	**Warm Ham-and-Cheese Toast** 1 cup skim milk or one container 2:90 strawberry yogurt with fiber (providing up to 90 calories) 1¾ cups fresh strawberries MEN: Add 1 whole egg plus 1 egg white *Morning Dividend**
Lunch	**Veggie Wraps**
Dinner	**Herb Pesto Tilapia Fillet** **Chilled Wedge Salad with Blue Cheese Dressing**
Reality Reward	**Brownies and Sliced Strawberries**

Morning Dividend—Choose one sweetener OR one creamer from the following:
1 teaspoon honey, 1 teaspoon white granulated sugar, or 1 teaspoon brown
sugar OR 2 tablespoons 2% milk, 1 tablespoon half-and-half, 1 tablespoon
soymilk creamer, 1 tablespoon nondairy liquid creamer, 2 teaspoons nondairy
powdered creamer

Recipe items are in boldface.

Day 2   Tuesday Menu

Breakfast   1 serving 2:90 calcium-fortified dry or hot cereal (providing up to 90 calories)

1 cup skim milk or one container 2:90 apple yogurt with fiber (providing 90 calories)

6 fresh apricots

3 slices Canadian bacon

MEN: Add 1 mozzarella string cheese (with no more than 4 grams of total fat per string); 1 whole egg plus 1 egg white *Morning Dividend*

Lunch   **Italian Flatbread Pizza**

Dinner   **Cannellini Beans and Broccoli Rabe**

Reality Reward   **Peanut Butter Chocolate Chip Cookies**

1 cup ice-cold skim milk

Day 3 · Wednesday Menu

Breakfast   **French Omelet with Tarragon**
2:90 English muffin
1 cup skim milk or one container 2:90 apple yogurt with
fiber (providing 90 calories)
3 small sliced plums
MEN: Add 1 mozzarella string cheese (with no more than
4 grams of total fat per string)
Morning Dividend

Lunch   **Asparagus-and-Mushroom Risotto**

Dinner   **Black Pepper Chicken with Oven-Roasted Tomatoes**

Reality Reward **Frozen Vanilla Yogurt with Cherries, Pistachios, and
Chocolate Chips**
1 cup ice-cold skim milk

Day 4   Thursday Menu

Breakfast

1 serving 2:90 calcium-fortified dry or hot cereal (providing up to 90 calories)

1 cup skim milk or one container 2:90 peach yogurt with fiber (providing up to 90 calories)

4 pitted dates

1 mozzarella string cheese (with no more than 4 grams of total fat per string)

MEN: Add 1 mozzarella string cheese (with no more than 4 grams of total fat per string)

Morning Dividend

Lunch   **Spaghetti Primavera**

Dinner   **Ginger-Teriyaki–Glazed Mahimahi**
Stir-fried Zucchini and Snow Peas

Reality Reward   **Pineapple Fritters**

Day 5   Friday Menu

Breakfast   **Egg-and-Chive Breakfast Sandwich**
1½ cups cantaloupe slices
1 cup skim milk or one container 2:90 peach yogurt with
fiber (providing up to 90 calories)
1 mozzarella string cheese (with no more than 4 grams of
total fat per string)
MEN: 1 whole egg plus 1 egg white
Morning Dividend

Lunch   **Soft Veggie Taco**
MEN: Add 12 almonds

Dinner   **Apricot-Citrus–Glazed Cornish Hen**
Sweet and Spicy Carrot Salad

Reality Reward   **Oatmeal-Raisin Cookies**
1 cup ice-cold skim milk

Day 6   Saturday Menu

Breakfast

1 serving 2:90 calcium-fortified dry or hot cereal (providing up to 90 calories)

1 cup skim milk or one container 2:90 strawberry yogurt with fiber (providing up to 90 calories)

1½ cups honeydew melon slices

1½ ounces any cheese (with more than 1 but no more than 3 grams of fat per ounce)

MEN: Add 4 slices Canadian bacon

Morning Dividend

Lunch

Saffron Paella

MEN: Add ¼ cup jicama sticks

Dinner

Sicilian Swordfish

Reality Reward

Mayan Hot Cocoa

1 dessert starch of your choice (see Equivalents Lists, page 381)

1 large fresh pear, sliced

¼ cup pistachios in the shell

Day 7   Sunday Menu

Breakfast	**Breakfast Burrito**
	1 cup skim milk or one container 2:90 peach yogurt with fiber (providing up to 90 calories)
	1 medium Asian pear
	MEN: Add 1 mozzarella string cheese (with no more than 4 grams of total fat per string)
	Morning Dividend
Lunch	**Spicy Jambalaya**
Dinner	**Lobster Salad with Lemon-Tarragon Aïoli**
Reality Reward	**Oatmeal-Raisin Cookies**
	1 cup ice-cold skim milk

Monday

Warm Ham-and-Cheese Toast

If you're on the run this morning, you can skip the broiling step in the recipe by simply sandwiching the ham and cheese between the slices of toasted bread.

   2 slices light 2:90 bread, toasted
   1 teaspoon light margarine
   Garlic powder, to taste
   Freshly ground black pepper, to taste
   ¾ ounce deli ham (with more than 1 but no more than 3 grams of fat per
      ounce)
   ¾ ounce Swiss cheese (with more than 1 but no more than 3 grams of fat
      per ounce)

Spread 1 teaspoon of margarine over each slice of toasted bread. Season both slices of bread with garlic powder and black pepper to taste. Layer the ham and cheese evenly on both slices of bread to make open-faced sandwiches.

Set a rack at the highest level of the oven and preheat to broil. Place the toast on a baking tray and place under the broiler until the cheese is melted, about 60 seconds.

Serves 1

CALORIES 180; FIBER 7g; FAT 5g; PROTEIN 16g; CARB 19g; SODIUM 480mg

Veggie Wraps

Sometimes simple dishes are the most appealing. This one fits that bill. Feel free to substitute ⅓ cup sliced red bell pepper for the broccoli and ½ cup sliced English cucumber for the zucchini if you want to avoid cooking.

Nonstick cooking spray

½ cup broccoli florets   MEN: 1 cup

½ cup chopped zucchini   MEN: 1 cup

Fresh lemon juice

Two 2:90 whole-wheat tortillas   MEN: Three tortillas

½ cup chopped tomatoes   MEN: 1 cup

½ cup shredded romaine lettuce   MEN: 1 cup

4 tablespoons mashed avocado   MEN: ½ cup

Freshly ground black pepper

Heat an 8-inch nonstick skillet over medium heat. Spray with nonstick cooking spray.

Add the broccoli and zucchini to the skillet and sauté for 3 to 4 minutes, or until softened. Season the vegetables with lemon juice to taste and toss to coat.

Microwave the tortillas for 10 to 15 seconds to soften. Place the tortillas on a plate and divide the broccoli sauté between the tortillas. Top each with equal amounts of the tomatoes, lettuce, and avocado, and season with black pepper to taste. Wrap and serve.

Serves 1

WOMEN: CALORIES 310; FIBER 21g; FAT 15g; PROTEIN 10g; CARB 38g; SODIUM 470mg

MEN: CALORIES 530; FIBER 35g; FAT 26g; PROTEIN 17g; CARB 64g; SODIUM 720mg

Herb Pesto Tilapia Fillet

Tilapia thrives in the warm waters of the tropics. Its low-fat flesh is sweet and sometimes it's tinged with swirls of pink. If you have trouble finding tilapia in your local market, use wild rainbow trout or halibut instead.

Nonstick cooking spray

One 6-ounce tilapia fillet (will yield 5 ounces cooked)

2 teaspoons minced fresh garlic

2 teaspoons extra-virgin olive oil

1 tablespoon chopped fresh flat-leaf parsley

1 tablespoon chopped fresh basil

1 teaspoon chopped fresh oregano

2 sprigs of fresh thyme

½ teaspoon freshly ground black pepper

3 thin lemon slices plus ½ lemon, cut into wedges

Preheat the oven to 375°F. Lay a 10 x 10-inch piece of aluminum foil on the counter. Spray the foil with the nonstick cooking spray. Place the tilapia fillet in the center of the foil.

In a small bowl, combine the garlic, olive oil, parsley, basil, oregano, thyme, and black pepper. Spread the mixture over the tilapia. Top with the lemon slices. Fold up the edges of the foil and crimp them together so no air or juices can escape.

Place in a baking dish and bake for 10 to 12 minutes. Carefully open the foil, allowing the steam to escape. Slide the fish and juices onto a plate and serve with the lemon wedges.

Serves 1

CALORIES 250; FIBER 0g; FAT 14g; PROTEIN 29g; CARB 0g; SODIUM 75mg

Chilled Wedge Salad with Blue Cheese Dressing

If retro is cool, then wedge salads are as hip as the 1950s. The steakhouse secret is to serve the wedge on a chilled plate—ten minutes in your freezer will do the trick.

½ cup iceberg lettuce, cut into a wedge shape   MEN: 1 cup

½ cup chopped tomato

¼ cup sliced cucumber   MEN: 1 cup

¼ cup sliced radishes   MEN: 1 cup

¼ cup grated carrot   MEN: ½ cup

¼ cup minced scallion   MEN: ½ cup

1 tablespoon fat-free blue cheese dressing

Freshly ground black pepper

Place the wedge of lettuce on the chilled plate. Top with the tomato, cucumber, radishes, carrot, and scallion. Drizzle the wedge with the dressing
and season with black pepper to taste.

Serves 1

WOMEN: CALORIES 70; FIBER 3g; FAT .5g; PROTEIN 2g; CARB 15g; SODIUM 180mg
MEN: CALORIES 120; FIBER 5g; FAT 1g; PROTEIN 4g; CARB 25g; SODIUM 240mg

Brownies and Sliced Strawberries

Here's a trick: If you're not filling all of the muffin cups with batter, pour
water into the unfilled cups so the pan won't warp in the oven.

⅓ cup non-fat dry milk powder

3½ tablespoons whole-wheat flour

2 tablespoons plus 1 teaspoon sugar substitute

1 tablespoon unsweetened cocoa powder

½ teaspoon baking powder

4 walnut halves, toasted and chopped

1 tablespoon light margarine

¼ cup water

1 teaspoon vanilla extract

Nonstick cooking spray

1¾ cups sliced strawberries

Preheat the oven to 375°F. In a medium bowl, mix together the dry milk,
flour, 2 tablespoons of the sugar substitute, the cocoa powder, baking powder, and walnuts. Place the margarine in a glass bowl and melt it in the microwave. Stir in the water and vanilla.

Pour the liquid ingredients into the dry and fold together until just
mixed. Spray 2 muffin cups with nonstick cooking spray and divide the batter between them. Bake for 10 minutes, or until a toothpick inserted into
the top of a brownie comes out clean.

While the brownies are cooling, toss together the strawberries and re-

maining 1 teaspoon sugar substitute. Place the brownies on a plate and top
with the sweetened strawberries.

Serves 1

CALORIES 370; FIBER 11g; FAT 12g; PROTEIN 16g; CARB 58g; SODIUM 230mg

Tuesday

Italian Flatbread Pizza

Authentic Italian pizza relies on fresh vegetables and seasonings more than
sauce and cheese. If you prefer a really crisp crust, bake the flatbread for 5
minutes before adding the toppings.

Nonstick cooking spray
One 2:90 flatbread or pita   MEN: Two
½ cup thinly sliced portobello mushrooms   MEN: 1 cup
½ cup thinly sliced red and yellow bell peppers   MEN: 1 cup
1 teaspoon minced fresh garlic
½ teaspoon dried oregano
⅛ teaspoon crushed red pepper flakes
½ cup prepared tomato sauce
½ cup fresh spinach leaves   MEN: 1 cup
5 pitted Kalamata olives, sliced
1 teaspoon olive oil   MEN: 3 teaspoons
1 tablespoon chopped fresh basil

Preheat the oven to 400°F. Heat an 8-inch nonstick skillet over medium-
high heat. Spray with nonstick cooking spray. Add the mushrooms and bell
peppers and sauté for 3 to 5 minutes, or until softened. Add the garlic,
oregano, and red pepper flakes, and sauté another minute.

Spread the pasta sauce evenly over the flatbread and top with the
spinach. Spoon the cooked mushroom mixture over the spinach and top
with the olives. Bake the flatbread for 10 minutes, or until golden-brown.

Remove the flatbread from the oven. Drizzle 2 teaspoons of the olive oil and sprinkle with the basil.

MEN: *Drizzle 1 teaspoon olive oil over each flatbread before baking.*

Serves 1

WOMEN: CALORIES 280; FIBER 8g; FAT 11g; PROTEIN 9g; CARB 42g; SODIUM 570mg

MEN: CALORIES 520; FIBER 16g; FAT 22g; PROTEIN 16g; CARB 74g; SODIUM 830mg

Cannellini Beans and Broccoli Rabe

This recipe is fast food at its healthiest. It can be prepared and on the table in ten minutes or less. Cannellini beans, often used by Italian chefs, are white kidney beans.

1 cup broccoli rabe or broccolini

½ cup chopped collard greens   MEN: 1 cup

2 teaspoons olive oil

¼ cup chopped yellow onion   MEN: ½ cup

1 teaspoon minced fresh garlic

1 cup rinsed and drained canned cannellini beans

2 teaspoons grated Parmesan cheese

⅛ teaspoon crushed red pepper flakes

Blanch the broccoli rabe and collard greens in boiling water until they turn bright green, about 3 minutes. Drain, then plunge into a bowl filled with ice water. Drain again. Set aside.

Heat an 8-inch nonstick skillet over medium-high heat. Add 1 teaspoon of the olive oil along with the onion and garlic, and cook for 2 minutes. Add the beans, broccoli rabe, and collard greens, and cook for another 2 minutes. Drizzle the remaining 1 teaspoon olive oil over the top and sprinkle with the Parmesan and crushed red pepper.

Serves 1

WOMEN: CALORIES 330; FIBER 12g; FAT 11g; PROTEIN 13g; CARB 43g; SODIUM 600mg

MEN: CALORIES 350; FIBER 13g; FAT 12g; PROTEIN 14g; CARB 48g; SODIUM 610mg

Peanut Butter Chocolate Chip Cookies

Revert to childhood and dip these delicious cookies in a tall glass of ice-cold milk. This recipe makes 2 servings, so save half for later this week.

3½ ounces 2:90 granola

8 pitted dates, chopped

4 teaspoons sugar subsitute

1 teaspoon ground cinnamon

1 teaspoon baking powder

2 tablespoons natural peanut butter

1 teaspoon chocolate mini-morsels

2 teaspoons vanilla extract

Nonstick cooking spray

Preheat the oven to 375°F. Spray a nonstick cookie sheet with nonstick cooking spray.

In a food processor, chop together the granola, dates, sugar substitute, cinnamon, and baking powder to a paste, about 45 seconds. Scrape the granola mixture into a medium bowl and stir in the peanut butter, chocolate morsels, and vanilla just until the dough holds together. Measure the dough by tablespoonfuls onto the prepared cookie sheet and press down on the dough. Bake for 10 minutes, or until lightly browned. Remove to a wire rack to cool slightly before serving.

Serves 2

CALORIES 300; FIBER 5g; FAT 11g; PROTEIN 7g; CARB 46g; SODIUM 180mg per serving

Wednesday

French Omelet with Tarragon

French chefs are often given eggs to cook when applying for a new job. The theory is that if they can properly cook an omelet, they have been well trained. A potential employer will look to see that the chef whips the eggs until frothy before cooking.

1 organic, cage-free whole large egg plus 1 egg white

½ tablespoon chopped fresh tarragon

Freshly ground black pepper

Nonstick cooking spray

Whip the eggs with a whisk until frothy, add the tarragon, and season with black pepper to taste.

Heat an 8-inch nonstick skillet over medium-high heat. Spray with nonstick cooking spray. Add the egg mixture to the skillet and scramble until it begins to set. Slide out of the pan onto a plate and flip over half to make an omelet.

Serves 1

CALORIES 100; FIBER 0g; FAT 6g; PROTEIN 10g; CARB 1g; SODIUM 125mg

Asparagus-and-Mushroom Risotto

Constant stirring, which releases the starch from the rice, is the key to creamy risotto. You can add any kind of fresh chopped herb you happen to have in your refrigerator.

2 teaspoons olive oil   MEN: 4 teaspoons, plus 2 for drizzling

½ cup sliced asparagus

½ cup sliced mushrooms   MEN: 1 cup

½ cup chopped scallions   MEN: 1 cup

1 tablespoon minced fresh garlic   MEN: 4 teaspoons

¼ cup Lundberg Wild Blend gourmet blend of wild rice and brown rice

    MEN: ⅓ cup

½ cup water   MEN: ⅔ cup

½ cup chopped tomatoes   MEN: 1 cup

2 teaspoons grated Parmesan cheese

Heat the oil in a medium saucepan over medium heat. Add the asparagus, mushrooms, scallions, and garlic, and sauté for 2 to 3 minutes, or until soft and aromatic.

Add the rice to the vegetable mixture, then add the water, stirring constantly until the water boils. Turn the heat down to a simmer and continue stirring until the water is completely absorbed. Add more water, in 1 tablespoon increments, until the rice is cooked. Stir in the tomatoes and Parmesan.

MEN: *Drizzle 2 teaspoons olive oil over the risotto before serving.*

Serves 1

WOMEN: CALORIES 320; FIBER 6.5g; FAT 10g; PROTEIN 9g; CARB 53g; SODIUM 25mg

MEN: CALORIES 340; FIBER 7.5g; FAT 10g; PROTEIN 9g; CARB 57g; SODIUM 35mg

Black Pepper Chicken with Oven-Roasted Tomatoes

This one-pot meal is both simple and sophisticated.

One 6-ounce boneless, skinless chicken breast (will yield 5 ounces cooked)

Freshly ground black pepper

5 ripe plum tomato slices   MEN: 10 slices

2 teaspoons olive oil

¼ cup chopped scallions

1 teaspoon fresh thyme leaves

½ cup baby spinach leaves   MEN: 1 cup

1 teaspoon balsamic vinegar

    MEN: ¼ cup sliced artichoke hearts (packed in water)

Preheat the oven to 450°F. Rinse the chicken breast and pat it dry. Place the chicken breast between 2 large pieces of plastic wrap and pound the breast with a meat mallet or a heavy-bottomed skillet until it is about ½-inch thick. Remove the chicken from the plastic wrap and season with lots of black pepper.

Arrange the tomato slices in a shallow roasting pan and drizzle with 1 teaspoon of the oil. Sprinkle with the chopped scallions, thyme, and black pepper to taste, and roast for 10 minutes. Turn the oven to broil. Remove the pan from the oven and place the chicken breast on top of the tomatoes. Return to the oven and broil for 3 minutes. Turn and broil for another 3 minutes, or until the chicken is no longer pink inside and the juices run clear.

Place the baby spinach on a plate. Remove the chicken from the oven and place over the spinach. Drizzle with the vinegar and remaining 1 teaspoon olive oil.

Serves 1

WOMEN: CALORIES 290; FIBER 1g; FAT 12g; PROTEIN 40g; CARB 4g; SODIUM 130mg

MEN: CALORIES 310; FIBER 2g; FAT 12g; PROTEIN 41g; CARB 8g; SODIUM 150mg

Frozen Vanilla Yogurt with Cherries, Pistachios, and Chocolate Chips

The ice cream parlor is never far away when making this parfait.

One container 2:90 vanilla yogurt with fiber (providing up to 90 calories)
18 fresh cherries, pitted and chopped
1 teaspoon semisweet chocolate mini-morsels
¼ cup pistachios with shells, shelled
1 teaspoon sugar substitute
1 teaspoon vanilla extract

Empty the yogurt into a shallow metal bowl and mix in the remaining ingredients. Freeze for 30 minutes, stir, and freeze another 15 minutes. Scoop into a parfait cup and serve.

Serves 1

CALORIES 310; FIBER 7g; FAT 9g; PROTEIN 12g; CARB 51g; SODIUM 105mg

Thursday

Spaghetti Primavera

Here's a chef's tip: Save some of the water the pasta was cooked in and add it back to the vegetables just before serving to moisten the veggies and pasta.

⅔ cup cooked 2:90 whole-wheat spaghetti (reserve ¼ cup of the cooking water)   MEN: 1 cup

2 teaspoons olive oil   MEN: 4 teaspoons, plus 2 for drizzling

¼ cup cauliflower florets   MEN: ½ cup

½ cup broccoli florets   MEN: 1 cup

½ cup thinly sliced carrots   MEN: 1 cup

1 tablespoon minced fresh garlic   MEN: 4 teaspoons

1 tablespoon chopped fresh flat-leaf parsley   MEN: 2 tablespoons

1 tablespoon chopped fresh basil   MEN: 2 tablespoons

1 teaspoon fresh thyme   MEN: 2 teaspoons

1 teaspoon fresh oregano   MEN: 2 teaspoons

Freshly ground black pepper

⅛ teaspoon crushed red pepper flakes

2 teaspoons grated Parmesan cheese

Heat the 2 teaspoons of olive oil in a large nonstick skillet over medium heat. Add the cauliflower, broccoli, carrots, and garlic, and sauté, stirring, until the vegetables are crisp-tender, about 5 minutes. Add the parsley, basil, thyme, oregano, black pepper to taste, and red pepper flakes. Add the pasta to the skillet along with a few tablespoons of the pasta water. Bring to a boil and add more water if needed. Stir in the Parmesan and serve.

MEN: *Drizzle 2 teaspoons olive oil over the spaghetti before serving.*

Serves 1

WOMEN: CALORIES 320; FIBER 8g; FAT 11g; PROTEIN 11g; CARB 49g; SODIUM 115mg

MEN: CALORIES 490; FIBER 12g; FAT 21g; PROTEIN 15g; CARB 66g; SODIUM 180mg

Ginger-Teriyaki–Glazed Mahimahi

As the mahimahi browns, the sugar in the marinade caramelizes, creating a wonderful aroma and flavor. Be careful not to burn the sugar, though, as it will turn bitter. Halibut also works well in this recipe.

1 tablespoon bottled teriyaki sauce

2 teaspoons sesame oil

2 teaspoons minced fresh ginger

2 teaspoons minced fresh garlic

1 teaspoon sugar substitute

⅛ teaspoon cayenne pepper

One 6-ounce mahimahi fillet (will yield 5 ounces cooked)

Nonstick cooking spray

In a small bowl, whisk together the teriyaki sauce, oil, ginger, garlic, sugar substitute, and cayenne. Set aside.

Place the mahimahi in the marinade and turn the fish to coat. Let marinate for 5 to 10 minutes.

Heat a large nonstick skillet over medium-high heat. Spray with nonstick cooking spray. Add the mahimahi and cook on one side for 2 minutes, or until golden-brown. Turn the fillet a quarter turn and cook another 2 minutes, or until that side is golden-brown. Turn and repeat the process on the remaining sides. Drizzle with a little marinade with every turn. Remove from the pan and serve.

Serves 1

CALORIES 260; FIBER 0g; FAT 12g; PROTEIN 32g; CARB 3g; SODIUM 470mg

Stir-fried Zucchini and Snow Peas

A simple stir-fry is a great accompaniment to an Asian-flavored fish or chicken dish.

Nonstick cooking spray

½ cup zucchini halved and cut crosswise into ¼-inch slices   MEN: 1 cup

½ cup snow peas   MEN: 1 cup

2 tablespoons chopped leek

1 tablespoon water   MEN: 2 tablespoons

Freshly ground black pepper

    MEN: ¼ cup chopped carrot

Heat a wok or large skillet over high heat and spray with nonstick cooking spray. Add the zucchini, snow peas, and leek and stir constantly for 2 minutes, turning the heat down to medium if the pan starts to smoke. Drizzle in the water. Continue stirring for another minute, or until the vegetables are softened. Sprinkle with black pepper to taste.

Serves 1

WOMEN: CALORIES 40; FIBER 2g; FAT 1.5g; PROTEIN 2g; CARB 6g; SODIUM 10mg

MEN: CALORIES 80; FIBER 4g; FAT 2g; PROTEIN 4g; CARB 14g; SODIUM 40mg

Pineapple Fritters

These fritters have an interesting mix of texture and flavor. The batter will stick better in some places than others, which gives them a real homemade look and feel.

⅓ cup non-fat dry milk powder

3½ tablespoons whole-wheat flour

1 teaspoon sugar substitute

¼ cup water

2 teaspoons canola oil

1⅛ cups canned pineapple rings (about 5 slices), packed in natural juices

2 teaspoons powdered sugar

In a small bowl, mix together the dry milk, flour, and sugar substitute. Add the water and blend until smooth.

Heat the oil in a large nonstick skillet over medium-high heat. Dip the pineapple rings in the batter and place them in the skillet. Fry until golden-brown on one side, about 2 minutes. Carefully turn the fritters over and cook another 2 minutes. Remove the fritters from the skillet and drain on paper towels. Arrange on a large plate and dust with the powdered sugar.

Serves 1

CALORIES 380; FIBER 6g; FAT 10g; PROTEIN 13g; CARB 64g; SODIUM 125mg

Friday

Egg-and-Chive Breakfast Sandwich

Fast-food breakfast sandwiches beware—there's a new kid on the block without the fat and sodium to worry about.

 1 organic, cage-free whole large egg plus 1 egg white
 2 teaspoons chopped fresh chives
 ⅛ teaspoon freshly ground black pepper
 Nonstick cooking spray
 2 slices light 2:90 bread, toasted

Whip the egg and egg white with a whisk until frothy and add the chopped chives and black pepper to taste.

Heat an 8-inch nonstick skillet over medium-high heat. Spray with nonstick cooking spray. Add the egg mixture to the skillet and scramble until begins to set. Slide out of the pan onto one slice of toast. Top with the second slice and cut in half diagonally.

Serves 1

CALORIES 190; FIBER 7g; FAT 8g; PROTEIN 15g; CARB 19g; SODIUM 380mg

Soft Veggie Taco

To make the rice *taquería* style, add a pinch of cumin, cayenne, and turmeric to the water before cooking.

⅓ cup cooked 2:90 rice

½ cup shredded romaine lettuce   MEN: 1 cup

¼ cup chopped yellow onion   MEN: ½ cup

½ cup chopped tomato   MEN: 1 cup

¼ cup chopped red and yellow bell peppers   MEN: ½ cup

8 large pitted black olives, sliced

2 tablespoons chopped fresh cilantro   MEN: 3 tablespoons

1 teaspoon olive oil

Hot sauce

One 2:90 whole-wheat tortilla   MEN: Two tortillas

In a small bowl, combine the cooked rice, lettuce, onion, tomato, bell peppers, olives, cilantro, olive oil, and hot sauce to taste.

Microwave the tortilla for 10 to 15 seconds to soften it. Place the tortilla(s) on a plate, fill, and wrap.

Serves 1

WOMEN: CALORIES 330; FIBER 11g; FAT 14g; PROTEIN 7g; CARB 47g; SODIUM 490mg

MEN: CALORIES 460; FIBER 20g; FAT 16g; PROTEIN 12g; CARB 71g; SODIUM 680mg

Apricot-Citrus–Glazed Cornish Hen

Cornish game hens are miniature chickens—just the right size for half a bird per serving. Treat the raw birds with the same care as you would with chicken.

2 tablespoons sugar-free apricot jam

1 tablespoon fresh lemon juice

½ teaspoon garlic powder

⅛ teaspoon freshly ground black pepper

2 teaspoons olive oil

One 6-ounce portion skinless Cornish hen (will yield 5 ounces cooked)

2 teaspoons chopped fresh basil

Preheat the oven to 400°F. In a small bowl, combine the jam, lemon juice, garlic powder, and black pepper.

Heat the olive oil in a medium nonstick skillet over medium-high heat. Place the hen in the skillet, top side down. Cook for 2 to 3 minutes, or until the hen is golden-brown. Brush the underside of the hen with a little bit of the glaze. Turn the hen over, brush on the remaining glaze, and place in the oven. Cook for 5 to 6 minutes, or until the meat is no longer pink inside and the juices run clear. Sprinkle with the basil.

Serves 1

CALORIES 300; FIBER 1g; FAT 14g; PROTEIN 24g; CARB 18g; SODIUM 90mg

Sweet and Spicy Carrot Salad

This crisp and cool salad tastes great with a roasted meat dish.

2 teaspoons fresh lime juice   MEN: 4 teaspoons

1 teaspoon sugar substitute   MEN: 2 teaspoons

⅛ teaspoon crushed red pepper

½ cup finely shredded carrot   MEN: 1 cup

¼ cup thinly sliced red onion   MEN: ½ cup

1 cup baby lettuce mix   MEN: 2 cups

In a small bowl, combine the lime juice, sugar substitute, and crushed red pepper. In a medium bowl, toss the carrot, onion, and lettuce together with the dressing.

Serves 1

WOMEN: CALORIES 50; FIBER 4g; FAT 0g; PROTEIN 2g; CARB 12g; SODIUM 60mg

MEN: CALORIES 100; FIBER 7g; FAT 0g; PROTEIN 3g; CARB 24g; SODIUM 120mg

Oatmeal-Raisin Cookies

Dip these cookies in a glass of ice-cold milk and reminisce about our fond childhood memories. This recipe makes 2 servings, so save half to eat later this week.

Two containers 2:90 vanilla yogurt with fiber (providing up to 90 calories)
½ cup 2:90 granola
6 tablespoons raisins
2 tablespoons light margarine, melted
4 teaspooons sugar substitute
2 teaspoons honey
2 teaspoons vanilla extract
1 teaspoon ground cinnamon
1 teaspoon baking powder
8 walnut halves, chopped
Nonstick cooking spray

Preheat the oven to 375°F. Spray a nonstick cookie sheet with nonstick cooking spray.

In a medium bowl, stir together all of the ingredients until well combined. Measure the dough by tablespoonfuls onto the prepared cookie sheet. Bake the cookies for 10 minutes, or until lightly browned. Remove to a wire rack to cool slightly before eating.

Serves 2

CALORIES 400; FIBER 5g; FAT 13g; PROTEIN 11g; CARB 64g; SODIUM 200mg

Saturday

Saffron Paella

Paella is the national dish of Spain. Chefs near the ocean add several kinds of seafood to the pan, while inland chefs rely on chicken and chorizo sausage. Despite regional variations, most paella includes saffron as the signature flavor. Because it is expensive, you may want to buy the smallest amount available. Saffron threads are more expensive than saffron powder.

Nonstick cooking spray

1 teaspoon olive oil   MEN: 3 teaspoons

2 tablespoons chopped leeks   MEN: ¼ cup

¼ cup chopped yellow onion   MEN: ½ cup

¼ cup chopped red and green bell peppers   MEN: ½ cup

¼ cup chopped carrots   MEN: ½ cup

4 teaspoons minced fresh garlic   MEN: 2 tablespoons

10 pitted green olives, sliced (high sodium)

1 teaspoon ground turmeric

⅛ teaspoon saffron

¼ cup uncooked Lundberg Wild Blend gourmet blend
of wild rice and brown rice

½ cup low-sodium natural vegetable broth
MEN: ½ cup corn

¼ cup water

Heat a medium nonstick skillet over medium-high heat. Spray with nonstick cooking spray and add 1 teaspoon of the olive oil. Add the leeks, onions, bell peppers, carrots, and garlic, and sauté for 5 minutes, or until softened. Add the olives, turmeric, and saffron, and cook for another minute.

Add the rice and stir to mix with the vegetables. Add the broth and water, stirring constantly until the liquid boils. Turn the heat down to low and cook uncovered for 15 minutes, or until the water is absorbed.

MEN: *Drizzle 2 teaspoons olive oil over the paella before serving.*

Serves 1

WOMEN: 290; FIBER 5g; FAT 14g; PROTEIN 5g; CARB 36g; SODIUM 880mg

MEN: CALORIES 480; FIBER 10g; FAT 24g; PROTEIN 9g; CARB 60g; SODIUM 950mg

Sicilian Swordfish

Many people prefer their fish medium to medium-rare. Salmon, halibut, and tuna work well this way. Swordfish, on the other hand, should be cooked through to medium-well.

Nonstick cooking spray
1 teaspoon olive oil
One 6-ounce swordfish fillet (will yield 5 ounces cooked)
1 cup ripe plum tomatoes sliced in half   MEN: 1½ cups
¼ cup chopped yellow onion   MEN: ½ cup
2 teaspoons minced fresh garlic   MEN: 1 tablespoon
5 pitted Kalamata olives, sliced
1 cup spinach leaves   MEN: 2 cups
1 teaspoon chopped fresh oregano

Heat a large nonstick skillet over medium-high heat. Spray with nonstick cooking spray and add the olive oil. Add the swordfish and cook on one side for 4 minutes, or until golden-brown. Turn the fillet over and add the tomatoes, onions, garlic, and olives to the skillet, forming a wreath around the fish. Cook for another 5 minutes, or until the vegetables are softened and aromatic.

Remove the swordfish from the skillet and add the spinach. Cook, stirring, until the spinach wilts, about 30 seconds. Spoon the vegetable mixture over the swordfish and garnish with the oregano.

Serves 1

WOMEN: CALORIES 340; FIBER 3g; FAT 16g; PROTEIN 33g; CARB 15g; SODIUM 480mg

MEN: CALORIES 380; FIBER 6g; FAT 17g; PROTEIN 35g; CARB 25g; SODIUM 510mg

Mayan Hot Cocoa

The ancient Mayans used cocoa beans for currency. The chocolate drink they called *chocolatl* was highly seasoned with native spices. The allspice and cayenne give this drink a kick.

1 cup skim milk

1 tablespoon unsweetened cocoa powder

1 tablespoon sugar substitute

½ teaspoon vanilla extract

¼ teaspoon ground cinnamon

Pinch of allspice (optional)

Pinch of cayenne pepper (optional)

Heat the milk in a small saucepan over medium-high heat until just at the boiling point. Remove from the heat and whisk in the cocoa powder, sugar substitute, vanilla, cinnamon, allspice, if using, and cayenne, if using.

Serves 1

CALORIES 100; FIBER 2g; FAT 1g; PROTEIN 9g; CARB 15g; SODIUM 130mg

Sunday

Breakfast Burrito

Here's another breakfast favorite from the Southwest. For those who crave spice, add a little chopped fresh jalapeño to get your morning started.

Nonstick cooking spray

¼ cup chopped tomatoes

1 tablespoon chopped fresh cilantro leaves

1 organic, cage-free whole large egg plus 1 egg white

One 2:90 tortilla

1 tablespoon chopped fresh jalapeño (optional)
Freshly ground black pepper
Hot sauce

Heat an 8-inch nonstick skillet over medium heat. Spray with nonstick cooking spray. Add the tomatoes and cilantro to the skillet and cook until the tomatoes soften and the cilantro becomes aromatic, about 30 seconds. Add the whole egg and egg white to the skillet and scramble until mixture begins to set.

Microwave the tortilla for 15 to 20 seconds to soften. Spoon the scrambled egg into the center of the tortilla. Add the chopped jalapeño, if using, and season with black pepper and hot sauce to taste. Roll up and serve.

Serves 1

CALORIES 190; FIBER 7g; FAT 9g; PROTEIN 13g; CARB 15g; SODIUM 350mg

Spicy Jambalaya

Jambalaya is the classic Cajun rice dish, not to be mistaken for gumbo, which has many similar ingredients but is a stew.

2 teaspoons canola oil
½ cup finely chopped celery   MEN: 1 cup
¼ cup finely chopped yellow onion   MEN: ½ cup
¼ cup finely chopped bell pepper   MEN: ½ cup
1 teaspoon finely chopped fresh garlic   MEN: 2 teaspoons
¼ cup prepared tomato sauce
⅔ cup uncooked 2:90 rice   MEN: ⅓ cup
¼ to ½ cup water   MEN: ½ to ¾ cup
⅛ teaspoon cayenne pepper
¼ cup finely chopped fresh flat-leaf parsley
    MEN: 2 teaspoons extra-virgin olive oil
Hot sauce

Heat the canola oil in a 2-quart stockpot over medium heat. Add the celery, onions, bell peppers, and garlic and sauté until the vegetables have softened, about 5 minutes. Add the tomato sauce and cook for another 2 minutes. Stir in the uncooked rice and ¼ cup of the water. Cook, covered, over very low heat until the rice is tender, about 20 minutes. Add more water if the jambalaya appears to be too dry. Stir in the parsley and hot sauce to taste.

MEN: *Drizzle 2 teaspoons of olive oil over jambalaya before serving.*

Serves 1

WOMEN: CALORIES 320; FIBER 8g; FAT 10g; PROTEIN 7g; CARB 54g; SODIUM 360mg

MEN: CALORIES 520; FIBER 13g; FAT 19g; PROTEIN 10g; CARB 83g; SODIUM 390mg

Lobster Salad with Lemon-Tarragon Aïoli

In case you're wondering, aïoli is a fancy word for seasoned mayonnaise. Throw that one around at the water cooler.

1 cup baby greens   MEN: 2 cups
5 ounces cooked lobster meat, chopped
½ cup thinly sliced celery   MEN: 1 cup
½ cup chopped tomato   MEN: 1 cup
¼ cup steamed snow peas   MEN: ½ cup
¼ cup diced avocado
1 tablespoon non-fat mayonnaise
1 tablespoon fresh lemon juice   MEN: 2 tablespoons
1 tablespoon chopped fresh tarragon
Freshly ground black pepper

Place the baby greens in the center of a large dinner plate. In a small bowl, mix together the remaining ingredients. Place the lobster salad in the center of the greens.

Serves 1

WOMEN: CALORIES 310; FIBER 8g; FAT 13g; PROTEIN 32g; CARB 19g; SODIUM 640mg

MEN: CALORIES 350; FIBER 11g; FAT 13g; PROTEIN 34g; CARB 29g; SODIUM 710mg

Week 4

Day 1 Monday Menu

Breakfast **Warm Ham-and-Cheese Toast**
1 cup skim milk or one container 2:90 strawberry yogurt
with fiber (providing up to 90 calories)
1¾ cups strawberries
MEN: Add 1 whole egg plus 1 egg white
Morning Dividend*

Lunch **Wild Rice Salad**
MEN: Add 8 toasted pecan halves

Dinner **Garlic Shrimp Scampi**
MEN: Add ½ cup jicama sticks

Reality Reward **Chocolate Hazelnut Granita with Raspberries**
1 dessert starch of your choice (see Equivalents Lists,
page 381)

---

*Morning Dividend—Choose one sweetener OR one creamer from the following:
1 teaspoon honey, 1 teaspoon white granulated sugar or 1 teaspoon brown
sugar OR 2 tablespoons 2% milk, 1 tablespoon half-and-half, 1 tablespoon
soymilk creamer, 1 tablespoon nondairy liquid creamer, 2 teaspoons nondairy
powdered creamer

Recipe items are in boldface.

Day 2   Tuesday Menu

Breakfast   1 serving 2:90 calcium-fortified dry or hot cereal (providing
up to 90 calories)
1 cup skim milk or one container 2:90 apple yogurt with
fiber (providing up to 90 calories)
6 fresh apricots
3 slices Canadian bacon
MEN: Add 1 mozzarella string cheese (with no more than
4 grams of total fat per string)
Morning Dividend

Lunch   **Vegetable Muffaletta Wraps**

Dinner   **Cajun Red Beans and Sausage**

Reality Reward   **Honey Spice Cake**
1 cup ice cold skim milk

Day 3   Wednesday Menu

Breakfast
Sunny-side-up Egg Salad
1 cup skim milk or one container 2:90 apple yogurt with
fiber (providing up to 90 calories)
3 small pitted and sliced plums
MEN: Add 1 whole hard-boiled egg plus 1 hard-boiled
egg white
Morning Dividend

Lunch
Vegetarian Taco Salad

Dinner
Halibut with Dijon-Caper Sauce
Green Beans with Lemon Zest
MEN: Add ½ cup jicama sticks

Reality Reward
Honey Spice Cake
1 cup ice-cold skim milk

Day 4   Thursday Menu

Breakfast
1 serving 2:90 calcium-fortified dry or hot cereal (providing up to 90 calories)
1 cup skim milk or one container 2:90 peach yogurt with fiber (providing up to 90 calories)
4 pitted dates
1½ ounces any cheese (with more than 1 but no more than 3 grams of fat per ounce)
MEN: Add 1½ ounces any cheese (with more than 1 but no more than 3 grams of fat per ounce)
Morning Dividend

Lunch
Chow Mein Stir-fry
MEN: Add 20 peanuts

Dinner
Duck à l'Orange with Roasted Cauliflower

Reality Reward
Strawberry Milkshake
12 cashews
1 dessert starch of your choice (see Equivalents Lists, page 381)

Day 5   Friday Menu

Breakfast   **Fresh Cantaloupe and Prosciutto**

1 slice regular 2:90 bread, toasted, with 2 tablespoons light margarine

1 cup skim milk or one container 2:90 peach yogurt with fiber (providing up to 90 calories)

MEN: Add 1 mozzarella string cheese (with no more than 4 grams of total fat per string)

Morning Dividend

Lunch   **Moroccan Couscous Tagine**

Dinner   **Flounder alla Fiorentina**

Reality Reward   **Chilled Apricot-Apple Crisp**

2 tablespoons hazelnuts

Day 6   Saturday Menu

Breakfast	1 serving 2:90 calcium-fortified dry or hot cereal (providing up to 90 calories) 1 cup skim milk or one container 2:90 strawberry yogurt with fiber (providing up to 90 calories) 1½ cups honeydew melon slices 1 mozzarella string cheese (with no more than 4 grams of total fat per string) MEN: Add 4 slices Canadian bacon (high sodium) *Morning Dividend*
Lunch	**Open-faced Wild Mushroom Lasagna**
Dinner	**Crab-and-Asparagus Casserole** MEN: Add ½ cup celery sticks, ½ cup carrot sticks, ½ cup sliced fennel
Reality Reward	**Chilled Apricot-Apple Crisp**

Day 7   Sunday Menu

Breakfast

1 serving 2:90 calcium-fortified dry or hot cereal (providing up to 90 calories)

1 cup skim milk or one container 2:90 peach yogurt with fiber (providing up to 90 calories)

1 medium Asian pear

1½ ounces any cheese (with more than 1 but no more than 3 grams of fat per ounce)

MEN: Add 1½ ounces any cheese (with more than 1 but no more than 3 grams of fat per ounce)

Morning Dividend

Lunch

Oven-Roasted Stuffed Red Bell Pepper

Dinner

Chicken Piccata

¾ cup sliced English cucumber

Reality Reward

Gingerbread Muffins

1 cup ice-cold skim milk

Monday

Wild Rice Salad

The rice takes forty-five minutes to cook, but it will hold for a few days in the refrigerator. Make it tonight for tomorrow's lunch.

2 teaspoons fresh lemon juice   MEN: 1 tablespoon

2 teaspoons extra-virgin olive oil

1 teaspoon minced fresh garlic

Freshly ground black pepper

⅔ cup cooked Lundberg Wild Blend gourmet blend
    of wild rice and brown rice

¼ cup thinly sliced scallions

1 cup baby spinach leaves   MEN: 2 cups

¼ cup thinly sliced carrots   MEN: ½ cup

¼ cup chopped tomato   MEN: ½ cup

¼ cup broccoli florets   MEN: ½ cup

1 tablespoon chopped fresh flat-leaf parsley

1 tablespoon chopped fresh chives

In a small bowl, whisk together the lemon juice, olive oil, garlic, and black pepper. In a second bowl, toss together the remaining ingredients, including the cooked rice. Dress the rice salad with the lemon juice mixture.

MEN: *Add ⅓ cup cooked soft wheat berries to the mixture in the first bowl.*

Serves 1

WOMEN: CALORIES 300, FIBER 6g, FAT 10g, PROTEIN 7g; CARB 50g; SODIUM 55mg

MEN: CALORIES 430; FIBER 12g; FAT 11g; PROTEIN 12g; CARB 78g; SODIUM 115mg

Garlic Shrimp Scampi

Shrimp scampi is a traditional Italian dish made with a garlic butter sauce. It's quick, easy, and you won't believe how delicious it is. Add more or less garlic depending on your taste.

Nonstick cooking spray

2 tablespoons light margarine

2 tablespoons chopped yellow onion   MEN: ¼ cup

½ cup thinly sliced scallions

¼ cup sliced mushrooms, cooked   MEN: ¾ cup

½ cup chopped tomato   MEN: 1 cup

6 ounces peeled and deveined shrimp (will yield 5 ounces cooked)

2 to 3 teaspoons minced fresh garlic   MEN: 3 to 4 teaspoons

2 teaspoons fresh lemon juice   MEN: 1 tablespoon

1 tablespoon white vinegar

2 tablespoons chopped fresh flat-leaf parsley

Freshly ground black pepper

Heat a large nonstick skillet over medium-high heat. Spray with nonstick cooking spray. Add the margarine and heat until melted. Add the onions and scallions and sauté until softened. Add the cooked mushrooms and tomato and sauté for another 2 minutes. Add the shrimp and garlic and sauté for 3 to 5 minutes, or until the shrimp turn pink, tossing several times. Add the lemon juice, vinegar, and parsley. Cook for another minute. Season with the black pepper to taste and toss well.

Serves 1

WOMEN: CALORIES 360; FIBER 3g; FAT 15g; PROTEIN 37g; CARB 20g; SODIUM 460mg

MEN: CALORIES 400; FIBER 5g; FAT 15g; PROTEIN 38g; CARB 31g; SODIUM 470mg

Chocolate Hazelnut Granita with Raspberries

This sweet treat is the perfect guilt-free ending to any meal. We like to call it healthful indulgence.

1 cup skim milk

1 tablespoon unsweetened cocoa powder

4 teaspoons sugar substitute

1 teaspoon vanilla extract

2 tablespoons finely chopped hazelnuts

1½ cups fresh raspberries

Pour the milk into a small saucepan and bring just to a boil over medium heat. Whisk in the cocoa and sugar substitute. Remove from the heat and stir in the vanilla and chopped hazelnuts.

Pour the milk mixture into an 8 x 8-inch shallow baking pan. Place in the freezer for 30 minutes. Remove from the freezer and quickly stir with a large spoon, being sure to scrape the bottom and sides. Smooth out the top. Return to the freezer and repeat the procedure twice more, stirring every 15 minutes. Cover with plastic wrap and let freeze until firm, about 1 hour more. Store in the freezer until ready to serve.

Place the raspberries in a small bowl and spoon the granita on top of the berries.

Serves 1

CALORIES 290; FIBER 3g; FAT 10g; PROTEIN 14g; CARB 49g; SODIUM 140mg

Tuesday

Vegetable Muffaletta Wraps

The muffaletta (also spelled "muffuletta") is one of New Orleans's signature sandwiches. It's fun to take one along with a sarsaparilla on a carriage ride.

8 large pitted black olives, chopped

3 chopped peperoncini

1 teaspoon olive oil   MEN: 3 teaspoons

1 teaspoon red wine vinegar

½ teaspoon minced fresh garlic   MEN: 1 teaspoon

½ teaspoon dried oregano   MEN: 1 teaspoon

¼ cup sliced yellow onion   MEN: ½ cup

¾ cup sliced red and green bell peppers   MEN: 1½ cups

Two 2:90 whole-wheat tortillas   MEN: Three tortillas

½ cup butter lettuce leaves   MEN: 1 cup

In a medium bowl, mix together the olives, peperoncini, olive oil, vinegar, garlic, oregano, onion, and bell peppers. Layer the lettuce leaves evenly over the tortillas and spoon the olive mixture evenly on top. Roll up and serve.

Serves 1

WOMEN: CALORIES 320; FIBER 17.5g; FAT 16g; PROTEIN 8g; CARB 38g; SODIUM 680mg

MEN: CALORIES 530; FIBER 28g; FAT 28g; PROTEIN 13g; CARB 62g; SODIUM 860mg

Cajun Red Beans and Sausage

Celery, green bell peppers, and yellow onions are the "holy trinity" in Cajun cooking, which means they form the flavor foundation for most dishes.

    Nonstick cooking spray
    2 teaspoons olive oil
    3 ounces sliced sausage (with 1 gram or less fat per ounce; will yield
        2½ ounces cooked)
    1 cup chopped celery   MEN: 2 cups
    ¼ cup chopped green bell pepper   MEN: ½ cup
    ¼ cup chopped yellow onion
    1 teaspoon minced fresh garlic   MEN: 2 teaspoons
    ½ cup rinsed and drained canned kidney beans
    ½ cup chopped tomato   MEN: 1 cup
    1 teaspoon chili powder
    Hot sauce

Heat a large nonstick skillet over medium-high heat. Spray with nonstick cooking spray. Add the olive oil, sausage, celery, bell pepper, onion, and garlic. Cook for 6 to 8 minutes, stirring often. Add the kidney beans, tomato, and chili powder, and cook another 3 minutes. Season with hot sauce to taste.

Serves 1

WOMEN: CALORIES 320; FIBER 9g; FAT 14g; PROTEIN 23g; CARB 30g; SODIUM 510mg

MEN: CALORIES 360; FIBER 11g; FAT 14g; PROTEIN 25g; CARB 40g; SODIUM 620mg

Honey Spice Cake

Follow the recipe the first time you make this cake, but then experiment with different spices, including ginger, mace, or even a pinch of cayenne pepper. This recipe makes 2 servings, so save half for later in the week.

Nonstick cooking spray
2 tablespoons light margarine
2 teaspoons honey
2 tablespoons sugar substitute
1 teaspoon ground cinnamon
¼ teaspoon ground allspice
7 tablespoons whole-wheat flour
2 teaspoons baking powder
6 tablespoons raisins
8 toasted walnut halves, chopped
2 teaspoons vanilla extract
10 tablespoons cold water

Preheat the oven to 375°F. Spray a round casserole dish (5 inches in diameter) with nonstick cooking spray.

In a medium bowl, cream together the margarine, honey, sugar substitute, cinnamon, and allspice until well blended. Stir in the flour, baking powder, raisins, and walnuts. Gently fold in the vanilla and water until a batter forms. Pour the batter into the prepared casserole dish and bake for 20 minutes, or until a knife inserted in the middle comes out clean. Let cool before serving.

Serves 2

CALORIES 310; FIBER 4g; FAT 12g; PROTEIN 6g; CARB 49g; SODIUM 110mg per single serving

Wednesday

Sunny-side-up Egg Salad

This is a foolproof method for hard boiling eggs. Say good-bye to that annoying green ring around the yolk.

   2 organic cage-free eggs (you will use 1 whole, plus 1 egg white)
   1 tablespoon non-fat mayonnaise
   Freshly ground black pepper
   One 2:90 whole-wheat English muffin, toasted

Place the eggs in a small saucepan with cool water to cover. Turn the heat on to medium and bring the water to a rolling boil. Turn off the heat, cover the saucepan with a tight-fitting lid, and let the eggs sit in the hot water for 13 minutes. Drain the eggs and immediately dip them in cool water until cool enough to handle. Peel the eggs and discard one yolk.

Finely chop the eggs. Place them in a small bowl and stir in the mayonnaise. Season with black pepper to taste. Spread the egg salad onto the toasted English muffin halves and serve "sunny-side-up."

   MEN: *Chop the additional egg and egg white from the menu list and add to the bowl before stirring in the mayonnaise. Or sprinkle it with pepper and eat as a mid-morning snack.*

Serves 1

CALORIES 190; FIBER 2g; FAT 7g; PROTEIN 16g; CARB 29g; SODIUM 480mg

Vegetarian Taco Salad

You can make this salad hot and spicy to your taste by adjusting the amount of hot sauce.

   ½ cup shredded romaine lettuce   MEN: 1½ cups
   ¼ cup thinly sliced onion   MEN: ½ cup

½ cup chopped tomato   MEN: 1 cup

¼ cup thinly sliced green and red bell peppers   MEN: ½ cup

2 tablespoons chopped avocado   MEN: 6 tablespoons

8 large pitted black olives, sliced

4 tablespoons chopped fresh cilantro

1½ tablespoons prepared salsa

Hot sauce

16 Garden of Eatin' Black Bean tortilla chips   MEN: 24 tortillas

In a large bowl, toss together all of the ingredients except the tortilla chips, and season with hot sauce to taste. Layer the tortilla chips on a plate and spoon the salad on top.

Serves 1

WOMEN: CALORIES 330; FIBER 10g; FAT 19g; PROTEIN 6g; CARB 39g; SODIUM 500mg

MEN: CALORIES 500; FIBER 16g; FAT 29g; PROTEIN 11g; CARB 65g; SODIUM 560mg

Halibut with Dijon-Caper Sauce

Here's one to impress your friends with, and it takes only fifteen minutes from start to finish.

Nonstick cooking spray

One 6-ounce halibut fillet (will yield 5 ounces cooked)

2 tablespoons light margarine

¼ cup chopped scallion   MEN: ½ cup

2 teaspoons minced fresh garlic   MEN: 1 tablespoon

1 teaspoon drained and chopped capers

1 teaspoon whole-grain Dijon mustard

1 tablespoon water

½ cup baby spinach leaves   MEN: 1 cup

Freshly ground black pepper

Heat a large nonstick skillet over medium-high heat. Spray with nonstick cooking spray. Add the halibut, top side down, to the skillet and cook for 4 to 5 minutes. Turn over the halibut and add the margarine, scallions, garlic, capers, mustard, and water. Cook for another 2 to 3 minutes, stirring twice, and remove the halibut from the skillet to a large plate.

Add the baby spinach to the skillet and cook until wilted, about 30 seconds. Stir together and season with black pepper to taste. Spoon the vegetables and sauce over the halibut.

Serves 1

WOMEN: CALORIES 305; FIBER 2g; FAT 15g; PROTEIN 37g; CARB 5g; SODIUM 510mg

MEN: CALORIES 315; FIBER 3g; FAT 15g; PROTEIN 37g; CARB 6g; SODIUM 530mg

Green Beans with Lemon Zest

1 cup green beans, ends trimmed

1 tablespoon lemon zest

1 tablespoon chopped fresh flat-leaf parsley   MEN: 2 tablespoons

¼ teaspoon garlic powder   MEN: ½ teaspoon

Freshly ground black pepper

Blanch the green beans in boiling water until they turn bright green, about 3 minutes. Drain and toss them in a bowl together with the lemon zest, parsley, garlic powder, and black pepper to taste.

Serves 1

CALORIES 35; FIBER 4g; FAT 0g; PROTEIN 1g; CARB 7g; SODIUM 0mg

Thursday

Chow Mein Stir-fry

Chow mein symbolizes American Chinese food. It's guaranteed to please even if you shy away from the exotic.

⅔ cup 2:90 cooked whole-wheat spaghetti   MEN: 1 cup

Nonstick cooking spray

2 teaspoons peanut oil

¼ cup chopped yellow onion   MEN: ½ cup

¼ cup thinly sliced carrot   MEN: ½ cup

¼ cup broccoli florets   MEN: ½ cup

½ cup sliced celery   MEN: 1 cup

½ cup bean sprouts

1 tablespoon minced fresh ginger   MEN: 4 teaspoons

1 teaspoon minced fresh garlic   MEN: 2 teaspoons

2 teaspoons naturally brewed low-sodium soy sauce

1 tablespoon rice vinegar

Heat a large nonstick skillet or wok over high heat. Spray with nonstick cooking spray. Add the oil, onions, carrots, broccoli, and celery, stirring often, for 3 to 4 minutes, until the vegetables soften. Add the bean sprouts, ginger, garlic, soy sauce, and vinegar. Cook for another minute. Spoon the vegetable mixture on top of the noodles.

Serves 1

WOMEN: CALORIES 340; FIBER 8g; FAT 12g; PROTEIN 12g; CARB 53g; SODIUM 490mg

MEN: CALORIES 470; FIBER 12g; FAT 12g; PROTEIN 17g; CARB 82g; SODIUM 570mg

Duck à l'Orange with Roasted Cauliflower

Unlike chicken, duck can be cooked to your preferred doneness. A rosy pink color is best, while well done tends to be a bit chewy.

2 teaspoons canola oil

1 teaspoon minced fresh garlic   MEN: 2 teaspoons

1 teaspoon minced fresh ginger   MEN: 2 teaspoons

1 tablespoon sugar-free orange marmalade

2 tablespoons orange zest

1 teaspoon sugar substitute

Nonstick cooking spray

One 6-ounce skinless domestic duck breast (will yield 5 ounces cooked)

¾ cup cauliflower florets   MEN: 1½ cups

¼ cup thinly sliced yellow onion   MEN: ½ cup

2 tablespoons thinly sliced leek   MEN: ¼ cup

Preheat the oven to 375°F. Heat the oil in a small saucepan over medium heat, add the garlic and ginger, stir, and cook for 2 minutes. Add the marmalade, orange zest, and sugar substitute. Stir and simmer for another 2 minutes. Turn the heat to low.

Heat a large ovenproof nonstick skillet over medium-high heat. Spray with nonstick cooking spray. Add the duck, top side down, to the skillet and cook for 4 to 5 minutes. Turn over the duck and place the cauliflower, onion, and leek around the duck. Spoon the orange sauce over the duck and roast in the oven for 8 to 10 minutes, or until reaches preferred doneness.

Remove the skillet from the oven and pour the remaining sauce over the duck.

Serves 1

WOMEN: CALORIES 340; FIBER 3g; FAT 16g; PROTEIN 30g; CARB 18g; SODIUM 110mg
MEN: CALORIES 380; FIBER 6g; FAT 16g; PROTEIN 32g; CARB 28g; SODIUM 135mg

Strawberry Milkshake

For a fancy garnish, place a strawberry on its side and make several slices about ⅛ inch apart from side to side. Press gently to fan the strawberry.

1¾ cups whole strawberries (reserve 1 for garnish)
One container 2:90 vanilla yogurt with fiber (providing up to 90 calories)
1 teaspoon sugar substitute
⅛ teaspoon ground nutmeg
3 or 4 ice cubes

Combine all of the ingredients in the jar of a blender. Cover and blend until smooth and frothy, about 30 seconds. Add a little water to thin the consistency if necessary.

Pour into a tall glass and garnish with the reserved strawberry.

Serves 1

CALORIES 180; FIBER 8g; FAT 1g; PROTEIN 8g; CARB 38g; SODIUM 95mg

Friday

Fresh Cantaloupe and Prosciutto

Melon and prosciutto is a classic sweet and salty combination.

1½ cups cantaloupe cut into spears
3 ounces prosciutto (with 1 but no more than 3 grams of fat per ounce),
    sliced into long strips
Freshly ground black pepper (optional)
1 teaspoon chopped fresh chives (optional)

Wrap the strips of prosciutto around the melon spears. Season with black pepper and chives to taste, if using.

Serves 1

CALORIES 200; FIBER 2.5g; FAT 5g; PROTEIN 23g; CARB 20g; SODIUM 510mg

Moroccan Couscous Tagine

A tagine is a Moroccan slow-cooked dish of meat and vegetables. This is a quick and easy vegetarian version that can be made ahead and refrigerated overnight. Reheat in the microwave or serve cold.

Nonstick cooking spray
¼ cup thinly sliced yellow onion   MEN: ½ cup
2 tablespoons thinly sliced leek   MEN: ¼ cup
¼ cup thinly sliced carrot   MEN: ½ cup
½ cup chopped tomato   MEN: 1 cup
⅓ cup cooked 2:90 whole-wheat couscous   MEN: ⅔ cup
½ teaspoon ground cumin
½ teaspoon ground coriander
½ teaspoon ground ginger   MEN: ¾ teaspoon

Freshly ground black pepper

12 almonds, slivered   MEN: 24 almonds

One 2:90 whole-wheat pita, halved and toasted

   MEN: 1 cup chopped romaine lettuce

Heat a large saucepan over medium-high heat. Spray with nonstick cooking spray. Add the onions, leeks, and carrots and sauté until crisp tender. Stir in the tomatoes and the cooked couscous, and cook for another 2 minutes. Stir in the cumin, coriander, ginger, and black pepper to taste, and mix well. Stir in the slivered almonds and spoon into the toasted pita bread.

MEN: Place the extra chopped vegetables on a plate and spoon the tagine ingredients over the top. Use the pita bread as "scoops" to eat with.

Serves 1

WOMEN: CALORIES 310; FIBER 9g; FAT 9g; PROTEIN 11g; CARB 52g; SODIUM 100mg

MEN: CALORIES 550; FIBER 17g; FAT 17g; PROTEIN 20g; CARB 90g; SODIUM 140mg

Flounder alla Fiorentina

Fiorentina refers to the spinach, which is in the style of Florence, Italy. Squeeze the fresh lemon juice directly into the skillet, and don't worry if a seed or two sneaks in.

Nonstick cooking spray

One 6-ounce flounder fillet (will yield 5 ounces cooked)

2 teaspoons olive oil

½ cup sliced red bell pepper   MEN: 1 cup

½ cup sliced zucchini   MEN: 1 cup

½ cup broccoli florets   MEN: 1 cup

½ cup baby spinach leaves   MEN: 1 cup

2 teaspoons fresh lemon juice   MEN: 1 tablespoon

1 teaspoon red wine vinegar   MEN: 2 teaspoons

Freshly ground black pepper

Dash of hot pepper sauce, or to taste

Preheat the oven to 375°F. Heat a large ovenproof nonstick skillet over medium-high heat. Spray with nonstick cooking spray. Add the flounder to the skillet and cook for 2 minutes. Turn over the flounder and add the olive oil, bell peppers, zucchini, and broccoli. Stir to coat the vegetables with the oil.

Roast the flounder and vegetables in the oven for 5 minutes. Remove the skillet from the oven and carefully lift out the flounder to a dinner plate. Add the baby spinach to the skillet and cook until wilted, about 30 seconds. Add the lemon juice, vinegar, black pepper to taste, and hot sauce. Arrange the vegetables next to the flounder on the plate.

Serves 1

WOMEN: CALORIES 290; FIBER 3g; FAT 13g; PROTEIN 35g; CARB 9g; SODIUM 170mg

MEN: CALORIES 330; FIBER 6g; FAT 14g; PROTEIN 38g; CARB 18g; SODIUM 190mg

Chilled Apricot-Apple Crisp

This recipe makes two servings, so save half for later this week.

Two containers 2:90 vanilla yogurt with fiber (providing up to 90 calories)

4 teaspoons sugar substitute

1 teaspoon vanilla extract

1 large unpeeled apple, cored and thinly sliced

12 dried apricot halves, chopped

½ cup 2:90 granola

4 tablespoons light or non-fat whipped topping

In a medium bowl, combine the yogurt, sugar substitute, and vanilla. Stir in the apples and apricots.

Spoon the mixture into a serving bowl and top with the granola and whipped topping.

Serves 2

CALORIES 290; FIBER 8g; FAT 1.5g; PROTEIN 10g; CARB 62g; SODIUM 105mg per single serving

Saturday

Open-faced Wild Mushroom Lasagna

There's no need to hassle with making a complicated layered lasagna when this open-faced version is just as delicious. You'll savor the time you save, too.

⅔ cup cooked 2:90 lasagna noodles (about 2 ounces cooked)
   MEN: 1 cup (about 3 ounces cooked)

2 teaspoons olive oil   MEN: 4 teaspoons

2 teaspoons minced fresh garlic   MEN: 1 tablespoon

½ cup sliced mushrooms (your choice of portobello, shiitake, or cremini)
   MEN: 1 cup

½ cup chopped tomato   MEN: 1 cup

½ cup spinach leaves   MEN: 1 cup

2 tablespoons chopped fresh flat-leaf parsley   MEN: 3 tablespoons

1 tablespoon chopped fresh basil   MEN: 2 tablespoons

½ tablespoon chopped fresh thyme

¼ teaspoon crushed red pepper flakes

⅛ teaspoon ground nutmeg

2 teaspoons grated Parmesan cheese

1 cup mixed greens

Preheat the oven to 400°F. Cook the lasagna noodles as per package instructions, drain, and reserve. Drizzle 2 teaspoons of olive oil in the bottom of a small round (5-inch-diameter) casserole dish.

Heat a medium nonstick skillet over medium-high heat. Spray with nonstick cooking spray. Add the garlic, mushrooms, and tomato and sauté for 4 minutes, stirring often. Add the spinach, parsley, basil, thyme, red pepper flakes, and nutmeg. Cook until the spinach is wilted, about 30 seconds.

Arrange the noodles on the bottom of the prepared casserole dish and spoon the tomato mixture on top. Sprinkle with the Parmesan and bake for 10 minutes, or until bubbling. Serve with the mixed greens.

MEN: *Drizzle the extra 2 teaspoons olive oil over the lasagna when it comes out of the oven.*

Serves 1

WOMEN: CALORIES 320; FIBER 10g; FAT 12g; PROTEIN 12g; CARB 43g; SODIUM 105mg

MEN: CALORIES 520; FIBER 15g; FAT 23g; PROTEIN 19g; CARB 66g; SODIUM 125mg

Crab-and-Asparagus Casserole

This entree can double as a party appetizer if you're having friends over for dinner. Serve it right out of the casserole dish and let your guests help themselves.

Nonstick cooking spray

½ cup asparagus cut into 1-inch lengths

2 tablespoons light margarine

1 teaspoon minced fresh garlic

¼ cup sliced mushrooms

¼ cup thinly sliced leek

5 ounces picked crabmeat

¼ teaspoon dry mustard

¼ teaspoon ground nutmeg

¼ teaspoon freshly ground black pepper

1 tablespoon chopped fresh flat-leaf parsley

1 teaspoon chopped fresh tarragon

2 teaspoons grated Parmesan cheese

Preheat the oven to 400°F. Spray a round casserole dish (5 inches in diameter) with nonstick cooking spray. Fill a nonstick skillet with water and bring to a boil.

Blanch the asparagus pieces until they turn bright green, about 3 minutes. Drain and set aside. Return the skillet to the stove over medium-high heat and add the margarine. Add the garlic, mushrooms, and leeks and sauté for 5 minutes, stirring often, until the vegetables have softened. Add the crabmeat, mustard, nutmeg, black pepper, parsley, tarragon, and cooked asparagus to the skillet and stir until combined.

Spoon the crab filling into the prepared casserole dish and top with the Parmesan. Bake for 10 minutes or until the cheese is golden-brown.

MEN: *Dip the celery, carrot, and fennel sticks from the menu list in the casserole as if it were a dip.*

Serves 1

CALORIES 320; FIBER 2g; FAT 14g; PROTEIN 42g; CARB 7g; SODIUM 830mg

Sunday

Oven-Roasted Stuffed Red Bell Pepper

Not like Mom used to make, this stuffed pepper is light and delicious.

1 medium red bell pepper   **MEN:** 2 medium
2 teaspoons olive oil   **MEN:** 4 teaspoons
½ cup well-drained chopped canned tomatoes   **MEN:** 1 cup
1 tablespoon chopped fresh mint   **MEN:** 2 tablespoons
1 tablespoon chopped fresh flat-leaf parsley   **MEN:** 2 tablespoons
⅔ cup cooked Lundberg Wild Blend gourmet blend of wild rice and brown
   rice   **MEN:** 1 cup
Freshly ground black pepper

Preheat the oven to 375°F. Slice off the top third of the bell pepper and reserve the top. Use a spoon to scoop out the pepper's ribs and seeds.

Add the olive oil, tomatoes, mint, and parsley to the cooked rice while it's still hot and season with black pepper to taste. Spoon the rice mixture into the prepared pepper and place the top back on as a cap. Place the stuffed pepper on a baking sheet and bake for about 30 minutes, or until the pepper can be easily pierced with a knife.

Serves 1

WOMEN: CALORIES 320; FIBER 7.5g; FAT 10g; PROTEIN 7; CARB 55g; SODIUM 340mg
MEN: CALORIES 550; FIBER 11.5g; FAT 20g; PROTEIN 12g; CARB 88g; SODIUM 690mg

Chicken Piccata

Piccata is an Italian favorite usually prepared with veal. Chicken is substituted here with the addition of lots of fresh tomatoes.

One 6-ounce boneless, skinless chicken breast (will yield 5 ounces cooked)
Freshly ground black pepper
Nonstick cooking spray
2 tablespoons light margarine
1¼ cups chopped tomatoes   MEN: 1¾ cups
Juice of 1 lemon
1 tablespoon drained capers
1 tablespoon chopped fresh flat-leaf parsley   MEN: 2 tablespoons
     MEN: ¾ cup broccoli
     MEN: ½ cup mushrooms

Slice the chicken breast diagonally into 3 medallions and place between 2 large sheets of plastic wrap. Pound the chicken with a meat mallet or the underside of a heavy skillet to ¼ inch thick. Season with black pepper to taste.

Heat a large nonstick skillet over high heat. Spray with nonstick cooking spray. Add the margarine and let it melt. Add the chicken pieces and sauté for about 2 minutes on each side, or until golden-brown. Arrange the cooked chicken on a dinner plate and keep warm.

Turn the heat down to medium and add the tomatoes, lemon juice, capers, and parsley. Cook for another 2 minutes, stirring often. Spoon the tomato mixture onto the chicken.

MEN: *Add the broccoli and mushrooms to the skillet with the tomatoes. Cover the skillet and cook an additional 3 minutes.*

Serves 1

WOMEN: CALORIES 340; FIBER 3g; FAT 14g; PROTEIN 41g; CARB 11g; SODIUM 590mg
MEN: CALORIES 430; FIBER 9g; FAT 15g; PROTEIN 48g; CARB 33g; SODIUM 630mg

Gingerbread Muffins

A little dried ginger goes a long way. If you like your gingerbread spicy, add a little more ginger to taste. Be cautious, though, only increasing it ¼ teaspoon at a time.

1 tablespoon light margarine, softened

1 teaspoon honey

1 tablespoon sugar substitute

½ teaspoon ground cinnamon

½ teaspoon ground ginger

3½ tablespoons whole-wheat flour

1 teaspoon baking powder

3 tablespoons raisins

4 toasted walnut halves, chopped

1 teaspoon vanilla extract

5 tablespoons cold water

2 tablespoons light or non-fat whipped topping

Preheat the oven to 375°F. Spray 2 muffin cups with nonstick cooking spray and fill any remaining cups in the tin half full with cool water (this will prevent the muffin pan from warping).

In a medium bowl, cream together the margarine, honey, sugar substitute, cinnamon, and ginger until well blended. Stir in the flour, baking powder, raisins, and walnuts. Gently fold in the vanilla and water until a batter forms. Pour the batter into the prepared muffin cups and bake for 15 to 20 minutes, or until knife inserted in middle of a muffin comes out clean. Let cool slightly before removing from the pan and top with whipped topping before serving.

Serves 1

CALORIES 310; FIBER 4g; FAT 11g; PROTEIN 6g; CARB 50g; SODIUM 110mg

Week 5

Day 1   Monday Menu

Breakfast   **Spiced Cottage Cheese and Pears**

1 slice regular 2:90 bread, toasted, with 1 tablespoon almond butter

MEN: Add 1 slice regular 2:90 bread

Morning Dividend*

Lunch   **Green Olive and White Albacore Tuna Sandwich**

1 cup skim milk or one container any 2:90 yogurt with fiber (providing up to 90 calories)

Dinner   **Flatbread Caesar**

MEN: Add 1 mozzarella string cheese (with no more than 4 grams of total fat per string)

Reality Reward   **Vanilla Bread Pudding with Raisins and Dates**

1 dessert starch of your choice (see Equivalents Lists, page 381)

½ cup ice-cold skim milk

---

*Morning Dividend—Choose one sweetener OR one creamer from the following: 1 teaspoon honey, 1 teaspoon white granulated sugar, or 1 teaspoon brown sugar OR 2 tablespoons 2% milk, 1 tablespoon half-and-half, 1 tablespoon soymilk creamer, 1 tablespoon nondairy liquid creamer, 2 teaspoons nondairy powdered creamer

Recipe items are in boldface.

Day 2   Tuesday Menu

Breakfast   **Scrambled Egg and Fresh Basil Sandwich**

3 small tangerines

MEN: Add ⅓ cup fruit muesli

Morning Dividend

Lunch   **Hoppin' John Pita Salad**

1 cup skim milk or one container any 2:90 yogurt with fiber
(providing up to 90 calories)

½ cup celery sticks

MEN: Add 1 cup carrot sticks and ½ cup celery sticks

Dinner   **Quick and Easy Vegetable Soup**

MEN: Add 1 small cooked skinless chicken leg
(about 1½ ounces)

Reality Reward   **Apple and Cheese Pita**

Day 3   Wednesday Menu

Breakfast
Waffle Sandwich with Ham and Syrup
¾ of a large fresh grapefruit
MEN: Add ¼ cup 2:90 granola
Morning Dividend

Lunch
Ham and Avocado Club Wrap
1 cup skim milk or one container any 2:90 yogurt with fiber
(providing up to 90 calories)

Dinner
Chinese Five-Spice Stir-fried Rice
MEN: Add 3 ounces chopped firm tofu and 20 peanuts

Reality Reward
Blueberry Vanilla Custard
1 dessert starch of your choice (see Equivalents Lists,
page 381)
¾ cup ice-cold skim milk

Day 4   Thursday Menu

Breakfast   **Herbed Cottage Cheese on an English Muffin**
4 pitted dates
8 walnut halves
MEN: Add ⅓ cup fruit muesli
Morning Dividend

Lunch   **Italian Sausage Sandwich**
1 cup skim milk or one container any 2:90 yogurt with fiber
(providing up to 90 calories)
MEN: Add ½ cup sliced carrots and 1 small sliced tomato

Dinner   **Middle Eastern Tabouli Salad**
MEN: Add 1 small cooked skinless chicken leg
(about 1½ ounces)

Reality Reward **Blueberry Vanilla Custard**
¾ cup ice-cold skim milk
1 dessert starch of your choice (see Equivalents Lists,
page 381)

Day 5   Friday Menu

Breakfast   **Cheese Toast with Oregano**
1½ cups honeydew melon slices
MEN: Add 1 cup 2:90 hot cereal
Morning Dividend

Lunch   **Chinese Chicken Pita**
1 cup skim milk or one container any 2:90 yogurt with fiber
(providing up to 90 calories)
MEN: Add ½ cup sliced cucumber and ½ cup sliced carrots

Dinner   **Angel-Hair Pasta with Fresh Herbs**
MEN: Add 1 mozzarella string cheese (with no more than
4 grams of total fat per string) and 8 pecan halves

Reality Reward **Chocolate-Banana Bread Pudding** (see pages 288–289)
½ cup ice-cold skim milk

Day 6   Saturday Menu

Breakfast	**Waffle Topped with Strawberries and Ricotta**
	12 cashews
	MEN: Add ¼ cup 2:90 granola
	Morning Dividend
Lunch	**Shrimp Curry with Rice**
	Chai Iced Tea
Dinner	**Oven-Roasted Potatoes and Vegetables**
	MEN: Add 1 small cooked skinless chicken leg
	(about 1½ ounces)
Reality Reward	**Italian Almond Cake with Figs**
	1 cup ice-cold skim milk

Day 7   Sunday Menu

Breakfast	**Warm Ham-and-Swiss Open-faced Sandwich** 1 large nectarine MEN: Add ¼ cup 2:90 granola *Morning Dividend*
Lunch	**Red Snapper Soft Taco** 1 cup skim milk or one container any 2:90 yogurt with fiber (providing up to 90 calories) MEN: Add ¼ cup carrot sticks
Dinner	**Eggplant Parmesan** MEN: Add 1 mozzarella string cheese (with no more than 4 grams of total fat per string) MEN: Add 12 almonds
Reality Reward	**Italian Almond Cake with Figs** 1 cup ice-cold skim milk

Monday

Spiced Cottage Cheese and Pears

You can either dice the pear and mix it into the cottage cheese or cut the pear into slices and serve it alongside the cottage cheese.

   ½ cup low-fat cottage cheese (containing up to 1% milkfat)

   1 large pear, diced

   ⅛ teaspoon ground nutmeg

   ⅛ teaspoon paprika

   ⅛ teaspoon ground cinnamon

In a small bowl, stir together the cottage cheese, pear, nutmeg, paprika, and cinnamon.

Serves 1

CALORIES 200; FIBER 6g; FAT 1.5g; PROTEIN 15g; CARB 35g; SODIUM 15mg

Green Olive and White Albacore Tuna Sandwich

Albacore is the cream of the canned tuna crop. Buy the "solid" or "fancy" grades, as they are the highest quality. "Chunks" and "flakes" are the lower-quality grades.

   2 ½ ounces canned white albacore tuna in water

   5 pitted green olives, chopped

   1 tablespoon chopped fresh chives   MEN: 2 tablespoons

   1 tablespoon chopped fresh flat-leaf parsley

   1 tablespoon reduced-fat mayonnaise

   1 teaspoon red wine vinegar

   Freshly ground black pepper

   ½ cup shredded romaine lettuce   MEN: 1 cup

1 cup chopped tomatoes   MEN: 2 cups

2 slices light 2:90 bread, toasted

   MEN: 1 cup sliced radishes

In a small bowl, combine the tuna, olives, chives, parsley, and mayonnaise. Add the vinegar and black pepper to taste. Spoon the tuna salad onto one slice of the bread. Top with the shredded lettuce, tomatoes, and the second slice of bread. Close the sandwich and cut it in half diagonally.

MEN: *Make a side salad with the extra tomatoes and radishes, and season with balsamic vinegar or lemon juice and freshly ground black pepper.*

Serves 1

WOMEN: CALORIES 300; FIBER 10g; FAT 12g; PROTEIN 23g; CARB 30g; SODIUM 800mg

MEN: CALORIES 360; FIBER 12g; FAT 8g; PROTEIN 25g; CARB 43g; SODIUM 860mg

Flatbread Caesar

This is a fork-and-knife sandwich.

One 2:90 flatbread or pita

Nonstick cooking spray

1 teaspoon garlic powder

½ teaspoon dried oregano

1 cup romaine lettuce cut into bite-size pieces   MEN: 2 cups

1 cup halved cherry or grape tomatoes   MEN: 2 cups

½ cup sliced red onion

4 tablespoons reduced-fat Caesar salad dressing

2 teaspoons grated Parmesan cheese

Freshly ground black pepper

   MEN: 2 teaspoons olive oil

   MEN: 1 teaspoon fresh lemon juice

Preheat the oven to 375°F. Spray the flatbread lightly with nonstick cooking spray and sprinkle with the garlic powder and oregano. Toast the flatbread in the oven for 5 to 7 minutes, or until toasted.

In a medium bowl, toss the lettuce, tomatoes, and red onions with the salad dressing and place on top of the toasted flatbread. Sprinkle with the Parmesan and season with black pepper to taste.

MEN: *Make a side salad with the extra lettuce and tomatoes. Toss the salad with the extra 2 teaspoons of olive oil and lemon juice to taste.*

Serves 1

WOMEN: CALORIES 260; FIBER 6g; FAT 10g; PROTEIN 7g; CARB 39g; SODIUM 460mg
MEN: CALORIES 340; FIBER 9g; FAT 20g; PROTEIN 9g; CARB 48g; SODIUM 480mg

Vanilla Bread Pudding with Raisins and Dates

Bread pudding is a bit like baked French toast. Use bread that's a little stale or toasted for the best results. Like its custard cousin, you can adjust the fruit and spices as long as the basic recipe is followed.

Nonstick cooking spray
1 slice regular 2:90 whole-wheat bread, torn into small pieces
2 teaspoons sugar substitute
1 teaspoon vanilla extract
1½ tablespoons golden raisins
2 dates, pitted and chopped
½ cup skim milk
1 organic, cage-free whole large egg plus 1 egg white, beaten
2 teaspoons powdered sugar, for sprinkling

Preheat the oven to 375°F. Spray a round casserole dish (5 inches in diameter) with nonstick cooking spray. In a medium bowl, combine the bread, sugar substitute, vanilla, raisins, and dates. Heat the milk in a small saucepan over medium-high heat until just at the boiling point. Pour the hot milk over the bread mixture and stir in the egg and egg white until well combined.

Pour the bread mixture into the prepared casserole dish and bake for 20 minutes, or until firm to the touch. Sprinkle with the powdered sugar and serve either hot or cold.

Serves 1

CALORIES 330; FIBER 5g; FAT 8g; PROTEIN 16g; CARB 53g; SODIUM 330mg

FOR CHOCOLATE-BANANA BREAD PUDDING

Substitute 1 teaspoon semi-sweet chocolate mini-morsels and 1 banana, cut into ¼-inch slices, for the raisins and dates. Add ⅛ teaspoon ground cinnamon. Remember to eat with ½ cup ice-cold skim milk.

CALORIES 320; FIBER 5g; FAT 9g; PROTEIN 19g; CARB 45g; SODIUM 380mg

Tuesday

Scrambled Egg and Fresh Basil Sandwich

Fresh basil and shallots give this egg sandwich a decidedly upscale taste.

- 5 egg whites
- 1 tablespoon chopped fresh basil leaves
- ⅛ teaspoon freshly ground black pepper
- 2 tablespoons light margarine
- 1 teaspoon minced shallots
- 2 slices light 2:90 bread

In a small bowl, whip the egg whites with a whisk until frothy, and add the basil and black pepper.

Heat an 8-inch nonstick skillet over medium-high heat. Melt 1 tablespoon of the margarine in the skillet. Add the shallots and sauté for 1 minute. Add the egg mixture and scramble until the curds just set. Toast the bread and spread with remaining 1 tablespoon margarine. Slide the eggs out of the pan onto one slice of the toast. Top with the second slice and cut in half diagonally.

Serves 1

CALORIES 260; FIBER 7g; FAT 11g; PROTEIN 24g; CARB 21g; SODIUM 500mg

Hoppin' John Pita Salad

Hoppin' John is a traditional southern New Year's Day black-eyed pea dish. This is a quick and easy chilled salad version for lunch.

½ cup cooked black-eyed peas

½ cup chopped yellow onion

1 teaspoon minced fresh garlic

1 tablespoon chopped fresh basil

1 tablespoon chopped fresh flat-leaf parsley

2 teaspoons olive oil

1 teaspoon cider vinegar

Freshly ground black pepper

Hot sauce

1 2:90 whole-wheat pita

In a medium bowl, combine the black-eyed peas, onions, garlic, basil, and parsley. Stir in the olive oil and vinegar and season with black pepper and hot sauce to taste. Stuff the salad into the toasted pita.

Serves 1

CALORIES 260; FIBER 7g; FAT 9g; PROTEIN 10g; CARB 39g; SODIUM 620mg

Quick and Easy Vegetable Soup

Get a jump-start on dinner by fortifying your favorite prepared soup with added vegetables and seasoning. It'll taste just like a hearty completely homemade meal.

2 teaspoons extra-virgin olive oil   MEN: 4 teaspoons

¼ cup chopped yellow onion   MEN: ½ cup

2 teaspoons minced fresh garlic

1 tablespoon chopped fresh jalapeño

¼ cup sliced carrot

½ cup broccoli florets   MEN: 1 cup

½ cup cauliflower florets

½ cup chopped tomato

½ cup natural chicken or vegetable broth

¾ cup prepared 2:90 vegetable soup

Freshly ground black pepper

1 tablespoon chopped fresh flat-leaf parsley

Heat 2 teaspoons of the olive oil in a medium saucepan over medium-high heat. Add the onions, garlic, and jalapeño and sauté for 3 minutes. Add the carrots, broccoli, and cauliflower, and cook another 2 minutes. Stir in the tomatoes, broth, and vegetable soup. Turn the heat to low, cover, and cook for 5 minutes. Season with the black pepper and sprinkle with the parsley.

MEN: *Stir in the cooked chicken meat from the menu list to your soup just before serving.*

Serves 1

WOMEN: CALORIES 210; FIBER 5g; FAT 11g; PROTEIN 7g; CARB 26g; SODIUM 210mg

MEN: CALORIES 320; FIBER 7g; FAT 21g; PROTEIN 8g; CARB 32g; SODIUM 220mg

Apple and Cheese Pita

The South has a long tradition of pairing apples with cheese. Here's a savory dessert that's a sweet way to end the day.

1 large unpeeled apple, cored and diced

1½ ounces any cheese (with more than 1 but no more than 3 grams of fat per ounce), diced

1 tablespoon non-fat mayonnaise

1 tablespoon fresh lemon juice

1 teaspoon paprika

One 2:90 whole-wheat pita, halved

In a medium bowl, mix together the apple and cheese with the mayonnaise and lemon juice. Sprinkle with paprika. Stuff into the pita halves.

Serves 1

CALORIES 270; FIBER 6g; FAT 5g; PROTEIN 18g; CARB 42g; SODIUM 360mg

Wednesday

Waffle Sandwich with Ham and Syrup

If you don't mind forfeiting your coffee dividend, the syrup is a wonderful accompaniment to this breakfast sandwich.

One 2:90 waffle

2½ ounces deli ham (with 1 gram or less fat per ounce)

8 toasted pecan halves, chopped

2 tablespoons sugar-free maple-flavored syrup (optional)

Toast the waffle and cut it in half. Arrange the ham over one half of the waffle and drizzle the maple syrup over the ham. Top with the other half of the waffle and sprinkle with the pecans. Drizzle the syrup on top, if desired. Eat with a fork and knife.

Serves 1

CALORIES 270; FIBER 3g; FAT 15g; PROTEIN 21g; CARB 16g; SODIUM 600mg

Ham and Avocado Club Wrap

Roll this wrap in wax paper for a quick and easy lunch on the go.

½ cup baby spinach leaves   MEN: 1 cup

¼ cup sliced cucumber   MEN: ½ cup

½ medium tomato, chopped   MEN: 1 medium

½ cup onion sprouts   MEN: 1 cup

Fresh lemon juice

Freshly ground black pepper

One 2:90 tortilla

1 tablespoon non-fat mayonnaise

2½ ounces deli ham (with 1 gram or less fat per ounce)

¼ cup sliced avocado

1 cup chopped romaine lettuce

2 tablespoons chopped fresh dill

In a medium bowl, toss together ½ cup spinach, ¼ cup cucumber, ½ chopped tomato, and ½ cup onion sprouts. Dress with lemon juice and black pepper to taste.

Microwave the tortilla for 10 to 15 seconds to soften it. Spread the mayonnaise over the tortilla and top with the ham, avocado, romaine and dill. Roll up and serve.

MEN: *Make a side salad with the extra spinach, cucumber, tomato, and onion sprouts. Add extra fresh dill to taste and drizzle with fresh lemon juice.*

Serves 1

WOMEN: CALORIES 310; FIBER 12g; FAT 17g; PROTEIN 24g; CARB 24g; SODIUM 710mg

MEN: CALORIES 350; FIBER 14g; FAT 17g; PROTEIN 26g; CARB 29g; SODIUM 730mg

Chinese Five-Spice Stir-fried Rice

Chinese five-spice powder is a traditional mixture of fennel, cloves, cinnamon, star anise, and Szechuan peppercorns. It's often called the "wonder powder" because it encompasses all five elements—sour, bitter, sweet, pungent, and salty. The spice blend is available in most supermarket spice aisles.

2 tablespoons rice vinegar

1 teaspoon Chinese five-spice powder   MEN: 1½ teaspoons

1 tablespoon minced fresh garlic   MEN: 4 teaspoons

1 tablespoon naturally brewed reduced-sodium soy sauce

Nonstick cooking spray

¼ cup sliced yellow onion   MEN: ½ cup

¼ cup sliced carrot   MEN: ½ cup

¼ cup diced leek   MEN: ½ cup

¼ cup sliced red bell pepper   MEN: ½ cup

¼ cup sliced celery   MEN: ½ cup

⅓ cup cooked 2:90 rice

12 toasted almonds, slivered

In a small bowl, combine the vinegar, five-spice powder, garlic, and soy sauce.

Heat a wok or large nonstick skillet over medium-high heat. Spray with nonstick cooking spray. Add the onions, carrots, leeks, bell peppers, and celery, in that order, cooking each vegetable for 15 seconds before adding the next. When all of the vegetables have been added to the wok, cook for 3 to 4 minutes, stirring constantly, until the vegetables are tender. Add the soy-sauce mixture, cooked rice, and almonds, and toss a few times to combine.

MEN: *Add the tofu and peanuts from the menu list to the stir-fry with the sauce.*

Serves 1

WOMEN: CALORIES 220; FIBER 5.5g; FAT 14g; PROTEIN 7g; CARB 19g; SODIUM 660mg

MEN: CALORIES 280; FIBER 9g; FAT 14g; PROTEIN 9g; CARB 32g; SODIUM 710mg

Blueberry Vanilla Custard

Custard, which is simply eggs and milk, is a great base for a variety of flavors, both sweet and savory. Substitute almost any fruit for favorable results. This recipe makes two servings, so save half for later this week.

Nonstick cooking spray
2¼ cups blueberries
2 organic, cage-free whole large eggs plus 2 egg whites
½ cup skim milk
2 tablespoons sugar substitute
2 teaspoons vanilla extract
2 teaspoons fresh lemon juice

Preheat the oven to 375°F. Spray a round (5-inch-diameter) casserole dish with nonstick cooking spray. Place 1 cup of the blueberries in the bowl of a food processor or blender and blend until smooth, about 30 seconds.

In a small bowl, whisk together the eggs, egg whites, milk, sugar substitute, vanilla, lemon juice, and pureed blueberries. Pour the custard mixture into the prepared casserole dish. Place the dish in a baking pan and pour hot water to come up about 1 inch. Bake for 45 to 60 minutes, or until the custard is just set (it should be wobbly to the touch). Let cool, cover with plastic, and refrigerate the custard for 3 to 24 hours before serving. Garnish with the remaining blueberries.

Serves 2

CALORIES 210; FIBER 4g; FAT 7g; PROTEIN 13g; CARB 27g; SODIUM 160mg per single serving

Thursday

Herbed Cottage Cheese on an English Muffin

A breakfast on the run can still be a healthy one.

½ cup low-fat cottage cheese (containing up to 1% milkfat)
1 tablespoon chopped fresh chives
1 tablespoon chopped fresh dill
One 2:90 whole-wheat English muffin, toasted

In a small bowl, combine the cottage cheese with the chives and dill. Spoon the mixture onto the toasted English muffin.

Serves 1

CALORIES 170; FIBER 2g; FAT 2.5g; PROTEIN 20g; CARB 29g; SODIUM 250mg

Italian Sausage Sandwich

Roll this flatbread sandwich and eat it like a burrito, or leave it flat and eat it with a fork and knife.

1 ounce cooked Italian sausage (with 1 gram or less fat per ounce), sliced

1 ounce of any cheese (with more than 1 but no more than 3 grams of fat per ounce), chopped

8 large pitted black olives, chopped

1 jar roasted red pepper, chopped

¾ cup thinly sliced red and yellow bell peppers

1 tablespoon chopped fresh flat-leaf parsley

1 teaspoon chopped fresh oregano

1 tablespoon reduced-fat mayonnaise

⅛ teaspoon crushed red pepper flakes

One 2:90 flatbread or pita

1 cup shredded romaine lettuce   MEN: 2 cups

In a small bowl, combine the sausage, cheese, olives, roasted pepper, raw peppers, parsley, oregano, mayonnaise, and red pepper flakes. Spoon the mixture onto the flatbread and top with the lettuce.

Serves 1

WOMEN: CALORIES 320; FIBER 3g; FAT 16g; PROTEIN 20g; CARB 31g; SODIUM 830mg

MEN: CALORIES 330; FIBER 5g; FAT 16g; PROTEIN 21g; CARB 32g; SODIUM 830mg

Middle Eastern Tabouli Salad

Tabouli is a bulghur wheat salad with a variety of crisp vegetables added for a cool crunch. You may find the word also spelled "tabbouleh."

2 tablespoons boxed natural tabouli wheat salad mix

1 tablespoon boiling water

1 tablespoon chopped fresh flat-leaf parsley   MEN: 2 tablespoons

1 cup shredded romaine lettuce   MEN: 2 cups

½ cup halved cherry tomatoes   MEN: 1 cup

½ cup sliced radishes   MEN: 1 cup

⅓ cup sliced red onion   MEN: ⅔ cup

2 teaspoons olive oil   MEN: 4 teaspoons

1 teaspoon fresh lemon juice   MEN: 2 teaspoons

In a medium bowl, stir the tabouli salad mix with the boiling water, cover, and let sit for several minutes to allow the grains to absorb the water. Add the remaining ingredients, and toss together.

MEN: *Chop the cooked chicken from the menu list and toss it with the salad.*

Serves 1

WOMEN: CALORIES 210; FIBER 7g; FAT 10g; PROTEIN 5g; CARB 29g; SODIUM 310mg

MEN: CALORIES 350; FIBER 9g; FAT 20g; PROTEIN 7g; CARB 41g; SODIUM 340mg

Friday

Cheese Toast with Oregano

Enjoy a spicy breakfast for a change of pace—the flavors will be sure to wake you up.

    1 slice regular 2:90 bread, toasted
    2 tablespoons light margarine
    2½ ounces any fat-free cheese (American, cheddar, or Swiss)
    1 teaspoon dried oregano
    ⅛ teaspoon paprika
    ⅛ teaspoon garlic powder (optional)
    Hot sauce

Preheat the broiler or toaster oven. Spread the margarine over the toasted bread and top with the cheese, oregano, paprika, and garlic powder, if using. Broil until the cheese is melted and bubbly. Cut the toast into quarters, like a pizza, and season with hot sauce to taste.

Serves 1

CALORIES 280; FIBER 3g; FAT 15g; PROTEIN 18g; CARB 19g; SODIUM 560mg

Chinese Chicken Pita

Adjust the spiciness of the chicken by adding more or less dry mustard to
your taste.

3 ounces boneless, skinless chicken breast, diced (will yield 2½ ounces
    cooked)
½ cup sugar snap peas, ends trimmed
¼ cup diced red bell pepper rings   MEN: ½ cup
2 tablespoons chopped fresh cilantro leaves
6 toasted almonds, chopped
1 teaspoon sugar substitute
1 tablespoon rice vinegar
1 teaspoon sesame oil
1 tablespoon bottled teriyaki sauce
1½ teaspoons dry mustard
One 2:90 whole-wheat pita, cut in half and toasted

Set a rack at the highest level of the oven and preheat to broil. Place the
chicken on a piece of foil and place under the broiler for 3 minutes. Turn
and broil for another 3 minutes, or until the chicken is no longer pink inside and the juices run clear.

Blanch the snap peas in boiling water until they turn bright green, about
3 minutes. Drain and rinse with cool water to chill. Chop into bite-size
pieces.

In a medium bowl, mix together the bell peppers, cilantro, almonds,
sugar substitute, vinegar, oil, teriyaki sauce, and mustard. Spoon into the
toasted pita pockets.

Serves 1

WOMEN: CALORIES 310; FIBER 6g; FAT 10g; PROTEIN 28g; CARB 27g; SODIUM 440mg
MEN: CALORIES 320; FIBER 7g; FAT 11g; PROTEIN 28g; CARB 30g; SODIUM 440mg

Angel-Hair Pasta with Fresh Herbs

Angel-hair pasta is very fine and needs less cooking time than spaghetti. Follow the package instructions closely and be careful—it's easy to overcook it.

2 teaspoons olive oil

¼ cup chopped yellow onion   MEN: ½ cup

2 teaspoons minced fresh garlic   MEN: 1 tablespoon

½ cup sliced mushrooms   MEN: 1 cup

¾ cup diced red and yellow bell peppers   MEN: 1½ cups

½ cup baby spinach leaves   MEN: 1 cup

1 teaspoon garlic powder

1 tablespoon chopped fresh flat-leaf parsley

1 tablespoon chopped fresh chives

1 tablespoon chopped fresh basil

⅓ cup cooked 2:90 whole-wheat angel-hair pasta

2 teaspoons grated Parmesan cheese

Heat the olive oil in a large nonstick skillet over medium heat. Add the onions, garlic, and mushrooms and sauté for 3 to 4 minutes, or until softened. Add the bell peppers and cook for another 2 to 3 minutes, or until softened. Add the spinach, garlic powder, parsley, chives, and basil, and cook until the spinach is wilted. Stir in the cooked pasta and Parmesan.

MEN: *Chop the string cheese and pecan halves from the menu list and sprinkle over the pasta just before serving.*

Serves 1

WOMEN: CALORIES 280; FIBER 5.5g; FAT 13g; PROTEIN 11g; CARB 33g; SODIUM 25mg

MEN: CALORIES 330; FIBER 10g; FAT 14g; PROTEIN 14g; CARB 45g; SODIUM 40mg

Saturday

Waffle Topped with Strawberries and Ricotta

Sit down and enjoy this breakfast with the newspaper. If you're in a hurry, slice the waffle into sticks, mix the strawberries into the ricotta mixture, and serve as a dip.

½ cup fat-free ricotta cheese
1 teaspoon sugar substitute
1 teaspoon vanilla extract
One 2:90 whole-wheat waffle
1¾ cups whole sliced strawberries

Combine the ricotta, sugar substitute, and vanilla in a small bowl. Toast the waffle and place it in the center of a dinner plate. Spoon the ricotta mixture over the waffle and top with the sliced strawberries.

Serves 1

CALORIES 280; FIBER 8g; FAT 4g; PROTEIN 14g; CARB 46g; SODIUM 340mg

Shrimp Curry with Rice

Curry is a word with many meanings. The two most common are "spice blend" and "gravy." However, curry isn't a single spice, as is often believed, but a mixture of several spices. The Chai Iced Tea is the perfect complement to this spicy curry dish.

½ cup skim milk
1 tablespoon tomato paste
1 teaspoon fresh lemon juice
1 teaspoon garam masala
½ teaspoon ground cumin

¼ teaspoon sugar substitute

⅛ teaspoon coconut extract

3 tablespoons finely chopped fresh cilantro

Nonstick cooking spray

2 teaspoons peanut oil

2 teaspoons minced fresh garlic

½ cup chopped yellow onion   MEN: 1 cup

¾ cup chopped tomato   MEN: 1½ cups

3 ounces shrimp, peeled and deveined (will yield 2½ ounces cooked)

⅓ cup cooked and cooled Lundberg Wild Blend gourmet blend of wild or
      premium brown rice

In a small bowl, combine the milk, tomato paste, lemon juice, garam masala, cumin, sugar substitute, coconut extract, and cilantro and mix well.

Heat a large nonstick skillet over medium-high heat. Spray with non-stick cooking spray. Add the oil, garlic, onions, and tomato, and sauté until soft. Add the shrimp and cook on each side for 2 minutes, or until opaque. Add the milk mixture, turn the heat to medium-low, and simmer for 5 minutes. Serve over the cooked rice. Serve with Chai Iced Tea (recipe follows).

Serves 1

WOMEN: CALORIES 310; FIBER 3g; FAT 13g; PROTEIN 25g; CARB 25g; SODIUM 230mg

MEN: CALORIES 370; FIBER 6g; FAT 14g; PROTEIN 27g; CARB 39g; SODIUM 240mg

Chai Iced Tea

If you have a cappuccino machine, steam the milk before mixing it in with the brewed tea.

4 ounces boiling water

1 chai tea bag

½ cup skim milk

1 teaspoon sugar substitute, or to taste

Pour the boiling water into a large mug. Add the tea bag and steep for 2 to 3 minutes. Remove the tea bag and pour in the milk. Sweeten with sugar substitute and pour in a tall glass filled with ice.

Serves 1

CALORIES 50; FIBER 0g; FAT 0g; PROTEIN 5g; CARB 7g; SODIUM 75mg

Oven-Roasted Potatoes and Vegetables

This is a rustic one-pan dinner. Put it in the oven and take your time setting the table, opening the mail, or completing other pre-dinner chores.

2 teaspoons extra-virgin olive oil   MEN: 4 teaspoons

¾ cup sliced red and green bell peppers   MEN: 1½ cups

½ cup sliced eggplant, peeled   MEN: 1 cup

¼ cup sliced yellow onion

1 small russet potato, ½-inch slices

1 teaspoon minced fresh garlic   MEN: 2 teaspoons

¼ teaspoon dried thyme   MEN: ½ teaspoon

¼ teaspoon dried oregano   MEN: ½ teaspoon

2 teaspoons grated Parmesan cheese

Preheat the oven to 400°F. Heat 2 teaspoons of the olive oil in an ovenproof nonstick skillet until hot. Add the bell peppers, eggplant, onions, potato, and garlic. Sauté for 2 minutes, stirring often, and place in the oven. Roast for 20 to 30 minutes, or until the vegetables are tender. Sprinkle with the Parmesan cheese.

MEN: *Chop the chicken from the menu list and stir it into the roasted potatoes when they come out of the oven. Drizzle the casserole with the extra 2 teaspoons of olive oil just before serving.*

Serves 1

WOMEN: CALORIES 250; FIBER 6.5g; FAT 11g; PROTEIN 6g; CARB 36g; SODIUM 70mg

MEN: CALORIES 390; FIBER 10g; FAT 21g; PROTEIN 7g; CARB 47g; SODIUM 70mg

Italian Almond Cake with Figs

The cuisine of Italy tends to be regionalized. A pastry chef from one region would consider this a staple on the menu while a chef from another region wouldn't include it on his. This recipe makes two servings, so save for later this week.

Nonstick cooking spray

7 tablespoons whole-wheat flour

10 teaspoons sugar substitute

2 teaspoons baking powder

2 organic, cage-free whole large eggs, separated

2 tablespoons lemon zest

⅔ teaspoon almond extract

½ teaspoon cream of tartar

4 teaspoons powdered sugar, for dusting

6 medium figs, sliced

Preheat the oven to 375°F. Spray a round casserole dish (10 inches in diameter) with nonstick cooking spray.

In a small bowl, combine the flour, sugar substitute, and baking powder. In a medium bowl, whisk together the egg yolks, lemon zest, and almond extract. Add the flour mixture to the egg-yolk mixture, adding a little flour at a time.

In a medium bowl, whisk the 2 egg whites with the cream of tartar with an electric mixer until they hold stiff peaks. Gently fold the whites into the batter. Spoon into the prepared casserole dish and bake for 15 to 20 minutes, or until a skewer inserted into the center comes out clean.

Let cool before removing from the pan, dust with the powdered sugar, and serve with the sliced figs.

Serves 2

CALORIES 300; FIBER 7g; FAT 7g; PROTEIN 14g; CARB 48g; SODIUM 125mg per single serving

Sunday

Warm Ham-and-Swiss Open-faced Sandwich

This sandwich can easily be made portable by using two slices of light 2:90 bread and serving it chilled.

    1 slice regular 2:90 bread, toasted
    2 tablespoons light margarine
    1½ ounces deli ham (with 1 gram or less fat per ounce)
    1 ounce fat-free Swiss cheese
    1 teaspoon chopped fresh chives

Preheat the broiler or toaster oven. Spread the margarine over the toasted bread and top with the ham, cheese, and chives. Broil until cheese is melted and bubbly. Cut the toast into quarters like a pizza.

Serves 1

CALORIES 310; FIBER 3g; FAT 16g; PROTEIN 24g; CARB 19g; SODIUM 740mg

Red Snapper Soft Taco

This taco tastes just like the ones they serve in little beachside *taquerías* on the Baja peninsula. The best part of a taco, though, is the abundance of toppings. Season the fish and veggies that fall from the tortilla with fresh lime juice and eat them like a salad.

    Nonstick cooking spray
    2 teaspoons minced fresh garlic
    One 3-ounce red snapper fillet (will yield 2½ ounces cooked),
        cut into bite-size pieces
    1 tablespoon fresh lime juice
    1 teaspoon chopped fresh thyme
    1 teaspoon chopped fresh oregano

One 2:90 whole-wheat tortilla

½ cup shredded romaine lettuce   MEN: 1 cup

½ cup chopped tomato   MEN: 1 cup

½ cup chopped scallions

¼ cup chopped jicama   MEN: ½ cup

¼ cup sliced avocado

3 tablespoons prepared salsa

2 sprigs of fresh cilantro

Heat an 8-inch nonstick skillet over medium-high heat. Spray with non-stick cooking spray. Add the garlic and sauté until golden. Add the red snapper and cook for 3 to 5 minutes, stirring often, until fish flakes apart. Add the lime juice, thyme, and oregano, and stir to coat.

Microwave the tortilla for 10 to 15 seconds to soften it. Spoon the fish mixture over the tortilla and top with the lettuce, tomatoes, scallions, jicama, avocado, salsa, and cilantro.

Serves 1

WOMEN: CALORIES 290; FIBER 13g; FAT 11g; PROTEIN 23g; CARB 28g; SODIUM 500mg

MEN: CALORIES 330; FIBER 17g; FAT 11g; PROTEIN 24g; CARB 36g; SODIUM 510mg

Eggplant Parmesan

This low-fat version of Eggplant Parmesan is light and delicious. The fresh oregano and basil lend a bright, aromatic flavor to the dish.

Nonstick cooking spray

⅛ cup chopped leek   MEN: ¼ cup

2 teaspoons finely chopped fresh garlic   MEN: 1 tablespoon

¼ cup chopped tomato   MEN: ½ cup

½ cup corn kernels   MEN: 1 cup

1 teaspoon sugar substitute   MEN: 2 teaspoons

1 teaspoon chopped fresh oregano   MEN: 2 teaspoons

2 teaspoons extra-virgin olive oil

1 cup peeled and sliced Japanese eggplant   MEN: 2 cups

2 teaspoons grated Parmesan cheese

1 tablespoon chopped fresh basil

Preheat the oven to 375°F. Spray a round casserole dish (5 inches in diameter) with nonstick cooking spray.

Heat a medium saucepan over medium-high heat. Spray with nonstick cooking spray. Add the leeks and garlic and cook for 2 minutes, or until softened. Add the tomatoes, corn, sugar substitute, and oregano and cook for about 10 minutes, or until tomatoes are soft and soupy.

Heat a nonstick skillet over medium-high heat. Add the olive oil, then the eggplant, and sauté on both sides until lightly browned and tender.

Arrange half of the eggplant in the bottom of the prepared casserole dish. Spoon the tomato mixture over the slices and arrange the remaining eggplant slices on top. Sprinkle with the Parmesan and bake for 20 minutes, or until bubbly. Remove from the oven, sprinkle with the basil, and serve from the casserole dish.

MEN: *Chop the string cheese from the menu list and sprinkle it over the eggplant a few minutes before it comes out of the oven.*

Serves 1

WOMEN: CALORIES 210; FIBER 3g; FAT 13g; PROTEIN 5g; CARB 21g; SODIUM 55mg

MEN: CALORIES 300; FIBER 6g; FAT 13g; PROTEIN 9g; CARB 43g; SODIUM 110mg

Week 6

Day 1   Monday Menu

Breakfast

Sausage Muffin
1¾ cups whole fresh strawberries
MEN: Add ⅓ cup fruit muesli
Morning Dividend*

Lunch

Cucumber-Dill Tea Sandwiches
1 cup skim milk or one container any 2:90 yogurt with fiber
(providing up to 90 calories)
½ cup celery sticks
MEN: Add ½ cup celery sticks; ½ cup carrot sticks;
and 1 medium tomato, sliced

Dinner

Tempura Vegetables
MEN: Add 12 almonds; ½ cup celery sticks; ½ cup carrot
sticks; and 1 medium tomato, sliced
MEN: Add 2 ounces unsalted edamame (Japanese
soybeans)

Reality Reward

Chocolate Espresso Mousse
½ cup ice-cold skim milk
1 dessert starch of your choice (see Equivalents Lists,
page 381)

---

*Morning Dividend—Choose one sweetener OR one creamer from the following:
1 teaspoon honey, 1 teaspoon white granulated sugar, or 1 teaspoon brown
sugar OR 2 tablespoons 2% milk, 1 tablespoon half-and-half, 1 tablespoon
soymilk creamer, 1 tablespoon nondairy liquid creamer, 2 teaspoons nondairy
powdered creamer

Recipe items are in boldface.

Day 2   Tuesday Menu

Breakfast   1 serving 2:90 calcium-fortified dry or hot cereal (providing
up to 90 calories)

1 large fresh peach

1 tablespoon natural cashew butter

½ cup low-fat cottage cheese containing up to 1% milkfat

MEN: Add 1 slice of regular bread

Morning Dividend

Lunch   **Hummus Wrap**

1 cup skim milk or one container any 2:90 yogurt with fiber
(providing up to 90 calories)

MEN: Add ½ cup celery sticks; ½ cup carrot sticks; and
1 medium tomato, sliced

Dinner   **Corn on the Cob with Cilantro-Chili Butter**

Butter Lettuce Salad with Dijon Vinaigrette

MEN: Add 1½ ounces cooked beefsteak and ½ cup celery
sticks

Reality Reward   **Chocolate Espresso Mousse**

½ cup ice-cold skim milk

1 dessert starch of your choice (see Equivalents Lists,
page 381)

Day 3   Wednesday Menu

Breakfast   **Waffle Sandwich with Ham and Syrup**
¾ large fresh grapefruit
MEN: Add ¼ cup 2:90 granola
Morning Dividend

Lunch   **Bean and Cheese Nachos**
1 cup skim milk or one container any 2:90 yogurt with fiber
(providing up to 90 calories)
MEN: Add ½ cup jicama sticks

Dinner   **Stir-fried Broccoli and Rice**
MEN: Add 3 ounces chopped firm tofu

Reality Reward   **Creamy Strawberry Tofu Dessert**
1 dessert starch of your choice (see Equivalents Lists,
page 381)

Day 4   Thursday Menu

Breakfast   **Apple–Peanut Butter Sandwich**

5 scrambled egg whites or ½ cup non-fat or low-fat cottage cheese (up to 1% milkfat)

MEN: Add 1 serving 2:90 dry cereal

Morning Dividend

Lunch   **Chinese Chicken Pita**

1 cup skim milk or 1 container any 2:90 yogurt with fiber (providing up to 90 calories)

MEN: Add ½ sliced cucumber and ½ cup sliced carrots

Dinner   **Polenta with Roasted Red Bell Pepper and Sage**

1 cup sliced radishes and 5 or 6 tomato slices

MEN: Add 1 small cooked skinless chicken leg (about 1½ ounces); ½ cup carrot sticks

Reality Reward   **Cherry-Almond Clafoutis**

Day 5   Friday Menu

Breakfast   1 serving 2:90 calcium-fortified dry or hot cereal (providing up to 90 calories)

5 scrambled egg whites with 4 tablespoons chopped avocado

1½ kiwis, sliced

MEN: Add 1 slice of regular bread

Morning Dividend

Lunch   **Quinoa Chili**

1 cup skim milk or one container any 2:90 yogurt with fiber (providing up to 90 calories)

MEN: Add ½ cup celery sticks; ½ cup carrot sticks; and 5 or 6 tomato slices

Dinner   **Spinach Pesto Fettuccine**

MEN: Add ½ cup carrot sticks and 1 mozzarella string cheese (with no more than 4 grams of total fat per string)

Reality Reward   **Cherry-Almond Clafoutis**

Day 6   Saturday Menu

Breakfast   **Ham-and-Cheese English Muffin**

1½ cups honeydew melon slices

MEN: Add 1 serving 2:90 hot cereal

Morning Dividend

Lunch   **Chicken Pasta Salad**

1 cup skim milk or one container any 2:90 yogurt with fiber
(providing up to 90 calories)

1 cup celery and ¼ cup carrots

½ cup jicama sticks and 5 to 6 slices tomato

Dinner   **Sizzling Vegetable Fajitas**

MEN: Add 3 ounces chopped firm tofu

Reality Reward   **Banana Flan**

1 cup ice-cold skim milk

1 dessert starch of your choice (see Equivalents Lists,
page 381)

Day 7   Sunday Menu

Breakfast   **Orange-Pecan Waffle**

MEN: Add ¼ cup 2:90 granola and 5 scrambled egg whites

Morning Dividend

Lunch   **Ham and Avocado Club Wrap**

1 cup skim milk or one container any 2:90 yogurt with fiber
(providing up to 90 calories)

Dinner   **Spanish Couscous**

MEN: Add 1 small cooked skinless chicken leg
(about 1½ ounces)

Reality Reward   **Chocolate Hazelnut Granita with Raspberries**

1 dessert starch of your choice (see Equivalents Lists,
page 381)

1 cup ice-cold skim milk

Monday

Sausage Muffin

Eat this sandwich with a fork and knife.

    One 2:90 English muffin, toasted
    2 tablespoons light margarine
    Nonstick cooking spray
    1 ounce chopped sausage (with 1 gram or less fat per ounce)
    1 ounce of any cheese (with more than 1 but no more than 3 grams of fat
        per ounce), chopped
    1 tablespoon chopped fresh flat-leaf parsley
    Freshly ground black pepper

Toast the English muffin and spread the margarine over both sides. Heat an
8-inch nonstick skillet over medium heat. Spray with nonstick cooking
spray. Add the sausage and cook for 5 minutes, or until cooked through.
Stir in the parsley and season with black pepper to taste.

  Spoon the sausage mixture over the toasted English muffin halves and
top with the cheese.

  Serves 1

CALORIES 290; FIBER 3g; FAT 16g; PROTEIN 22g; CARB 28g; SODIUM 770mg

Cucumber-Dill Tea Sandwiches

Cut the crusts off the bread and you'll feel like you're having high tea.

    1 medium tomato, sliced
    ¼ cup thinly sliced red onion
    Balsamic vinegar
    Freshly ground black pepper
    2 slices light 2:90 bread

2 tablespoons reduced-fat mayonnaise

2½ ounces smoked turkey deli meat (with 1 gram or less fat per ounce)

10 cucumber slices

½ teaspoon white vinegar

1 tablespoon chopped fresh dill

4 small sprigs of dill, for garnish

Arrange the tomato slices in a circle on the center of a large plate. Arrange the red onion slices on top and drizzle with balsamic vinegar and black pepper to taste.

Spread both slices of the bread with the mayonnaise. Top one slice of bread with the turkey and cucumbers. Sprinkle with the white vinegar and dill. Top with the second slice of bread and slice the sandwich into quarters. Top each quarter with a small sprig of dill and arrange next to the tomato salad.

Serves 1

CALORIES 280; FIBER 9g; FAT 13g; PROTEIN 20g; CARB 28g; SODIUM 860mg

Tempura Vegetables

This is a challenging recipe because the batter needs to be the right consistency for it to stick to the vegetables. The bread crumbs tend to absorb water, so you might need to add more water to the batter as you're cooking. Panko are Japanese-style bread crumbs.

½ cup panko (Japanese bread crumbs)

2 teaspoons cornstarch

1 teaspoon minced fresh ginger

1 teaspoon minced fresh garlic

1 teaspoon rice vinegar

About 6 tablespoons ice-cold water

2 teaspoons canola oil

Nonstick cooking spray

4 broccolini stalks

2 scallions, sliced ½-inch thick

½ cup broccoli florets

½ cup cauliflower florets

Combine the panko and cornstarch in the bowl of a food processor and pulse 5 or 6 times. Add the ginger, garlic, vinegar, and 4 tablespoons of water. Pulse another 5 or 6 times.

Heat an 8-inch nonstick skillet over medium-low heat. Add the canola oil and spray with the nonstick cooking spray.

Pulse the food processor again and add more water, 1 tablespoon at a time, to form a batter. Scrape the batter into a small bowl and place it next to the stove.

Dip a few vegetables into the batter and place in the skillet. Turn up the heat to medium and cook until crisp, carefully turning to cook all sides. Place the finished vegetables on a paper towel–lined plate and repeat the cooking process with the remaining vegetables, spraying the skillet with more nonstick cooking spray as needed.

Serves 1

CALORIES 250; FIBER 4g; FAT 12g; PROTEIN 6g; CARB 32g; SODIUM 85mg

Chocolate Espresso Mousse

You can make the mousse a day ahead since it's best when completely chilled. This recipe makes two servings, so save half for later this week.

1 cup light soymilk

4 tablespoons sugar substitute

2 tablespoons unsweetened cocoa powder

2 tablespoons instant espresso granules

2 teaspoons vanilla extract

12 ounces organic silken tofu

3 cups raspberries

In a medium saucepan, combine the soymilk, sugar substitute, cocoa powder, espresso granules, and vanilla. Whisk together and turn the heat to medium-low. Continue whisking until the milk mixture is hot and frothy.

Place the tofu in the bowl of a food processor. Pour in the milk mixture and process for 90 seconds. Pour the mousse into a serving bowl, cover with plastic, and refrigerate for 3 to 24 hours. Serve topped with the raspberries.

Serves 2

CALORIES 230; FIBER 2g; FAT 6g; PROTEIN 13g; CARB 41g; SODIUM 55mg per single serving

Tuesday

Hummus Wrap

This spicy hummus makes a great dip or sandwich spread. It can be stored in an airtight container in the fridge for three to four days.

½ cup canned drained chick peas

1 teaspoon extra-virgin olive oil

1 teaspoon garlic powder

2 to 3 teaspoons fresh lemon juice, or to taste

Pinch of cayenne pepper, or more to taste

Freshly ground black pepper

One 2:90 tortilla wrap

½ cup shredded romaine lettuce

5 pitted Kalamata olives, sliced (high sodium)

1½ tablespoons chopped peperoncini (high sodium)

1 teaspoon red wine vinegar

1 tablespoon chopped fresh flat-leaf parsley

½ cup carrot sticks

Combine the chickpeas, olive oil, garlic powder, lemon juice, cayenne, and black pepper to taste in the bowl of a food processor and blend for 60 to 90 seconds, until smooth, scraping down the sides occasionally.

Microwave the tortilla for 10 to 15 seconds to soften it. Spread the hummus over the wrap and top with the lettuce, olives, and peperoncini. Sprinkle with the vinegar and top with the parsley. Roll up and serve with the carrot sticks on the side.

Serves 1

CALORIES 320; FIBER 15g; FAT 14g; PROTEIN 10g; CARB 39g; SODIUM 730mg

Corn on the Cob with Cilantro-Chili Butter

For an even more flavorful butter, grate about ½ teaspoon of fresh lime zest into the mix.

1 medium ear of corn   MEN: 2 ears
2 tablespoons light margarine   MEN: 4 tablespoons
1 tablespoon chopped fresh cilantro   MEN: 2 tablespoons
⅛ teaspoon chili powder   MEN: ¼ teaspoon
1 teaspoon fresh lime juice   MEN: 2 teaspoons
Pinch of cayenne pepper   MEN: 2 pinches

Fill a medium saucepan with water and bring to a simmer over high heat. Carefully place the corn in the water and cook for 3 to 5 minutes. Drain. In a small bowl, combine the remaining ingredients. Slather the margarine mixture over the hot ear(s) of corn.

MEN: *Season the beef from the menu list with fresh lime juice and a pinch each of freshly ground black pepper and chili powder before broiling.*

Serves 1

WOMEN: CALORIES 210; FIBER 4g; FAT 12g; PROTEIN 5g; CARB 27g; SODIUM 220mg
MEN: CALORIES 430; FIBER 8g; FAT 23g; PROTEIN 9g; CARB 54g; SODIUM 430mg

Butter Lettuce Salad with Dijon Vinaigrette

This salad is as fresh and crisp as summer, but available year round.

2 teaspoons extra-virgin olive oil

1 teaspoon red wine vinegar

1 teaspoon Dijon mustard

1 teaspoon fresh minced garlic

Freshly ground black pepper

1 cup butter lettuce torn into bite-size pieces   MEN: 2 cups

1 cup diced tomato   MEN: 1½ cups

1 cup sliced radishes

¼ cup sliced red onion

In a small bowl, whisk together the olive oil, vinegar, mustard, and garlic until frothy. Season with black pepper to taste.

In a medium salad bowl, toss together the lettuce, tomatoes, radishes, and red onions. Dress the salad with the vinaigrette.

Serves 1

WOMEN: CALORIES 170; FIBER 3g; FAT 10g; PROTEIN 4g; CARB 19g; SODIUM 190mg

MEN: CALORIES 200; FIBER 5g; FAT 11g; PROTEIN 6g; CARB 24g; SODIUM 200mg

Wednesday

Bean and Cheese Nachos

This plate of nachos is the perfect size for a hearty lunch. If you're not at home, you can heat the beans and melt the cheese in a microwave.

One 90-calorie serving black bean tortilla chips, about 16 chips

¼ cup cooked black beans

1 ounce fat-free cheddar cheese, cut into strips

½ cup shredded romaine lettuce   MEN: 1 cup

½ medium tomato, sliced   MEN: 1 medium

¼ cup chopped avocado

2 tablespoons chopped fresh cilantro leaves

Hot sauce

Set a rack at the highest level of the oven and preheat to broil. Arrange the chips on a pie tin or other ovenproof plate. Layer the black beans and cheese on top of the chips and broil until the cheese has melted, about 45 seconds. Top with the lettuce, tomato, avocado, and cilantro. Season with hot sauce to taste.

Serves 1

WOMEN: CALORIES 285; FIBER 9g; FAT 13g; PROTEIN 19g; CARB 26g; SODIUM 430mg

MEN: CALORIES 300; FIBER 10g; FAT 13g; PROTEIN 19g; CARB 28g; SODIUM 430mg

Stir-fried Broccoli and Rice

The aromatics—garlic, ginger, and chili flakes—are the keys to a flavorful stir-fry. Make sure to cook them for the full thirty seconds, stirring constantly, to get the full effect of their flavor.

Nonstick cooking spray

½ cup sliced yellow onion

½ cup sliced carrots

1 cup sliced mushrooms

1 cup broccoli florets   MEN: 2 cups

2 teaspoons minced fresh garlic   MEN: 1 tablespoon

1 teaspoon minced fresh ginger   MEN: 2 teaspoons

¼ teaspoon crushed red pepper flakes   MEN: ½ teaspoon

⅓ cup cooked 2:90 rice

1 tablespoon naturally brewed reduced-sodium soy sauce

12 almonds, sliced   MEN: 24 almonds

Heat a wok or large nonstick skillet over medium-high heat. Spray with nonstick cooking spray. Add the onions, carrots, mushrooms, and broccoli, in that order, cooking each vegetable for 15 seconds before adding the next. When all of the vegetables have been added to the wok or skillet, cook for another 3 to 4 minutes, stirring constantly, until the vegetables are tender. Add the garlic, ginger, red pepper flakes, and soy sauce, and cook for another 30 seconds. Serve the stir-fry over the rice and garnish with the almonds.

MEN: *Add the tofu from the menu list to the stir-fry when adding the aromatics.*

Serves 1

WOMEN: CALORIES 290; FIBER 9g; FAT 9g; PROTEIN 13g; CARB 45g; SODIUM 670mg

MEN: CALORIES 400; FIBER 13g; FAT 17g; PROTEIN 18g; CARB 50g; SODIUM 690mg

Creamy Strawberry Tofu Dessert

The longer you freeze this strawberry dessert, the more it tastes like ice cream. Much longer than an hour in the freezer, though, and it will freeze too hard to eat with a spoon.

6 ounces soft organic firm silken organic tofu

One container 2:90 vanilla yogurt with fiber (providing up to 90 calories)

1 tablespoon sugar substitute

1 teaspoon vanilla extract

1¾ cups sliced strawberries

Combine the tofu, yogurt, sugar substitute, vanilla, and half the strawberries in the bowl of a food processor and process for 60 seconds, until smooth.

Place the remaining strawberries in a medium bowl and pour in the pureed tofu mixture. Stir together and chill in the freezer for 30 to 60 minutes, stirring occasionally.

Serves 1

CALORIES 280; FIBER 8g; FAT 5g; PROTEIN 16g; CARB 43g; SODIUM 105mg

Thursday

Apple–Peanut Butter Sandwich

Take a bite and this sandwich will be sure to remind you of your youth.

  1 tablespoon natural peanut butter
  2 slices light 2:90 bread, toasted
  1 large unpeeled Granny Smith apple, cored and thinly sliced
  1 teaspoon sugar substitute
  ½ teaspoon ground cinnamon

Spread the peanut butter evenly on both slices of the toast. Top one piece of toast with the apple slices, and sprinkle with the sugar substitute and cinnamon. Top with the second slice of bread. Close the sandwich and cut it in half diagonally.

Serves 1

CALORIES 270; FIBER 12g; FAT 9g; PROTEIN 9g; CARB 45g; SODIUM 240mg

Polenta with Roasted Red Bell Pepper and Sage

Cooking polenta is similar to cooking risotto—it takes a lot of attention and stirring to achieve the right texture. Make sure to add the mushroom liquid a little at a time for a consistency and flavor that suits your taste.

  ½ cup water
  ½ ounce dried porcini mushrooms
  Nonstick cooking spray
  ½ cup chopped onion
  2 teaspoons minced fresh garlic
  ¼ cup polenta
  1 roasted red bell pepper (from a jar), chopped
  2 tablespoons light margarine

1 teaspoon chopped fresh sage, plus 2 or 3 fresh sage leaves, for garnish

2 teaspoons grated Parmesan cheese

> MEN: 2 teaspoons olive oil

In a small saucepan, bring ¼ cup of the water to a simmer. Add the dried mushrooms, cover, turn off the heat and let steep for 15 minutes.

Heat an 8-inch nonstick skillet over medium-high heat. Spray with nonstick cooking spray. Add the onions and garlic and sauté until softened, about 2 minutes. Add the polenta and stir until it's coated with the onions and garlic. Add the remaining ½ cup of water and cook, stirring constantly, until the water is absorbed.

Strain the mushrooms, reserving the liquid, and dice the mushrooms into small pieces. Add the mushroom pieces to the polenta and stir in the reserved mushroom liquid, 1 tablespoon at a time, until the polenta is soft.

Stir in the bell pepper, margarine, sage, and Parmesan until well mixed. Garnish with the fresh sage leaves.

> MEN: *Chop the cooked chicken from the menu list and sprinkle it over the polenta, and drizzle the extra olive oil over the polenta just before serving.*

Serves 1

WOMEN: CALORIES 230; FIBER 5g; FAT 2.5g; PROTEIN 6g; CARB 45g; SODIUM 80mg

MEN: CALORIES 310; FIBER 5g; FAT 12g; PROTEIN 6g; CARB 45g; SODIUM 80mg

Cherry-Almond Clafoutis

Clafoutis is a classic French dessert that's half pudding and half cake. Cherries are the traditional fruit of choice, but you're welcome to substitute any other kind of berry. This recipe makes two servings, so save half for later this week.

Nonstick cooking spray

36 fresh cherries, pitted and halved

2 tablespoons sugar substitute

7 tablespoons whole-wheat flour

2 organic, cage-free whole large eggs plus 2 egg whites

⅔ cup non-fat dry milk

2 tablespoons cold water

½ teaspoon almond extract

4 teaspoons powdered sugar, for garnish

Preheat the oven to 375°F. Spray a round casserole dish (5 inches in diameter) with nonstick cooking spray.

In a small bowl, toss the cherries with 2 teaspoons of the sugar substitute.

In a medium bowl, combine the remaining sugar substitute, the flour, eggs, egg white, and dry milk. Stir in the cold water and almond extract. Mix well to form a smooth batter.

Arrange the cherries on the bottom of the prepared casserole dish and pour the batter over the cherries. Bake for 25 to 30 minutes, or until puffed and lightly browned. Let cool and sprinkle with the powdered sugar.

Servings: 2

CALORIES 380; FIBER 6g; FAT 8g; PROTEIN 27g; CARB 66g; SODIUM 320mg per single serving

Friday

Quinoa Chili

Quinoa is an ancient Incan grain that is a complete protein. You might have to look in a specialty market or natural food store to find it, but the extra trip will be worth your while.

⅓ cup cooked organic quinoa

2 teaspoons extra-virgin olive oil

2 teaspoons minced fresh garlic

½ cup chopped red onion

1 teaspoon chili powder

1 teaspoon ground cumin

1 teaspoon garlic powder

¼ teaspoon cayenne pepper (optional)

¼ cup canned tomatoes, no added salt   MEN: ½ cup

½ cup cooked kidney or pinto beans

Fresh lime juice

Hot sauce

Heat a medium saucepan over medium-high heat. Add the olive oil, then the garlic and red onions and sauté for 2 minutes, stirring often. Add the chili powder, cumin, garlic powder, and cayenne, if using, and stir until aromatic, about 30 seconds. Stir in the beans and ¼ cup of the tomatoes and beans. Reduce the heat to medium-low and simmer for 10 minutes. Add the quinoa and cook for another 2 to 3 minutes, stirring often. Season with lime juice and hot sauce to taste.

MEN: *Spoon the remaining ¼ cup of chopped tomatoes over the chili just before serving.*

Serves 1

WOMEN: CALORIES 320; FIBER 12g; FAT 10g; PROTEIN 11g; CARB 49g; SODIUM 10mg

MEN: CALORIES 330; FIBER 13g; FAT 10g; PROTEIN 11g; CARB 51g; SODIUM 15mg

Spinach Pesto Fettuccine

Pesto is usually made with basil, but it can be made with any fresh herbs. If you like marjoram and oregano, stir a few leaves of each into the pesto.

Nonstick cooking spray

1 teaspoon minced fresh garlic

½ cup sliced mushrooms

1 cup finely chopped broccoli florets

1 cup finely chopped cauliflower florets

½ cup baby spinach leaves

⅓ cup cooked 2:90 fettuccine

4 teaspoons prepared pesto   MEN: 8 teaspoons

2 teaspoons grated Parmesan cheese

Heat a large nonstick skillet over medium-high heat. Spray with nonstick cooking spray. Add the garlic and mushrooms and sauté for 5 minutes, or until the mushrooms have softened. Add the broccoli and cauliflower and continue cooking until they have softened. Add up to ¼ cup of water if necessary. Add the spinach and cook for 30 seconds, or until wilted. Stir in the cooked fettuccine, 4 teaspoons of the pesto, and Parmesan, and continue cooking to warm through.

MEN: *Spoon the extra 4 teaspoons of pesto over the pasta, and chop the string cheese from the menu list and sprinkle it on the pesto.*

Serves 1

WOMEN: CALORIES 230; FIBER 8g; FAT 8g; PROTEIN 12g; CARB 32g; SODIUM 190mg

MEN: CALORIES 290; FIBER 8g; FAT 14g; PROTEIN 14g; CARB 33g; SODIUM 310mg

Saturday

Ham-and-Cheese English Muffin

You can eat this breakfast muffin open-faced or wrapped in a napkin, the way short-order cooks do.

One 2:90 English muffin

2 tablespoons light margarine

1½ ounces deli ham (with 1 gram or less fat per ounce)

1 ounce fat-free cheddar or Swiss cheese

1 teaspoon chopped fresh chives

Set a rack at the highest level of the oven and preheat to broil. Toast the English muffin and spread with the margarine. Top with the ham and cheese and place under the broiler until the cheese is melted and bubbly. Top with the fresh chives.

Serves 1

CALORIES 310; FIBER 2g; FAT 16g; PROTEIN 26g; CARB 27g; SODIUM 790mg

Chicken Pasta Salad

The flavors of the Mediterranean come together in this chicken dish. Serve it hot in a pasta bowl or chill it and serve as a salad.

Nonstick cooking spray

3 ounces boneless, skinless chicken breast, cut into 1-inch pieces (will
    yield 2½ ounces cooked)

1 teaspoon garlic powder

½ teaspoon chopped fresh thyme

¼ teaspoon freshly ground black pepper

⅓ cup cooked 2:90 whole-wheat bow-tie pasta

1 cup baby spinach leaves

½ cup chopped English cucumber

5 pitted Kalamata olives, chopped

1 teaspoon extra-virgin olive oil

1 teaspoon white wine vinegar

1 tablespoon chopped fresh basil

1 teaspoon lemon zest

Heat an 8-inch nonstick skillet over medium-high heat. Spray with non-stick cooking spray. Season the chicken with the garlic powder, thyme, and black pepper. Add the chicken pieces to the skillet and cook for about 2 minutes per side, or until the juices run clear.

Add the cooked pasta, spinach, cucumber, olives, olive oil, and vinegar to the skillet. Stir together to wilt the spinach, and sprinkle with the basil and lemon zest.

Serves 1

CALORIES 290; FIBER 3g; FAT 13g; PROTEIN 22g; CARB 24g; SODIUM 380mg

Sizzling Vegetable Fajitas

The sizzle of fajitas makes them fun to serve. It's optional, though, if you're in a hurry.

2 teaspoons extra-virgin olive oil   MEN: 4 teaspoons

¼ cup sliced red onion   MEN: ½ cup

2 teaspoons minced fresh garlic   MEN: 1 tablespoon

¾ cup sliced red and green bell peppers   MEN: 1½ cups

½ cup sliced zucchini   MEN: 1 cup

¼ cup sliced button mushrooms   MEN: ½ cup

2 tablespoons chopped fresh cilantro leaves   MEN: 3 tablespoons

2 teaspoons non-fat sour cream

Hot sauce (optional)

One 2:90 tortilla

Preheat the oven to 450°F. Place a cast-iron skillet over high heat until it starts to smoke. Place the skillet in the oven to continue heating.

Heat the olive oil in an 8-inch nonstick skillet over medium-high heat. Add the red onions and garlic and sauté for 3 minutes, or until softened. Add the bell peppers, zucchini, and mushrooms and cook another 3 minutes, or until tender-crisp.

With great care, remove the hot cast-iron skillet from the oven and place on the stove. Spoon the vegetable mixture into the skillet for the fajita sizzle. Garnish with the cilantro, sour cream, and hot sauce to taste. Microwave the tortilla for 10 to 15 seconds to soften it and serve alongside.

MEN: *Add the tofu from the menu list to the skillet when adding the peppers.*

Serves 1

WOMEN: CALORIES 230; FIBER 10.5g; FAT 12g; PROTEIN 6g; CARB 26g; SODIUM 240mg

MEN: CALORIES 370; FIBER 15g; FAT 22g; PROTEIN 9g; CARB 39g; SODIUM 250mg

Banana Flan

Flan is one of Spain's signature classics. This healthier version skips the caramel but adds a nutritious banana for flavor and texture.

Nonstick cooking spray
6 ounces soft organic silken tofu
1 banana, sliced
2 teaspoons fresh lemon juice
2 teaspoons sugar substitute
1 teaspoon vanilla extract
¼ teaspoon ground cinnamon

Preheat the oven to 375°F. Spray a round casserole dish (5 inches in diameter) with nonstick cooking spray.

Puree all of the ingredients together in a food processor until smooth. Pour the mixture into the prepared casserole dish and bake for 25 minutes, or until just set (it should be wobbly to the touch). Remove from the oven, cool, then cover with plastic and refrigerate for at least 2 hours before serving.

Serves 1

CALORIES 180; FIBER 3g; FAT 5g; PROTEIN 9g; CARB 28g; SODIUM 10mg

Sunday

Orange-Pecan Waffle

This recipe fits the bill in the morning.

One 2:90 whole-wheat or multigrain waffle
1 tablespoon light margarine
1 large orange, peeled and sliced
4 toasted pecan halves, chopped
1 tablespoon orange zest
1 teaspoon sugar substitute

Toast the waffle and spread with the margarine. Top with the orange slices, pecans, and orange zest. Sprinkle with the sugar substitute.

Serves 1

CALORIES 270; FIBER 7g; FAT 13g; PROTEIN 5g; CARB 36g; SODIUM 310mg

Spanish Couscous

Olive oil, garlic, and onions are the base for most Spanish dishes. The aroma will whet your appetite and prepare you for a hearty dinner with lots of tomatoes, peppers, and fresh marjoram.

2 teaspoons olive oil   MEN: 4 teaspoons

2 teaspoons chopped fresh garlic   MEN: 1 tablespoon

¼ cup chopped yellow onion

½ cup chopped scallions

¾ cup chopped red and green bell peppers   MEN: 1½ cup

½ teaspoon ground cumin

½ teaspoon chili powder   MEN: 1 teaspoon

1 cup chopped tomatoes

1 tablespoon tomato paste

⅓ cup cooked organic whole-wheat couscous

1 teaspoon chopped fresh marjoram, plus more to taste

Freshly ground black pepper

Heat the olive oil in an 8-inch nonstick skillet over medium-high heat. Add the garlic, onions, scallions, and bell peppers, and sauté for 3 to 5 minutes, or until softened. Turn the heat to medium-low and add the cumin and chili powder. Cook, stirring for 30 seconds. When the spices are aromatic, add the tomatoes and tomato paste. Cook, stirring, for another 3 minutes. Add the cooked couscous, marjoram, and black pepper to taste.

Serves 1

WOMEN: CALORIES 290; FIBER 10.5g; FAT 11g; PROTEIN 7g; CARB 46g; SODIUM 45mg

MEN: CALORIES 400; FIBER 13g; FAT 2g; PROTEIN 8g; CARB 53g; SODIUM 45mg

Week 7

Day 1   Monday Menu

Breakfast

Cinnamon Toast Sandwich with Dried Plums
1 cup skim milk or one container 2:90 strawberry yogurt
with fiber (providing up to 90 calories)
MEN: Add 1 serving 2:90 dry cereal
*Morning Dividend**

Lunch

Turkey and Watercress Sandwich
½ cup jicama sticks
MEN: Add: ½ cup celery sticks; ½ cup carrot sticks;
5 or 6 slices of tomato; 2 tablespoons chopped avocado

Dinner

Parmesan Chicken
Cooked Mixed Greens
1 cup skim milk or one container any 2:90 yogurt with fiber
(providing up to 90 calories)
MEN: Add 4 chopped and toasted pecan halves

Reality Reward

Key Lime Cheesecake

Morning Dividend—Choose one sweetener OR one creamer from the following:
1 teaspoon honey, 1 teaspoon white granulated sugar, or 1 teaspoon brown sugar
OR 2 tablespoons 2% milk, 1 tablespoon half & half, 1 tablespoon soymilk creamer,
1 tablespoon nondairy liquid creamer, 2 teaspoons nondairy powdered creamer

Recipe items are in boldface.

Day 2   Tuesday Menu

Breakfast   1 serving 2:90 calcium-fortified dry or hot cereal (providing up to 90 calories)

1 cup skim milk or one container 2:90 apple yogurt with fiber (providing 90 calories)

1 tablespoon natural peanut butter

1 large orange

MEN: Add ¼ cup 2:90 granola

Morning Dividend

Lunch   **Tuscan Panino**

Ten 2:90 potato chips (low-fat gourmet baked potato chips, such as Kettle Krisps) or 8 Garden of Eatin' Black Bean tortilla chips

MEN: Add 2 tablespoons chopped avocado; ½ cup celery sticks; ½ cup carrot sticks; and 5 or 6 tomato slices

Dinner   **Snapper Vera Cruz**

1 cup skim milk or one container any 2:90 yogurt with fiber (providing up to 90 calories)

MEN: Add 6 almonds

Reality Reward   **Orange Panna Cotta**

1 dessert starch of your choice (see Equivalents Lists, page 381)

Day 3   Wednesday Menu

Breakfast	**Apricot-Pecan Oatmeal** MEN: Add 1 slice of regular bread *Morning Dividend*
Lunch	**Toasted Tuna and Avocado Sandwich** MEN: Add ½ cup celery sticks; ½ cup carrot sticks; 5 or 6 tomato slices; 2 tablespoons chopped avocado
Dinner	**Shrimp Cocktail Salad** 1 cup skim milk or one container any 2:90 yogurt with fiber (providing up to 90 calories) MEN: Add 2 tablespoons chopped avocado
Reality Reward	**Chocolate Milkshake** 1 medium Asian pear

Day 4   Thursday Menu

Breakfast

1 serving 2:90 calcium-fortified dry or hot cereal (providing up to 90 calories)

1 cup skim milk or one container 2:90 peach yogurt with fiber (providing up to 90 calories)

8 walnut halves

1½ cups cantaloupe slices

MEN: Add ¼ cup 2:90 granola

Morning Dividend

Lunch

BBQ Veggie Burger

Ten 2:90 potato chips (low-fat gourmet baked potato chips, such as Kettle Krisps) or 8 Garden of Eatin' Black Bean tortilla chips

MEN: Add 1 mozzarella string cheese (with no more than 4 grams of total fat per string) and 2 tablespoons chopped avocado

Dinner

Cuban Black Bean Soup

1 cup skim milk or one container any 2:90 yogurt with fiber (providing up to 90 calories)

Reality Reward

Blackberry Cheescake (see pages 340–342)

Day 5   Friday Menu

Breakfast   **Cashew Butter Waffle**
                 1 cup skim milk or one container 2:90 peach yogurt with
                 fiber (providing up to 90 calories)
                 MEN: Add 1 serving 2:90 hot cereal
                 Morning Dividend

Lunch   **Manhattan Hot Dog with Sauerkraut**
                 Ten 2:90 potato chips (low-fat gourmet baked potato chips,
                 such as Kettle Krisps) or 8 Garden of Eatin' Black Bean
                 tortilla chips
                 MEN: Add 1 mozzarella string cheese (with no more than
                 4 grams of total fat per string); 2 tablespoons chopped
                 avocado; ½ cup celery sticks; ½ cup carrot sticks;
                 5 or 6 tomato slices

Dinner   **Paprika Chicken**
                 ½ cup skim milk or one container 2:90 peach yogurt with
                 fiber (providing up to 90 calories)
                 MEN: Add 4 pecan halves

Reality Reward   **Chocolate-Banana Cake**
                 ½ cup low-fat cottage cheese (up to 1% milkfat)

Day 6   Saturday Menu

Breakfast

1 serving 2:90 calcium-fortified dry or hot cereal (providing up to 90 calories)

1 cup skim milk or one container 2:90 strawberry yogurt with fiber (providing up to 90 calories)

1½ cups honeydew melon slices

12 cashews

MEN: Add 1 serving 2:90 dry cereal

Morning Dividend

Lunch

Canadian Bacon Pizza

MEN: Add ½ cup celery sticks; ½ cup carrot sticks; 5 or 6 tomato slices; 1 mozzarella string cheese (with no more than 4 grams of total fat per string); and 10 peanuts

Dinner

Swordfish Kebabs

1 cup skim milk or one container any 2:90 yogurt with fiber (providing up to 90 calories)

MEN: Add 4 pecan halves

Reality Reward

Chocolate-Banana Cake

½ cup low-fat cottage cheese

Day 7   Sunday Menu

Breakfast

Cherry-Almond Granola Parfait (see pages 216–217)

MEN: Add ¼ cup 2:90 granola

Morning Dividend

Lunch

Greek-Style Pasta

MEN: Add 6 cashews

Dinner

Dijon Flounder

1 cup skim milk or one container any 2:90 yogurt with fiber
(providing up to 90 calories)

MEN: Add 4 pecan halves

Reality Reward

Chocolate Milkshake

1 medium Asian pear

Monday

Cinnamon Toast Sandwich with Dried Plums

Cinnamon and raisins are always a great combination. The dried plums lend a unique tart flavor, giving a new twist to the combo.

    2 slices light 2:90 bread
    2 tablespoons light margarine
    2 teaspoons ground cinnamon
    2 teaspoons sugar substitute
    4½ dried plums, pitted and chopped

Preheat the broiler. Toast the bread and spread with the margarine. Mix the cinnamon with the sugar substitute and sprinkle on the toast. Place the toast under the broiler until a glaze forms. Remove the toast from the broiler and top one slice with the chopped dried plums. Top with the second slice of bread. Close the sandwich and cut in half diagonally.

Serves 1

CALORIES 260; FIBER 10g; FAT 11g; PROTEIN 5g; CARB 42g; SODIUM 440mg

Turkey and Watercress Sandwich

Watercress is a member of the mustard family, which means its flavor is sharp and peppery.

    1 cup watercress (thick stems removed)
    2 teaspoons fresh lemon juice
    ¼ teaspoon freshly ground black pepper
    1 tablespoon reduced-fat mayonnaise
    2 slices regular 2:90 bread
    1½ ounces deli turkey meat (with more than 1 but no more than 3 grams of
        fat per ounce)   MEN: 3 ounces
    4 tomato slices
    ¼ cup sliced spring onions or scallions

Combine the watercress, lemon juice, and pepper in the bowl of a food processor and blend until the watercress is finely chopped. Add the mayonnaise and pulse to combine to make a pesto.

Spread equal amounts of the pesto over each slice of bread. Top 1 slice of bread with the turkey, tomato slices, and spring onions. Cover with the second slice of bread and cut the sandwich in half diagonally.

Serves 1

WOMEN: CALORIES 300; FIBER 7g; FAT 8g; PROTEIN 19g; CARB 42g; SODIUM 750mg

MEN: CALORIES 340; FIBER 7g; FAT 10g; PROTEIN 28g; CARB 42g; SODIUM 990mg

Parmesan Chicken

This Parmesan chicken for the heart- and waistline-conscious is a refreshing change of pace. It's great with the Cooked Mixed Greens (recipe follows) served alongside.

2 teaspoons grated Parmesan cheese

1 teaspoon paprika

⅛ teaspoon cayenne pepper

½ teaspoon garlic powder

3 ounces boneless, skinless chicken breast, cut into strips
   (will yield 2½ ounces cooked)

Nonstick cooking spray

1 tablespoon light margarine

In a medium bowl, combine the Parmesan, paprika, cayenne, and garlic powder. Rub the mixture onto the chicken pieces and set aside.

Heat an 8-inch nonstick skillet over medium-high heat. Spray with nonstick cooking spray. Add the margarine and let it melt. Arrange the chicken pieces in the skillet and cook for 2 to 3 minutes per side, or until golden-brown on both sides.

MEN: *Sprinkle the chicken with the chopped pecans from the menu list just before serving.*

Serves 1

CALORIES 160; FIBER 0g; FAT 9g; PROTEIN 21g; CARB 0g; SODIUM 160mg

Cooked Mixed Greens

Chard is a member of the beet family and kale is a sibling of cabbage. Both pack a respectable punch of iron and vitamins A and C.

1 cup Swiss chard, woody stems trimmed
½ cup kale, woody stems trimmed
1½ cups mustard greens, woody stems trimmed   MEN: 3 cups
Nonstick cooking spray
2 teaspoons minced fresh garlic   MEN: 4 teaspoons
1 teaspoon white wine vinegar   MEN: 2 teaspoons
Hot sauce

Chop the chard, kale, and mustard greens into bite-size pieces and blanch for 5 minutes in a pot of boiling water. Drain and set aside.

Heat an 8-inch nonstick skillet over medium-high heat. Spray with non-stick cooking spray. Add the garlic and sauté for 1 minute, then add the blanched greens. Sprinkle with the vinegar and hot sauce to taste and cook until heated through.

Serves 1
WOMEN: CALORIES 60; FIBER 4g; FAT 2g; PROTEIN 4g; CARB 9g; SODIUM 110mg
MEN: CALORIES 80; FIBER 7g; FAT 2g; PROTEIN 6g; CARB 13g; SODIUM 135mg

Key Lime Cheesecake

Key limes have a unique flavor that distinguishes them from other limes. Sometimes they're a challenge to find, though, so substitute regular limes if necessary.

Nonstick cooking spray
½ teaspoon unflavored gelatin
2 tablespoons cool water
⅓ cup Kellogg's All-Bran Bran Buds cereal
2 tablespoons sugar substitute

2 tablespoons light margarine, melted

½ cup low-fat cottage cheese (containing up to 1% milkfat)

1 teaspoon vanilla extract

1 teaspoon Key lime juice

1 teaspoon lime zest

1½ cups raspberries

Spray a round casserole dish (5 inches in diameter) with nonstick cooking spray.

In a small bowl, whisk together the gelatin and water and let sit until the gelatin is dissolved, about 5 minutes. In a small bowl, crush the cereal to a lumpy powder and mix with 1 tablespoon of the sugar substitute and the melted margarine. Press the cereal mixture into the bottom of the prepared casserole dish to form a crust.

In the bowl of a food processor, combine the cottage cheese, remaining 1 tablespoon sugar substitute, the vanilla, lime juice, lime zest, and dissolved gelatin. Pulse several times to combine, then run the processor until the mixture is smooth, about 60 seconds.

Pour the cottage cheese mixture over the crust and wrap tightly with plastic wrap. Refrigerate for at least 2 hours before serving. Top with the raspberries just before serving.

Serves 1

CALORIES 360; FIBER 12g; FAT 14g; PROTEIN 22g; CARB 55g; SODIUM 400mg

FOR CHOCOLATE-CHERRY CHEESECAKE

Substitute 1 teaspoon chocolate extract and 1 teaspoon unsweetened cocoa powder for the lime juice and lime zest. After pulsing the processor to combine the cottage cheese mixture, add ¼ cup of fresh cherries and run until mixture is smooth, about 60 seconds. Top with 1½ cup fresh cherries and whipped topping just before serving.

CALORIES 360; FIBER 17g; FAT 15g; PROTEIN 18g; CARB 52g; SODIUM 420mg

FOR BLACKBERRY CHEESECAKE

Reduce amount of sugar substitute in cottage cheese mixture to 1 teaspoon. Substitute 1 teaspoon fresh lemon juice for lime juice and lime zest. Add ¼ cup blackberries (substitute frozen blackberries with no sugar added when blackberries aren't in season) after pulsing to combine the cottage cheese mixture, and run the processor until smooth, about 60 seconds. Top with ⅛ cup blackberries and whipped topping just before serving.

CALORIES 350; FIBER 13g; FAT 14g; PROTEIN 19g; CARB 49g; SODIUM 420mg

Tuesday

Tuscan Panino

Panini are pressed sandwiches, traditionally made in a panini press to help marry the flavors.

    2 teaspoons prepared pesto
    2 slices regular 2:90 bread
    1 mozzarella string cheese (no more than 4 grams
        of total fat per serving), cut lengthwise into ¼-inch slices   MEN: 2 string
        cheeses
    1 roasted red bell pepper (from a jar, packed in water)
    1 cup spinach leaves
    3 or 4 fresh basil leaves
    Nonstick cooking spray
    Aged balsamic vinegar
    Freshly ground black pepper
    5 or 6 tomato slices
    Balsamic vinegar, to taste

Spread 1 teaspoon of the pesto over each slice of bread. Layer the next 4 ingredients onto the bread in the following order: mozzarella slices, roasted bell pepper, spinach, and basil. Top with the second slice of bread.

Heat an 8-inch nonstick skillet over medium-low heat. Spray with nonstick cooking spray. Place the panino in the skillet and press it down gently by placing a clean second skillet on top of the panino. Grill for 2 minutes, turn it over, and press again with the skillet. Grill for another 2 minutes, or until golden-brown.

Remove the panino from the skillet, open it, and drizzle with vinegar and black pepper to taste.

MEN: *Drizzle the sliced tomatoes and avocado from the menu list with balsamic vinegar.*

Serves 1

WOMEN CALORIES 300; FIBER 8g; FAT 9g; PROTEIN 17g; CARB 43g; SODIUM 700mg

MEN CALORIES 350; FIBER 8g; FAT 12g; PROTEIN 23g; CARB 44g; SODIUM 880mg

Snapper Veracruz

Expect a tangy array of onions, tomatoes, olives, peppers, and capers when a dish is called "Veracruz." Use halibut if snapper isn't available.

Nonstick cooking spray

One 3-ounce red snapper fillet

1 tablespoon fresh lime juice, plus more to taste

1 teaspoon chili powder

¼ cup chopped scallions   MEN: ½ cup

1 teaspoon olive oil

½ cup chopped tomato   MEN: 1 cup

¼ cup chopped red and green bell peppers   MEN: ¾ cup

5 pitted green olives, chopped

2 teaspoons drained capers, chopped

¼ cup baby spinach leaves   MEN: ½ cup

1¼ cups mustard greens, cooked

Freshly ground black pepper

Heat an 8-inch nonstick skillet over medium-high heat. Spray with non-stick cooking spray. Place the snapper fillet in the skillet and add with the lime juice and chili powder.

Cook the fillet for 2 minutes on each side. Move the fish to the side of the pan and add the scallions. Cook for 2 minutes, stirring once. Add the olive oil, tomatoes, bell peppers, olives, and capers. Cook for another 2 to 3 minutes, or until the vegetables are crisp-tender.

Remove the fish from the skillet and place on a dinner plate over a bed of the baby spinach and cooked mustard greens. Spoon the vegetables over the fish and season with lime juice and black pepper to taste.

Serves 1

WOMEN: CALORIES 230; FIBER 4g; FAT 11g; PROTEIN 21g; CARB 13g; SODIUM 570mg

MEN: CALORIES 280; FIBER 5g; FAT 12g; PROTEIN 22g; CARB 23g; SODIUM 590mg

Orange Panna Cotta

Panna cotta means "cooked cream" in Italian and is typically served with fruit and cookies. This version is simplified for easy home cooking.

¼ teaspoon unflavored gelatin

1 tablespoon cold water

½ cup low-fat cottage cheese (containing up to 1% milkfat)

2 teaspoons sugar substitute

1 teaspoon vanilla extract

1 tablespoon orange zest

1 large orange, peeled and sliced

8 toasted pecan halves, chopped

Sprinkle the gelatin over the cold water. Let stand for 5 minutes.

In the bowl of a food processor, combine the cottage cheese, sugar substitute, and vanilla and process until the mixture is very smooth, about 60 seconds, scraping down the sides of the bowl as needed.

Add the gelatin, orange zest, and half of the orange slices. Pulse the food processor a few times to mix. Spoon the mixture into a small bowl, cover, and chill in the refrigerator for at least 1 hour. Garnish with the pecans and remaining orange slices.

Serves 1

CALORIES 260; FIBER 6g; FAT 10g; PROTEIN 17g; CARB 29g; SODIUM 15mg

Wednesday

Apricot-Pecan Oatmeal

Having a big bowl of oatmeal is a great way to start the day. Buy plain rolled oats and doctor your oatmeal to customize the flavors to your taste.

1 serving 2:90 rolled oatmeal
1 cup skim milk
12 dried apricots halves, chopped
Pinch of ground nutmeg
8 toasted pecan halves, chopped

In a medium saucepan over medium heat combine all of the ingredients except the pecans. Bring the mixture to a boil, cover, reduce the heat to low, and simmer for about 5 minutes, stirring occasionally, until the oats are soft and the milk is absorbed. Spoon into a bowl and top with the toasted pecans.

Serves 1

CALORIES 370; FIBER 6g; FAT 10g; PROTEIN 15g; CARB 55g; SODIUM 150mg

Toasted Tuna and Avocado Sandwich

This is a tuna sandwich deli-style!

1½ ounces canned light tuna, drained   MEN: 3 ounces
¾ cup thinly sliced red and yellow bell peppers
¼ cup chopped scallions
2 tablespoons chopped avocado
1 teaspoon reduced-fat mayonnaise
1 teaspoon Dijon mustard
1 teaspoon prepared horseradish
1 teaspoon fresh lemon juice

Freshly ground black pepper

2 slices regular 2:90 bread, toasted

½ cup mixed baby lettuce leaves

In a medium bowl, mix together the tuna, bell peppers, scallions, avocado, mayonnaise, mustard, horseradish, and lemon juice. Season with black pepper to taste.

Spread the tuna mixture on 1 slice of the toasted bread. Top with the lettuce. Cover with the second slice of toast and slice the sandwich in half diagonally.

Serves 1

WOMEN: CALORIES 320; FIBER 9g; FAT 6g; PROTEIN 21g; CARB 50g; SODIUM 730mg

MEN: CALORIES 370; FIBER 9g; FAT 8g; PROTEIN 31g; CARB 50g; SODIUM 900mg

Shrimp Cocktail Salad

Cooking shrimp in their shells will help the shrimp keep their natural shape and size. The dressing can be made in advance to save time before dinner.

1 tablespoon prepared cocktail sauce

2 teaspoons prepared horseradish

Juice of ½ lemon

2 teaspoons olive oil

Hot sauce

2 cups water

1 tablespoon white wine vinegar

2 cloves garlic, crushed

3 ounces unpeeled shrimp (will yield 2½ ounces cooked)

¼ cup shredded iceberg or romaine lettuce   MEN: ½ cup

¼ cup chopped cucumber   MEN: ½ cup

¼ cup sliced radishes   MEN: ½ cup

¼ cup sliced celery   MEN: 1 cup

½ cup chopped scallions

½ cup halved cherry tomatoes   MEN: 1 cup

In a small bowl, whisk together the cocktail sauce, horseradish, lemon juice, olive oil, and hot sauce to taste. Cover and chill until ready to serve.

Combine the water, vinegar, and garlic in a large saucepan and bring to a boil. Add the shrimp, cover, and cook over low heat for 2 minutes, or until the shrimp are pink and firm. Drain and rinse immediately in cold water to stop the cooking. Peel the shrimp and refrigerate.

In a medium bowl, toss the lettuce, cucumber, radishes, celery, scallions, and tomatoes with the half dressing. Place the salad in a large wine glass, arrange the shrimp around the rim, and drizzle with the remaining dressing.

Serves 1

WOMEN: CALORIES 250; FIBER 5g; FAT 12g; PROTEIN 19g; CARB 17g; SODIUM 380mg

MEN: CALORIES 290; FIBER 6g; FAT 12g; PROTEIN 21g; CARB 26g; SODIUM 470mg

Chocolate Milkshake

It might seem odd to add cottage cheese to a milkshake, but it gives this milkshake its creamy texture.

1 frozen fudge bar, stick removed, cut into 3 pieces

½ cup low-fat cottage cheese (containing up to 1% milkfat)

1 teaspoon vanilla extract

1 tablespoon natural peanut butter

1 tablespoon unsweetened cocoa powder

1 tablespoon sugar substitute

2 or 3 ice cubes

Combine all of the ingredients in a blender and blend until smooth. Pour into a tall frosted glass.

Serves 1

CALORIES 300; FIBER 4g; FAT 13g; PROTEIN 22g; CARB 27g; SODIUM 75mg

Substitute 1 medium banana for peanut butter and unsweetened cocoa powder. Substitute 1 teaspoon chocolate extract for vanilla extract.

CALORIES 260; FIBER 3g; FAT 5g; PROTEIN 18g; CARB 39g; SODIUM 75mg

Thursday

BBQ Veggie Burger

If you like a spicier barbecue sauce, mix in a pinch of chipotle chili powder. Chipotles are smoked jalapeño chiles. The powder can be found in most upscale supermarkets.

Nonstick cooking spray
1 veggie burger patty
One 2:90 hamburger bun
1 tablespoon reduced-fat mayonnaise
1 tablespoon barbecue sauce (containing no fat and with about 15 calories per tablespoon)
½ cup shredded iceberg lettuce   MEN: 1 cup
2 tomato slices   MEN: 4 tomato slices
¼ cup chopped scallions   MEN: ½ cup
Freshly ground black pepper
½ cup sliced yellow and red bell peppers   MEN: 1 cup
½ cup sliced cucumber   MEN: 1 cup
Lemon juice, to taste

Heat an 8-inch nonstick skillet over medium heat. Spray with nonstick cooking spray. Cook the veggie burger patty for 3 to 4 minutes on each side, or until heated through.

Spread both sides of the bun with the mayonnaise. Place the cooked veggie burger on the bottom half of the bun, spread with the barbecue sauce, and top with ½ cup lettuce, 2 tomato slices, and ¼ cup scallions. Season with black pepper to taste and top with the top half of the bun.

MEN AND WOMEN: *Make a side salad with the extra veggies that don't fit on your burger. Dress the salad with lemon juice and freshly ground black pepper.*

Serves 1

WOMEN: CALORIES 270; FIBER 8g; FAT 3.5g; PROTEIN 11g; CARB 55g; SODIUM 780mg

MEN: CALORIES 320; FIBER 10g; FAT 3.5g; PROTEIN 12g; CARB 65g; SODIUM 790mg

Cuban Black Bean Soup

This soup is best when start you with dried black beans. If you use canned beans, make sure they are low in sodium.

Nonstick cooking spray

1 teaspoon olive oil   MEN: 2 teaspoons

¼ cup chopped red onion   MEN: ½ cup

¼ cup chopped red and green bell peppers   MEN: ½ cup

½ cup chopped celery   MEN: 1 cup

1 tablespoon minced garlic   MEN: 4 teaspoons

⅛ teaspoon cayenne pepper

¼ teaspoon ground cumin

1 teaspoon chili powder   MEN: 2 teaspoons

½ cup chopped tomato   MEN: 1 cup

½ cup cooked black beans

½ cup natural (fat-free, reduced sodium) chicken broth

1 tablespoon apple cider vinegar

2 tablespoons fresh orange juice

1 tablespoon fresh chopped cilantro   MEN: 2 tablespoons

Heat the olive oil in a heavy soup pot over medium-high heat. Spray with nonstick cooking spray. Add the olive oil, red onions, bell peppers, celery, and garlic. Cook, stirring frequently, for 5 minutes, or until the vegetables have softened. Add the cayenne, cumin, and chili powder. Stir well and cook for 30 seconds. Add the tomatoes and black beans and cook for another 2 minutes. Add the chicken broth and vinegar, bring to a boil, then reduce the heat to low and simmer, covered, for 10 minutes.

Stir in the orange juice and cilantro just before serving.

Serves 1

WOMEN: CALORIES 220; FIBER 8g; FAT 8g; PROTEIN 10g; CARB 33g; SODIUM 530mg

MEN: CALORIES 310; FIBER 9g; FAT 13g; PROTEIN 12g; CARB 45g; SODIUM 580mg

Friday

Cashew Butter Waffle

The flavors and nutrients in the waffle will help you get your day off to a great start.

   1 tablespoon cashew butter

   One 2:90 whole-wheat or multigrain waffle, toasted

   2 pitted dates, chopped

   1½ tablespoons raisins

   1 teaspoon sugar substitute

   ½ teaspoon ground cinnamon

Heat the cashew butter for 10 to 15 seconds in the microwave to soften it. Spread the cashew butter evenly over the waffle and sprinkle with the chopped dates, raisins, sugar substitute, and cinnamon. Cut into quarters.

Serves 1

CALORIES 270; FIBER 3g; FAT 11g; PROTEIN 6g; CARB 42g; SODIUM 220mg

Manhattan Hot Dog with Sauerkraut

This hot dog can be boiled or broiled depending on your taste and time. Boiling the dog will make it taste like it came from a corner cart in midtown Manhattan. Add the salad and a fork and knife for an uptown feel.

   1 tablespoon reduced-fat mayonnaise

   2 teaspoons German-style coarse-grain mustard

   ¼ cup chopped onion

½ cup chopped celery

¾ cup chopped green bell pepper

1 teaspoon chopped fresh flat-leaf parsley

One 2:90 hot dog bun

One 1-ounce hot dog (with between 1 and 3 grams of fat per ounce)

1 ounce cheese (with more than 1 gram but no more than 3 grams of fat
    per ounce), chopped

2 tablespoons prepared low-sodium sauerkraut

In a small bowl, combine the mayonnaise, mustard, onion, celery, bell pepper, and parsley.

Fill a small saucepan with water, bring to a boil, add the hot dog, and boil for 5 minutes, or until heated through. Drain.

Spread the inside of the bun with the salad mixture and top with the hot dog and cheese. Garnish with the sauerkraut.

Serves 1

CALORIES 250; FIBER 7g; FAT 5g; PROTEIN 23g; CARB 34g; SODIUM 910mg

Paprika Chicken

Paprika chicken is Hungary's most popular dish. Paprika is like curry powder in that home cooks and chefs alike have their own personal blends. Some are spicy and others are sweet.

3 ounces boneless, skinless chicken breast, cut into 1-inch pieces (will
    yield 2½ ounces cooked)

1 teaspoon freshly ground black pepper

Nonstick cooking spray

1 teaspoon canola oil

½ cup sliced button mushrooms   MEN: 1 cup

¼ cup chopped yellow onion   MEN: ½ cup

2 teaspoons minced garlic

1 cup chopped tomatoes   MEN: 2 cups

1 tablespoon paprika

¼ cup prepared tomato sauce

½ cup water

¼ cup plain non-fat yogurt

2 tablespoons chopped fresh flat-leaf parsley

Season the chicken pieces with the black pepper.

Heat a medium saucepan over medium-high heat. Spray with nonstick cooking spray, then add the oil. When the oil is hot, add the chicken pieces and brown each side, turning once. Transfer to a bowl. Add the mushrooms, onions, garlic, and tomatoes to the saucepan and cook for 3 to 5 minutes, or until softened.

Stir in the paprika, tomato sauce, water, and yogurt. Return the chicken pieces to the saucepan and simmer, covered, over low heat until the chicken is tender, about 5 minutes. Sprinkle with the parsley.

Serves 1

WOMEN: CALORIES 250; FIBER 3g; FAT 8g; PROTEIN 26g; CARB 24g; SODIUM 110mg

MEN: CALORIES 310; FIBER 6g; FAT 9g; PROTEIN 29g; CARB 37g; SODIUM 130mg

Chocolate-Banana Cake

Chocolate and bananas are a combination made in kid heaven. Revert to your childhood and enjoy this cake with the vigor of youth.

1 tablespoon light margarine

1 tablespoon unsweetened cocoa powder

1 tablespoon sugar substitute

1 teaspoon vanilla extract

1 teaspoon chocolate extract

¼ cup water

3½ tablespoons whole-wheat flour

½ teaspoon baking powder

4 toasted walnut halves, chopped

1 medium banana, sliced

Preheat the oven to 375°F. Spray a round casserole dish (5 inches in diameter) with nonstick cooking spray.

In a medium microwaveable bowl, combine the margarine and cocoa powder. Melt for 10 to 15 seconds in the microwave. Stir in the sugar substitute, vanilla, chocolate extract, and water. Fold in the flour, baking powder, walnuts, and banana slices.

Spoon the batter into the prepared casserole dish and bake for 15 to 20 minutes, or until a skewer inserted into the center comes out clean. Allow the cake to cool slightly, and then eat it from the casserole dish.

Serves 1

CALORIES 290; FIBER 7g; FAT 11g; PROTEIN 6g; CARB 44g; SODIUM 105mg

Saturday

Canadian Bacon Pizza

Get ready! This pizza is piled high with tasty toppings. If you choose to broil it at the end, keep a close eye on it so your hard work doesn't burn.

Nonstick cooking spray
One 2:90 whole-wheat or flatbread pita
½ cup prepared tomato sauce
4 slices Canadian bacon, chopped
¼ cup baby spinach leaves
½ cup thinly sliced mushrooms
¼ cup chopped green bell pepper
½ cup chopped scallions
8 large pitted black olives, sliced (high sodium)
2 teaspoons grated Parmesan cheese
½ teaspoon dried oregano
½ teaspoon dried basil
Crushed red pepper flakes (optional)

Preheat the oven to 450°F. Spray a nonstick baking sheet with nonstick cooking spray. Place the flatbread on the baking sheet. Spread the tomato sauce over the crust, leaving a 1-inch border around the rim.

Heat an 8-inch nonstick skillet over medium heat. Spray with nonstick cooking spray. Add the bacon, spinach, mushrooms, bell pepper, scallions, and olives, and cook for 8 to 10 minutes, or until the vegetables have softened.

Spoon the bacon mixture on top of the tomato pasta sauce and sprinkle with the Parmesan, oregano, basil, and red pepper flakes, if using.

Place in the oven and bake for 8 to 10 minutes, or until the flatbread is crisp. If you like, turn the oven to broil for the last couple of minutes to crisp the top.

Serves 1

CALORIES 380; FIBER 3g; FAT 11g; PROTEIN 17g; CARB 64g; SODIUM 900mg

Swordfish Kebabs

There are as many tasty choices to skewer on a stick as there are ways to spell "kebab." The only limit is your imagination. The hot kebabs will wilt and dress the bed of baby spinach.

1 teaspoon extra-virgin olive oil

1 tablespoon minced fresh garlic   MEN: 4 teaspoons

2 tablespoons fresh lime juice   MEN: 3 tablespoons

½ teaspoon freshly ground black pepper

One 3-ounce swordfish fillet, cut into 1-inch pieces

½ cup cherry tomatoes, halved   MEN: 1 cup

¼ cup green bell pepper, cut into 1-inch pieces   MEN: ½ cup

½ cup button mushrooms   MEN: 1 cup

½ cup zucchini, cut into 1-inch pieces   MEN: 1 cup

1 cup baby spinach leaves   MEN: 2 cups

In a medium bowl, whisk together the olive oil, garlic, lime juice, and black pepper. Add the swordfish pieces, cover, and marinate for at least 10 minutes and up to 2 hours.

Set a rack at the highest level of the oven and preheat to broil. Soak two bamboo skewers in water to cover for 10 minutes.

Thread the swordfish and vegetables on the bamboo skewers, alternating the pieces according to color. Place the skewers on a pie plate and drizzle with any remaining marinade. Broil for 4 to 5 minutes on each side, or until the swordfish is cooked through. Place the baby spinach on a plate and serve the hot skewers on the spinach.

MEN: *Make a third skewer with the extra vegetables.*

Serves 1

WOMEN: CALORIES 190; FIBER 3g; FAT 9g; PROTEIN 20g; CARB 9g; SODIUM 115mg

MEN CALORIES 290; FIBER 6g; FAT 9g; PROTEIN 24g; CARB 19g; SODIUM 150mg

Sunday

Greek-Style Pasta

Dishes like this get better with age, and this one is equally delicious served either hot or cold. Cook it the night before to get a jump start on lunch.

Nonstick cooking spray

1 cup sliced zucchini   MEN: 1½ cups

1 cup halved cherry tomatoes   MEN: 2 cups

½ cup baby spinach leaves   MEN: 1 cup

⅔ cup cooked 2:90 penne

1 ounce reduced-fat feta cheese (with no more than 4 grams of total fat per ounce)   MEN: 2 ounces

1 teaspoon chopped fresh flat-leaf parsley

3 or 4 chopped fresh basil leaves   MEN: 6 to 8 leaves

1 teaspoon garlic powder   MEN: 1½ teaspoons

½ teaspoon dried oregano   MEN: 1 teaspoon

1 teaspoon extra-virgin olive oil

1 teaspoon fresh lemon juice

Heat an 8-inch nonstick skillet over medium-high heat. Spray with non-stick cooking spray. Add the zucchini and sauté for 2 to 3 minutes, or until softened. Add the tomatoes and spinach and cook for another 2 to 3 minutes. Stir in the cooked pasta, feta cheese, parsley, and basil. Add the garlic powder, oregano, olive oil, and lemon juice and stir to combine.

Serves 1

WOMEN: CALORIES 340; FIBER 8g; FAT 11g; PROTEIN 17g; CARB 52g; SODIUM 410mg

MEN: CALORIES 430; FIBER 10g; FAT 14g; PROTEIN 25g; CARB 63g; SODIUM 810mg

Dijon Flounder

Flounder fillets are very thin and delicate, so keep a watchful eye while cooking and a gentle hand when lifting the fillet from pan to plate.

1 tablespoon Dijon mustard

1 tablespoon reduced-fat mayonnaise

1 teaspoon chopped fresh flat-leaf parsley   MEN: 2 teaspoons

¼ teaspoon freshly ground black pepper   MEN: ½ teaspoon

Nonstick cooking spray

One 3-ounce flounder fillet (will yield 2½ ounces cooked)

1 cup halved cherry tomatoes   MEN: 2 cups

½ cup sliced zucchini   MEN: 1 cup

3 spears asparagus, cut into 1-inch pieces   MEN: 6 spears

2 tablespoons water

Juice of ½ lemon

Set a rack at the highest level of the oven and preheat to broil.

In a small bowl, whisk together the mustard, mayonnaise, parsley, and black pepper. Spray a small baking pan with nonstick cooking spray, place the flounder in the pan, and brush with the mustard mixture. Broil the flounder for 3 to 4 minutes, until it flakes to the touch, watching carefully so that it doesn't burn.

Heat an 8-inch nonstick skillet over medium heat. Spray with nonstick cooking spray. Add the tomatoes, zucchini, asparagus, and water and cook for 5 minutes, or until the vegetables are tender. Spoon the vegetables over the flounder and drizzle with the lemon juice.

Serves 1

WOMEN: CALORIES 170; FIBER 4g; FAT 3.5g; PROTEIN 22g; CARB 16g; SODIUM 570mg

MEN: CALORIES 230; FIBER 7g; FAT 4g; PROTEIN 25g; CARB 28g; SODIUM 590mg

Week 8

Day 1   Monday Menu

Breakfast
Apricot-Pecan Oatmeal
MEN: Add 1 slice regular bread
Morning Dividend*

Lunch
Canadian Bacon Pizza
MEN: Add ½ cup celery sticks; ½ cup carrot sticks; 5 or 6 tomato slices; 1 mozzarella string cheese (with no more than 4 grams of total fat per string); and 10 peanuts

Dinner
Vegetarian Cassoulet
1 cup skim milk or one container any 2:90 yogurt with fiber (providing up to 90 calories)

Reality Reward
Banana-Chocolate Milkshake (see pages 347–348)
¼ cup pistachios in the shell

---

*Morning Dividend—Choose one sweetener OR one creamer from the following: 1 teaspoon honey, 1 teaspoon white granulated sugar, or 1 teaspoon brown sugar OR 2 tablespoons 2% milk, 1 tablespoon half-and-half, 1 tablespoon soymilk creamer, 1 tablespoon nondairy liquid creamer, 2 teaspoons nondairy powdered creamer

Recipe items are in boldface.

Day 2   Tuesday Menu

Breakfast	1 serving 2:90 calcium-fortified dry or hot cereal (providing up to 90 calories) 1 cup skim milk or one container 2:90 apple yogurt with fiber (providing up to 90 calories) 2 tablespoons flaxseeds 6 fresh apricots MEN: Add 1 slice of regular bread *Morning Dividend*
Lunch	**Toasted Tuna and Avocado Sandwich** MEN: Add ½ cup celery sticks; ½ cup carrot sticks; 5 or 6 slices of tomato; and 2 tablespoons chopped avocado
Dinner	**Caribbean Jerk Chicken** 1 cup skim milk or one container any 2:90 yogurt with fiber (providing up to 90 calories) MEN: Add 10 peanuts
Reality Reward	**Cranberry-Almond Bars** ½ cup non-fat or low-fat cottage cheese

Day 3   Wednesday Menu

Breakfast   **Gingerbread Waffle**
1 cup skim milk or one container 2:90 peach yogurt with
fiber (providing up to 90 calories)
1 tablespoon flaxseeds
MEN: Add ¼ cup 2:90 granola
Morning Dividend

Lunch   **Mushroom and Cheese Quesadilla**
with Fresh Guacamole Dip
MEN: Add 1 mozzarella string cheese (with no more than
4 grams of total fat per string); 2 tablespoons chopped
avocado; ½ cup celery sticks; ½ cup carrot sticks; and
5 or 6 tomato slices

Dinner   **Seafood Provençal**
1 cup skim milk or one container of any 2:90 yogurt with
fiber (providing up to 90 calories)
MEN: Add ½ cup celery sticks and 6 whole almonds

Reality Reward   **Cranberry-Almond Bars**
½ cup non-fat or low-fat cottage cheese (up to 1% milkfat)

Day 4   Thursday Menu

Breakfast   1 serving 2:90 calcium-fortified dry or hot cereal (providing
                 up to 90 calories)
                 1 cup skim milk or one container 2:90 apple yogurt with
                 fiber (providing up to 90 calories)
                 12 mixed nuts
                 7 ounces unsweetened applesauce
                 MEN: Add 1 slice of regular bread
                 Morning Dividend

Lunch   **Moo-Shu Chicken Wraps**
                 MEN: Add 10 peanuts

Dinner   **Ham-Wrapped Vegetables with Black Olive Tapenade**
                 1 cup skim milk or one container any 2:90 yogurt with fiber
                 (providing up to 90 calories)
                 MEN: Add 2 tablespoons chopped avocado and ½ cup
                 cooked okra

Reality Reward   **Panna Cotta with Dates**
                 12 cashews
                 1 dessert starch of your choice (see Equivalents Lists,
                 page 381)

Day 5   Friday Menu

Breakfast   **Grilled Banana Sandwich**

1 cup skim milk or one container 2:90 vanilla yogurt with
fiber (providing up to 90 calories)

MEN: Add 1 cup 2:90 dry cereal

Morning Dividend

Lunch   **Turkey and Watercress Sandwich**

½ cup jicama sticks

MEN: Add ½ cup celery sticks; ½ cup carrot sticks; 5 or 6
tomato slices; and 2 tablespoons chopped avocado

Dinner   **Vegetarian Stir-fry with Garlic Sauce**

1 cup skim milk or one container any 2:90 yogurt with fiber
(providing up to 90 calories)

MEN: Add 10 peanuts

Reality Reward   **Chocolate-Cherry Cheesecake** (see pages 340–341)

Day 6   Saturday Menu

Breakfast   1 serving 2:90 calcium-fortified dry or hot cereal (providing
up to 90 calories)
1 cup skim milk or one container 2:90 strawberry yogurt
with fiber (providing up to 90 calories)
1½ cups honeydew melon slices
2 tablespoons flaxseeds
MEN: Add ⅓ cup fruit muesli
Morning Dividend

Lunch   **Classic Hamburger**
Ten 2:90 potato chips (low-fat gourmet baked potato chips,
such as Kettle Krisps) or 8 Garden of Eatin' Black Bean
tortilla chips
MEN: Add ½ cup celery sticks; ½ cup carrot sticks;
1 mozzarella string cheese (with no more than 4 grams of
total fat per string); and 2 tablespoons chopped avocado

Dinner   **Spicy Cajun Shrimp Gumbo**
1 cup skim milk or one container of any 2:90 yogurt with
fiber (providing up to 90 calories)
MEN: Add 4 pecan halves

Reality Reward   **Fresh Peaches and Smoked Ham**
12 cashews
1 dessert starch of your choice (see Equivalents Lists,
page 381)

Day 7   Sunday Menu

Breakfast   1 serving 2:90 calcium-fortified dry or hot cereal (providing
up to 90 calories)
1 cup skim milk or one container 2:90 peach yogurt with
fiber (providing up to 90 calories)
1 tablespoon natural peanut butter
1 medium Asian pear
MEN: Add ⅓ cup fruit muesli
Morning Dividend

Lunch   **Salmon Croquettes**
MEN: Add 1 mozzarella string cheese (with no more than
4 grams of total fat per string) and 6 cashews

Dinner   **Lobster Thermidor over Warm Spinach Salad**
MEN: Add 4 pecan halves

Reality Reward   **Banana-Chocolate Milkshake** (see pages 347–348)
¼ cup pistachios in the shell

Monday

Vegetarian Cassoulet

Cassoulet is French for comfort food. It's warm and hearty, perfect for a chilly evening.

Nonstick cooking spray

1 teaspoon olive oil   MEN: 2 teaspoons

½ cup sliced scallions

2 teaspoons minced fresh garlic   MEN: 1 tablespoon

½ cup cooked navy beans

¼ cup sliced mushrooms   MEN: ½ cup

1 bay leaf

½ cup chopped Swiss chard   MEN: 1 cup

½ cup baby spinach leaves   MEN: 1 cup

1 tablespoon white wine vinegar

⅛ teaspoon ground white pepper   MEN: ¼ teaspoon

2 tablespoons chopped fresh flat-leaf parsley   MEN: 3 tablespoons

1 teaspoon chopped fresh thyme   MEN: 2 teaspoons

   MEN: ½ cup cooked collard greens

Preheat the oven to 375°F. Spray a round casserole dish (5 inches in diameter) with nonstick cooking spray.

Heat an 8-inch nonstick skillet over medium heat. Add the olive oil, scallions, garlic, beans, mushrooms, and bay leaf. Cook for 5 minutes, stirring often. Add the Swiss chard, spinach, vinegar, and pepper. Turn the heat to low and cook for another 5 minutes, stirring often, until the Swiss chard is wilted.

Spoon the mixture into the prepared casserole dish and bake for 15 minutes, or until bubbling. Remove the bay leaf and garnish with the parsley and thyme.

MEN: *Place the cooked collard greens on a large plate and spoon the cassoulet on top of the greens just before serving.*

Serves 1

WOMEN: CALORIES 180; FIBER 8g; FAT 7g; PROTEIN 8g; CARB 24g; SODIUM 65mg

MEN: CALORIES 240; FIBER 9g; FAT 12g; PROTEIN 10g; CARB 27g; SODIUM 120mg

Tuesday

Caribbean Jerk Chicken

Jerked meat dishes are traditionally very spicy. This version is more flavorful than hot, but if you like to eat fire, add more hot sauce and a pinch of cayenne pepper.

1 tablespoon chili sauce

2 teaspoons sugar substitute

2 tablespoons fresh lime juice

2 teaspoons minced fresh garlic

2 teaspoons minced fresh ginger

1 teaspoon hot sauce

⅛ teaspoon ground allspice

3 ounces boneless, skinless chicken breast, cut into 1-inch pieces
   (will yield 2½ ounces cooked)

Nonstick cooking spray

1 teaspoon peanut oil

¾ cup thinly sliced red and green bell peppers   MEN: 1½ cups

¼ cup chopped scallions   MEN: ½ cup

2 tablespoons chopped yellow onion   MEN: ½ cup

Measure the chili sauce, sugar substitute, lime juice, garlic, ginger, hot sauce, and allspice into a large resealable plastic bag. Add the chicken. Press the air out of the bag and seal tightly. Turn the bag to distribute the marinade. Refrigerate for 4 to 24 hours, turning occasionally.

Heat an 8-inch nonstick skillet over medium heat. Spray with nonstick cooking spray and add the oil. Remove the chicken from the marinade and discard the remaining marinade. Add the chicken and sauté for 3 minutes on each side, or until the juices run clear. Add the bell peppers, scallions, and onions, and cook for another 5 minutes, stirring often, until the vegetables have softened.

Serves 1

WOMEN: CALORIES 210; FIBER 1g; FAT 8g; PROTEIN 21g; CARB 16g; SODIUM 65mg

MEN: CALORIES 270; FIBER 3g; FAT 8g; PROTEIN 23g; CARB 30g; SODIUM 75mg

Cranberry-Almond Bars

These bars are packed with a delicious blend of dried fruit, granola, and almond butter. Who knew something so nutritious could taste so good? This recipe makes two servings, so save half for later this week.

½ cup 2:90 granola

6 tablespoons dried cranberries

4 tablespoons sugar substitute

1 teaspoon baking powder

2 tablespoons natural almond butter

Nonstick cooking spray

Preheat the oven to 375°F. In the bowl of a food processor, combine the granola, cranberries, sugar substitute, and baking powder and process for about 45 seconds to form a coarse paste. Scrape the granola mixture into a medium bowl and cream together with the almond butter just until the dough holds together.

Spray a nonstick baking sheet with nonstick cooking spray. With wet hands, compress the dough very tightly into four small rectangular bars. Place the bars on the prepared baking sheet and bake for 10 minutes, or until lightly browned. Remove carefully to a wire rack to cool slightly before eating.

Serves 2

CALORIES 270; FIBER 4g; FAT 12g; PROTEIN 5g; CARB 40g; SODIUM 140mg per single serving

Wednesday

Gingerbread Waffle

If you're willing to give up your coffee dividend, top with 2 tablespoons sugar-free syrup for a more decadent breakfast.

    1 tablespoon light margarine, softened
    ⅛ teaspoon ground cinnamon
    ⅛ teaspoon ground ginger
    Pinch of ground nutmeg
    Pinch of ground cloves
    1 teaspoon sugar substitute
    One 2:90 whole-wheat or multigrain waffle, toasted
    3 tablespoons raisins
    2 tablespoons sugar-free maple-flavored syrup (optional)

In a small bowl, cream together the margarine with the spices and sugar substitute, using a small wooden spoon. Spread the creamed margarine over the waffle and sprinkle with the raisins and syrup, if using.

Serves 1

CALORIES 230; FIBER 2g; FAT 8g; PROTEIN 3g; CARB 37g; SODIUM 320mg

Mushroom and Cheese Quesadilla with Fresh Guacamole Dip

The trick to a great quesadilla is to cook it slowly, so the veggie and cheese flavors melt together and the tortillas get golden and crispy.

    2 tablespoons chopped avocado
    ½ cup chopped tomato
    2 tablespoons chopped fresh cilantro leaves
    Fresh lime juice

Nonstick cooking spray

¾ cup chopped green and red bell peppers

¾ cup sliced mushrooms

¾ cup baby spinach leaves

Two 2:90 whole-wheat tortillas

1½ ounces cheddar cheese (with more than 1 but no more than 3 grams of fat per ounce)

Hot sauce

In a medium bowl, combine the avocado, tomatoes, cilantro, and lime juice to taste. Mix and smash the mixture together with a fork.

Heat an 8-inch nonstick skillet over medium-high heat. Spray with non-stick cooking spray. Add the bell peppers and mushrooms and sauté for 3 minutes, stirring often. Add the spinach and cook for another 30 seconds, or until wilted. Continue cooking until most of the vegetable liquid has evaporated. Spoon the vegetable mixture into a bowl.

Wipe out the skillet and spray again with nonstick cooking spray. Add 1 tortilla to the skillet. Top with the cheese and cooked vegetables. Top with the second tortilla. Cook over medium heat for 2 to 3 minutes, or until the tortilla has toasted. Flip the quesadilla and toast for 2 to 3 minutes on the other side. Remove the quesadilla from the skillet, cut it into quarters, and spoon the guacamole on each quarter. Drizzle a little hot sauce over the guacamole.

Serves 1

CALORIES 360; FIBER 19g; FAT 13g; PROTEIN 25g; CARB 38g; SODIUM 640mg

Seafood Provençal

An aromatic blend of garlic, tomatoes, mushrooms, and wine is a trademark of dishes prepared à la provençal, or in the style of southern France.

1 tablespoon light margarine

½ cup chopped scallions

1 tablespoon chopped fresh garlic   MEN: 4 teaspoons

¼ cup chopped tomato

¾ cup sliced mushrooms   MEN: 1½ cups

½ cup baby spinach leaves   MEN: 1 cup

One 3-ounce swordfish fillet (will yield 2½ ounces when cooked)

1 tablespoon white wine vinegar   MEN: 4 teaspoons

2 tablespoons chopped fresh basil leaves   MEN: 3 tablespoons

Heat an 8-inch nonstick skillet over medium heat. Spray with nonstick cooking spray and add the margarine. When the margarine has melted, add the scallions and garlic and cook for 2 minutes. Stir in the tomatoes, mushrooms, and spinach, and cook for another 5 minutes, or until the vegetables are softened. Add the swordfish, cover the skillet, and continue cooking for another 6 to 8 minutes. Stir in the vinegar and basil just before serving.

Serves 1

WOMEN: CALORIES 200; FIBER 4g; FAT 9g; PROTEIN 19g; CARB 9g; SODIUM 230mg

MEN: CALORIES 210; FIBER 5g; FAT 9g; PROTEIN 21g; CARB 11g; SODIUM 240mg

Thursday

Moo-Shu Chicken Wraps

The moo-shu filling can be made ahead and refrigerated overnight. Carry the wraps with you to work and heat the filling in the microwave.

1 teaspoon sesame oil

1 tablespoon rice vinegar   MEN: 4 teaspoons

2 teaspoons minced fresh ginger   MEN: 1 tablespoon

2 teaspoons minced fresh garlic   MEN: 1 tablespoon

2 ounces boneless, skinless, dark chicken meat, sliced into thin strips
   (will yield 1½ ounces when cooked)   MEN: 4 ounces (will yield 3 ounces
   when cooked)

Nonstick cooking spray

¼ cup shredded cabbage   MEN: ½ cup

¼ cup sliced button mushrooms   MEN: ½ cup

⅓ cup chopped broccoli   MEN: 1 cup

1 cup chopped celery

½ cup chopped scallions

Two 2:90 whole-wheat tortillas

1 tablespoon reduced-sodium teriyaki sauce

Measure the sesame oil, vinegar, ginger, and garlic into a large resealable plastic bag. Add the chicken. Press the air out of the bag and seal tightly. Turn the bag to distribute the marinade. Refrigerate for 4 to 24 hours, turning occasionally.

Remove the chicken from marinade and discard the marinade. Heat an 8-inch nonstick skillet over high heat. Spray with nonstick cooking spray. Add the marinated chicken and stir-fry until golden-brown, about 3 to 5 minutes. Add the cabbage, mushrooms, broccoli, celery, and scallions and stir-fry another 3 to 5 minutes, or until the vegetables have softened.

Microwave the tortillas for 10 to 15 seconds to soften them. Spread equal amounts of the teriyaki sauce onto each tortilla and spoon equal amounts of the chicken filling onto each. Roll up and serve.

Serves 1

WOMEN: CALORIES 350; FIBER 17g; FAT 13g; PROTEIN 21g; CARB 37g; SODIUM 840mg

MEN: CALORIES 440; FIBER 18g; FAT 15g; PROTEIN 34g; CARB 34g; SODIUM 910mg

Ham-Wrapped Vegetables with Black Olive Tapenade

Tapenade is a thick paste typically made with olives and capers as its base. Fresh herbs, vegetables, and a dash of vinegar are typically added for a chef's signature flavor.

1 teaspoon Dijon mustard

8 large pitted black olives, chopped

1 teaspoon drained capers

¾ cup finely chopped green and red bell peppers   MEN: 1 cup

1 tablespoon chopped fresh basil leaves   MEN: 2 tablespoons

1 tablespoon chopped fresh flat-leaf parsley

1 tablespoon red wine vinegar

¼ teaspoon freshly ground black pepper

Nonstick cooking spray

3 asparagus spears, stem ends trimmed   MEN: 9 spears

2 broccolini stalks   MEN: 4 stalks

2½ ounces deli ham (with 1 gram or less fat per ounce)

Set a rack at the highest level of the oven and preheat to broil.

In a small bowl, combine the mustard, olives, capers, bell peppers, basil, parsley, vinegar, and black pepper to make the tapenade.

Spray a nonstick baking sheet with nonstick cooking spray. Place the asparagus and Broccolini with 2 tablespoons water on the prepared baking sheet and place under the broiler for 2 to 3 minutes, or until the vegetables begin to soften.

Remove the vegetables from the broiler. Lay the ham slices on a cutting board, place a few vegetable spears on each, and wrap. Arrange the wraps on the baking sheet, seam side down, spoon equal amounts of the tapenade on each roll and broil for another minute, or until the tapenade is hot.

MEN: *Serve the chopped avocado and the cooked okra from the menu list with the ham roll-ups.*

Serves 1

WOMEN: CALORIES 210; FIBER 2g; FAT 11g; PROTEIN 22g; CARB 12g; SODIUM 900mg

MEN: CALORIES 250; FIBER 3g; FAT 11g; PROTEIN 25g; CARB 20g; SODIUM 990mg

Panna Cotta with Dates

Since panna cotta is neutral in taste, feel free to experiment with your favorite fruit for your own signature flavor.

¼ teaspoon unflavored gelatin

1 tablespoon cool water

4 pitted dates, halved

½ cup low-fat cottage cheese (containing up to 1% milkfat)

2 teaspoons sugar substitute

1 teaspoon vanilla extract

In a small bowl, whisk together the gelatin and water and let sit until the gelatin is dissolved, about 5 minutes. Place half of the dates in the bowl of a food processor, and pulse 4 to 5 times to chop. Add the cottage cheese, sugar substitute, vanilla, and dissolved gelatin. Run until the mixture is very smooth, about 60 seconds, scraping down the sides of the bowl as needed.

Spoon the mixture into a small bowl, cover, and chill in the refrigerator for at least 1 hour. Garnish with the remaining dates.

Serves 1

CALORIES 170; FIBER 2g; FAT 1g; PROTEIN 15g; CARB 26g; SODIUM 15mg

Friday

Grilled Banana Sandwich

This sandwich is simple to prepare but requires some care when turning it over. If some of the banana sticks to the skillet, simply scoop it up with the spatula and put it on top of the bread.

1 medium ripe banana

1 teaspoon sugar substitute

Nonstick cooking spray

1 tablespoon light margarine

1 slice regular 2:90 bread

4 toasted walnut halves, chopped

In a small bowl, mash the banana with a fork until it's very soft and smooth. Stir in the sugar substitute and spread the mixture over the bread.

Heat an 8-inch nonstick skillet over medium-high heat. Add the margarine. When the margarine has melted, carefully place the bread, banana side down, in the skillet. Cook for 3 to 5 minutes, until bananas are soft, and turn over with a metal spatula. Cook another 2 minutes to grill the bread. Sprinkle with the toasted walnuts.

Serves 1

CALORIES 270; FIBER 6g; FAT 13g; PROTEIN 6g; CARB 38g; SODIUM 290mg

Vegetarian Stir-fry with Garlic Sauce

Tempeh is a high-protein meat substitute similar to tofu. Look for it in the refrigerated case of the natural foods section of your local supermarket.

1 tablespoon minced fresh ginger   MEN: 4 teaspoons

2 teaspoons minced fresh garlic   MEN: 1 tablespoon

½ teaspoon crushed red pepper flakes

1 teaspoon peanut oil

2½ ounces tempeh

½ cup snow peas, ends trimmed   MEN: 1 cup

¼ cup shredded cabbage   MEN: ½ cup

1 tablespoon naturally brewed reduced-sodium soy sauce

1 tablespoon cider vinegar

1 tablespoon water

¼ cup bean sprouts   MEN: ½ cup

1 tablespoon chopped fresh cilantro leaves   MEN: 2 tablespoons

In a small bowl, combine the ginger, garlic, and red pepper flakes.

Heat a wok or nonstick skillet over high heat. Spray with nonstick cooking spray and add the oil. Add the tempeh, snow peas, and cabbage, and cook for 3 to 4 minutes, stirring constantly, until the cabbage is softened. Add the ginger mixture and cook for another 30 seconds. Add the soy sauce, vinegar, and water, and bring to a boil. Turn off the heat and stir in the bean sprouts and cilantro.

Serves 1

WOMEN: CALORIES 190; FIBER 2g; FAT 11g; PROTEIN 13g; CARB 14g; SODIUM 330mg
MEN: CALORIES 240; FIBER 4g; FAT 12g; PROTEIN 18g; CARB 20g; SODIUM 340mg

Saturday

Classic Hamburger

Eat this hamburger with all the fixings hot off the skillet.

2 teaspoons mustard

2 teaspoons ketchup

1 teaspoon reduced-fat mayonnaise

Nonstick cooking spray

2 ounces 90% fat-free ground round beef (will yield 1½ ounces when
cooked)

One 2:90 hamburger bun

¾ large dill pickle, sliced into rounds

4 tomato slices

½ cup shredded iceberg lettuce

¼ cup sliced scallions

In a small bowl, combine the mustard, ketchup, and mayonnaise.

Heat an 8-inch nonstick skillet over medium-high heat. Spray with nonstick cooking spray. Form the beef into a patty and place in the skillet. Cook for 2 minutes on each side, or until reaches desired doneness.

While the hamburger is cooking, spread both sides of the bun with the mustard mixture. Place the cooked patty on the bottom half of the bun, layer the pickles, tomato slices, lettuce, and scallions on the patty, and top with the top half of the bun.

Serves 1

CALORIES 260; FIBER 5g; FAT 9g; PROTEIN 19g; CARB 30g; SODIUM 530mg

Spicy Cajun Shrimp Gumbo

Okra is the essential ingredient in gumbo. It thickens and flavors the stew, giving it the Creole signature.

1 teaspoon canola oil

2 tablespoons chopped yellow onion   MEN: ¼ cup

2 teaspoons minced fresh garlic   MEN: 1 tablespoon

½ cup chopped celery   MEN: 1 cup

¼ cup chopped red and green bell peppers   MEN: ½ cup

½ cup sliced okra   MEN: 1 cup

⅛ teaspoon cayenne pepper   MEN: ¼ teaspoon

1 tablespoon chopped fresh flat-leaf parsley   MEN: 2 tablespoons

1 bay leaf

¼ cup canned chopped tomatoes, drained

½ cup water

3 ounces shrimp, peeled and deveined (will yield 2½ ounces cooked)

Freshly ground black pepper

Hot sauce

Heat the oil in a medium saucepan over medium heat. Add the onions, garlic, celery, bell peppers, and okra, and cook for 5 minutes, stirring often. Add the cayenne, parsley, and bay leaf, and cook for 30 seconds. Stir in the tomatoes and water and bring to a boil. Add the shrimp, turn the heat to low, cover, and cook for 3 to 5 minutes, or until shrimp are pink. Season with black pepper and hot sauce to taste.

Serves 1

WOMEN: CALORIES 180; FIBER 5g; FAT 6g; PROTEIN 20g; CARB 13g; SODIUM 200mg

MEN: CALORIES 220; FIBER 10g; FAT 7g; PROTEIN 22g; CARB 21g; SODIUM 260mg

Fresh Peaches and Smoked Ham

Peaches are the new melon. Here's a new way to eat the classic melon and prosciutto.

1 large fresh peach, pitted and cut into quarters

2½ ounces smoked ham (with 1 gram or less fat per ounce),
    sliced into 4 long strips

4 fresh basil leaves

Freshly ground black pepper

Balsamic vinegar

Wrap the strips of smoked ham around the peach quarters and tuck in a basil leaf. Secure the ham to the peach with a toothpick. Season with black pepper to taste and finish with a drizzle of vinegar.

Serves 1

CALORIES 180; FIBER 3g; FAT 4.5g; PROTEIN 20g; CARB 19g; SODIUM 390mg

Sunday

Salmon Croquettes

Panko are Japanese bread crumbs that stay crisp even after cooking. Using panko in this recipe eliminates the need for an egg batter and lots of oil.

¾ cup arugula leaves   MEN: 1½ cup

¾ cup sliced radishes   MEN: 1½ cup

1 cup halved cherry tomatoes   MEN: 2 cups

2 tablespoons chopped fresh dill   MEN: 3 tablespoons

1½ ounces canned salmon

1 teaspoon reduced-fat mayonnaise

2 tablespoons fresh lemon juice

1 cup 2:90 panko (Japanese bread crumbs)

Nonstick cooking spray

1 teaspoon canola oil

1 tablespoon balsamic vinegar

Freshly ground black pepper

On a large plate, toss together the arugula, radishes, cherry tomatoes, and 1 tablespoon of the dill. Place the plate in the refrigerator until ready to serve.

In a small bowl, mix together the salmon, mayonnaise, 1 tablespoon of the lemon juice, the panko, and remaining 1 tablespoon dill. Heat an 8-inch nonstick skillet over medium-high heat. Spray with nonstick cooking spray and add the oil. When the pan is hot, form the salmon mixture into two small patties and place them in the skillet. Cook, turning once, until golden-brown. Remove the croquettes from the skillet and place on top of the salad. Drizzle with the vinegar and remaining 1 tablespoon lemon juice and season with black pepper to taste.

Serves 1

WOMEN: CALORIES 380; FIBER 4g; FAT 10g; PROTEIN 18g; CARB 58g; SODIUM 310mg

MEN: CALORIES 410; FIBER 6g; FAT 12g; PROTEIN 18g; CARB 63g; SODIUM 400mg

Lobster Thermidor over Warm Spinach Salad

This classic dish dates back to the French Revolution. It was one of Napoleon's favorites. Of course, his chefs used heavy cream rather than skim milk.

1¼ cups baby spinach leaves   MEN: 2½ cups

½ cup thinly sliced fennel   MEN: 1 cup

⅓ cup chopped scallions   MEN: ½ cup

1 tablespoon light margarine

½ cup evaporated skim milk

2 teaspoons Dijon mustard

1 tablespoon chopped fresh tarragon

⅛ teaspoon ground nutmeg

⅛ teaspoon paprika   MEN: ¼ teaspoon

⅛ teaspoon cayenne pepper

2½ ounces cooked lobster meat (crawfish can be used as an alternative)

1 tablespoon chopped fresh flat-leaf parsley   MEN: 2 tablespoons

On a small plate, toss together the spinach, fennel, and scallions. Place the plate in the refrigerator until ready to serve.

In a medium saucepan over medium heat, heat the margarine and evaporated milk, mustard, and tarragon, stirring until margarine is melted and combined. Stir in the nutmeg, paprika, and cayenne, and cook for 2 minutes or until the broth simmers. Add the lobster meat and cook for another minute, or until the lobster is heated through.

Spoon the lobster over the spinach salad. Drizzle the remaining sauce over the lobster. The warm lobster will slightly wilt the greens. Garnish with the parsley and serve.

Serves 1

WOMEN: CALORIES 260; FIBER 3g; FAT 6g; PROTEIN 26g; CARB 26g; SODIUM 830mg

MEN: CALORIES 290; FIBER 6g; FAT 6g; PROTEIN 28g; CARB 32g; SODIUM 880mg

Equivalents Lists

These guidelines will help you choose foods that are equivalent to one serving size from each food group.

Starches

Women should have four servings of starches a day, and men five. Each serving of starch must contain at least 2 grams of dietary fiber for every 90-calorie serving.

One 90-calorie portion of the following starches is equivalent to one starch serving:
Light bread
Regular bread
Pita bread
Bagels
Dry cereals (calcium-fortified)
Cereal bars
Hot cereals
Toasted wheat bran
Wheat germ
Oat bran

Flatbread
Waffles
Whole-wheat tortillas
Chips
Whole-wheat wraps (serving size: 35 grams)
Crackers or whole-wheat matzo
Popcorn (with no saturated or trans fats; can be high in sodium,
    so check food labels)
Rice cakes (regular or mini)
Bread crumbs (with no artificial colors, flavors, or preservatives)
Whole-wheat flour
Organic polenta
Hummus

**One 90-calorie portion of the following starches is equivalent to one
starch serving:**
Fruit muesli
Granola (look for a label indicating "original")
Fudge bars
Cookies
Cinnamon flatbread crackers
Cereal bars
Ice cream bars

**The following portions of grains are equivalent to one 2:90 starch
serving:**
Cooked organic whole-wheat couscous, ⅓ cup
Cooked organic quinoa (Inca Red has the most fiber), ⅓ cup
Cooked organic bulgur wheat, ⅓ cup
Cooked Kashi breakfast pilaf, ⅓ cup
Cooked Lundberg Wild Blend gourmet blend of wild and premium
    brown rice, ⅓ cup
Cooked whole oat groats, ⅓ cup
Cooked roasted buckwheat (kasha), ⅓ cup
Cooked pearl barley, ⅓ cup
Cooked hulled barley, ⅓ cup

Cooked hard red winter wheat berries, ⅓ cup

Cooked soft wheat berries, ⅓ cup

Dry natural Tabouli wheat salad mix, 2 tablespoons

Whole-wheat pasta/noodles, cooked al dente, ⅓ cup (1 ounce dry
pasta equals ⅓ cup cooked)

The following portions of starchy vegetables and fruits are equivalent to one 2:90 serving:

Corn kernels, ½ cup

1 medium ear of corn (8 inches long)

Green peas, ½ cup

1 small sweet potato, plain, with skin (5 ounces, or about
5 inches long)

1 small potato, baked, with skin (5 ounces, or about 5 inches long)

Baked winter squash (acorn, butternut, pumpkin, turban, spaghetti,
golden nugget, red kuri, kabocha, heart of gold, sweet dumpling,
or delicata), chopped, 1 cup

Mixed vegetables (with corn and peas), ⅔ cup

Plantain, sliced, ½ cup

The following amounts of other starches are equivalent to one 2:90 serving:

Baked beans, vegetarian style, ¼ cup

Tomato-based pasta sauce, ½ cup (should provide 3 grams of fiber
and no saturated fat for every ½ cup serving)

Soup, ¾ cup (bean, mixed vegetable, or homemade soup containing
pasta or rice that meets the 2:90 rule)

Fruits

Women and men both should have two servings of fruit each day. Avoid dried fruits that contain added sugars or syrups. Fresh or frozen fruit is best, but make sure that frozen fruit is without added juices, sugars, or syrups. You may use fruits to make smoothies occasionally; however, juicing is not recommended, since juice contains little or no fiber.

The following amounts are equivalent to approximately 90 calories, or one serving.

Fruit	Fiber Content (grams per 90-calorie serving)
Raspberries, 1½ cups	11
Blackberries, 1⅛ cup	10
Passion fruit, 3½ ounces	10
Boysenberries, 1¼ cups	9
Cranberries, fresh 1¾ cups	9
Guavas, 2	9
Kumquats, 7	8.3
Currants, 1⅓ cups	6.9
Star fruit slices, 2 cups	6
Strawberries, whole, 1¾ cups	5.1
Tangerines, 3 small	4.5
Orange, 1 large	4.3
Asian pear, 1 medium	4
Apple, 1 large, with skin	4
Annona, ½ of a 3-inch fruit	4
Papaya slices, 1½ cups	4
Kiwis, 1½	4
Apricots, fresh, 6 whole	3.7
Mulberries, 1½ cups	3.6
Figs, 3 medium	3.6
Applesauce, unsweetened, 7 ounces	3.6
(Should provide 2 grams of fiber for every 50-calorie serving; the only ingredients should be apples, water, and ascorbic acid to maintain color.)	
Blueberries, 1⅛ cups	3.5
Grapefruit, large, ¾	3.4
Apricot halves, dried, 12	3
Cherries, fresh, 18	3
Nectarine, 1 large	3
Peach, fresh, 1 large	3

Dates, 4 whole or pitted	2.8
Banana, 1 medium (6 inches)	2.7
Plums, 3 small (2 inches)	2.7
Pineapple, 1⅛ cups	2.7
Mango, ¾ cup	2.5
Cantaloupe, 1½ cups	2.4
Honeydew melon, 1½ cups	2
Lychees, ¾ cup	2
Plums, dried, 4½	2
Prunes, 7 breakfast size	2
Tamarinds, 18	2
*Grapes, 25 small	1.2
*Raisins, 3 tablespoons	1.2
*Watermelon, 2 cups	1.2

Vegetables

Women should have one serving of vegetables daily, and men two. To make sure you receive the right amount of fiber for the day, one serving of vegetables should include three selections from the following chart.

Raw Vegetables	Fiber Content (grams per 30-calorie serving)
3 cups chopped endive	4.8
¾ cup sliced yambean (jicama)	4.5
1 cup chopped escarole	4
1 cup broccoli sprouts	4
2 cups diced celery	3.8
1 cup green beans	3.7
2 cups chopped turnip greens	3.6
3 cups cos or romaine lettuce, shredded	3.6
36 celtuce leaves	3.6

*Do not meet 2:90 Rule.

2¼ cups grape leaves	3
¾ cup chopped kohlrabi	3
2 cups chopped chives	3
¾ cup bamboo shoots	3
1½ cups radish slices	2.9
4 cups butter, Boston, or Bibb lettuce	2.8
1 cup sliced fennel	2.7
1 cup chopped spring onions or scallions	2.6
1 cup cauliflower florets	2.5
¾ cup chopped bell peppers	2.4
4 cups chopped iceberg lettuce	2.4
3 cups loose-leaf lettuce	2.4
3 cups alfalfa sprouts	2.4
1 cup chopped broccoli	2.4
½ cup snow peas or sugar-snap peas	2.3
⅕ bunch broccoli rabe	2.3
1 cup chopped tomatoes	2.2
1 cup diced rhubarb	2.2
1½ cups chopped spinach	2.1
1½ cups chopped cabbage	2.1
½ cup chopped carrots	2
1 cup onion sprouts	2
4½ cups arugula leaves	1.8
1 medium tomato	1.6
2 cups mushroom slices	1.6
1 cup summer squash slices (all varieties)	1.6
1½ cups cucumber slices	1.5
½ cup chopped raw onions	1.4
6 cups watercress	1.2
3 cups radicchio	1.2
1½ cups zucchini slices	1.2
8 broccolini stalks	1
¼ cup water chestnuts	1
½ cup chopped leeks	0.8
1 cup bean sprouts	0.6

Cooked Vegetables	Fiber Content (grams per 30-calorie serving)
1 cup chopped turnip greens	5
1½ cups chopped mustard greens	4.2
1½ cups chopped bok choy	4
1 cup shredded cabbage	3.6
½ medium artichoke	3.5
1 cup cauliflower (1-inch pieces)	3.4
1 cup turnip cubes	3.2
¾ cup chayote pieces	3.2
½ cup Brussels sprouts	3.2
½ cup sliced okra	3
¾ cup spinach leaves	3
¾ cup Italian beans	3
¾ cup wax beans	3
¾ cup chopped broccoli	3
⅓ cup artichoke hearts	2.9
¾ cup chopped Swiss chard	2.8
½ cup chopped collard greens	2.7
1 cup diced celery	2.4
1½ cups zucchini slices	2.1
2 cups bamboo shoots	2
½ cup sliced carrots	2
½ cup mushroom pieces	2
⅔ cup green beans or yellow snap beans	2
¾ cup cooked eggplant (1-inch cubes)	2
¾ cup chopped kale	2
¾ cup summer squash slices, all varieties	2
1½ cups pumpkin flowers	1.8
1½ cups squash flowers	1.8
⅔ cup asparagus (about 6 spears)	1.8
¾ cup chopped bell peppers	1.5
½ cup beet slices	1
½ cup kohlrabi slices	1
¾ cup chopped leeks	0.9
¼ cup chopped onions	0.8

Dairy

Women and men both should have two servings of dairy a day. The following foods and amounts are equivalent to approximately 90 calories, or one serving:

Fat-free (skim) milk, 1 cup
1% milk, 1 cup
Light soymilk, 1 cup
Plain, vanilla, or unsweetened soymilk, ¾ cup
Fat-free buttermilk, 1 cup
Low-fat buttermilk, ¾ cup
Evaporated non-fat milk, ½ cup
Non-fat dry milk powder, ⅓ cup
Plain non-fat yogurt, ¾ cup
1 container any flavored 2:90 yogurt (providing at least 2 grams
    of fiber for every 90 calories)
Low-fat plain kefir, ¾ cup
Non-fat plain kefir, 1 cup

Primary Proteins

Women and men both should have two servings of primary proteins every day. The following amounts are equivalent to approximately 90 calories, or one serving:

Poultry (2½ ounces cooked, or 3 ounces raw)
    Chicken breast (one skinless chicken breast is approximately
        3 ounces)
    Cornish hen (no skin)
    Turkey breast (no skin)

Fish (2½ ounces cooked, or 3 ounces raw)

Anchovies, fresh

Cod

Flounder

Grouper

Haddock

Halibut

Mahimahi

Rainbow trout, wild

Snapper

Sole

Swordfish

Tilapia

Tuna, fresh

Tuna, canned in water (low-sodium if desired)

Whitefish

Shellfish (2½ ounces cooked, or 3 ounces raw)

Clams

Crab (for imitation crabmeat, one serving is equivalent to ½ cup)

Lobster

Scallops

Shrimp

Game (2½ ounces cooked, or 3 ounces raw)

Duck or pheasant (skinless)

Venison

Buffalo

Ostrich

Other meats

Goat (roasted), 2½ ounces

Deli meats with 1 gram or less fat per ounce, 2½ ounces

Hot dogs with 1 gram or less fat per ounce, 2½ ounces

Sausage with 1 gram or less fat per ounce, 2½ ounces

4 slices 95% fat-free extra-lean turkey bacon

Cheese
Fat-free cheese, 2½ ounces

Fat-free or low-fat cottage cheese (containing up to 1% milk fat),
½ cup

Non-fat ricotta cheese, ½ cup

Other
Seasoned wheat gluten vegetarian stir-fry strips, 2½ ounces

Cooked beans (garbanzo, black, pinto, lima beans, kidney, cannellini,
white, split, lentils, black-eyed peas), vegetarian style, ½ cup

5 egg whites (or approximately ⅔ cup any egg-white product)

Secondary Proteins

Women should have one serving of secondary proteins daily, and men should have two. The following foods and amounts are equivalent to approximately 90 calories, or one serving:

Poultry (1½ ounces cooked, or 2 ounces raw)
Chicken, dark meat, skinless (one cooked drumstick is
approximately 1½ ounces; one cooked leg is approximately 3½
ounces; one cooked thigh is approximately 2 ounces; 1 cooked
wing is approximately 1 ounce)

Goose, skinless

Turkey, dark meat, skinless

Fish
Arctic char, 1½ ounces cooked (2 ounces raw)

Catfish, 1½ ounces cooked (2 ounces raw)

Herring (uncreamed or smoked), 1½ ounces cooked (2 ounces raw)

Mackerel, 1½ ounces cooked (2 ounces raw)

Oysters, 9 medium

Salmon, fresh (wild Atlantic) or canned, 1½ ounces cooked
(2 ounces raw)

Sardines, 3 canned medium

Sardines, fresh, 1½ ounces cooked (2 ounces raw)
Tuna, canned, in oil, drained, 1½ ounces

Beef (USDA Select or Choice grades of lean beef with visible fat trimmed, best if grass-fed; 1½ ounces cooked, or 2 ounces raw)
Cube steak
Ground round
Porterhouse steak
Roast (rib, rump, chuck)
Round, sirloin, and flank steak
T-bone steak
Tenderloin (filet mignon)

Lamb (Roast, chop, leg), 1½ ounces cooked (2 ounces raw)

Pork (fresh ham; canned, cured, or boiled ham; tenderloin; center-l chop), 1½ ounces cooked (2 ounces raw)

Rabbit, 1½ ounces cooked (2 ounces raw)

Veal (Lean chop, roast), 1½ ounces cooked (2 ounces raw)

Other meats
Deli meats with more than 1 but no more than 3 grams of fat per ounce, 1½ ounces
2¼-ounce hot dog with more than 1 but no more than 3 grams of per ounce
4 slices Canadian bacon
6 slices Schneider's Canadian bacon (lower in fat and sodium)

Cheese
Any cheese with more than 1 but no more than 3 grams of fat per ounce, 1½ ounces
1 mozzarella string cheese with no more than 4 grams of total fat per serving
Grated Parmesan, 3½ tablespoons

Reduced-fat feta with no more than 4 grams of total fat per ounce,
    1 ounce

Other

Edamame (soybeans), 2 ounces

Organic plain tofu (firm, soft, or lite firm), 3 ounces

Silken organic tofu, 6 ounces

Tempeh, 1¾ ounces

1 veggie burger patty (such as Gardenburger veggie medley or
    Morningstar Farms garden veggie patties)

1 whole egg plus 1 egg white (limit whole eggs to 3 per week, use
    organic, cage-free eggs if possible)

Fats

Women should have three servings of fat daily, and men four. The following foods and corresponding portions are equivalent to approximately 90 calories, or one serving:

Oils (2 teaspoons of the following)

Flaxseed or linseed oil (add after cooking)

Wheat germ oil

Canola oil

Olive oil

Peanut oil

Avocado oil

Toasted pumpkin seed oil

Hazelnut oil

Sesame oil

Macadamia nut oil

Peanut oil

Walnut oil

Grapeseed oil
Corn oil
Safflower oil
Soybean oil
Sunflower oil

Butters and condiments

Natural peanut butter, 1 tablespoon
Cashew butter, 1 tablespoon
Almond butter, 1 tablespoon
Almond paste, 1 tablespoon
Soy nut butter, 1 tablespoon
Light margarine (with no trans fat), 2 tablespoons
Mayonnaise (reduced-fat), 2 tablespoons
Miracle Whip salad dressing, reduced-fat, 2 tablespoons
Salad dressing, reduced-fat, 4 tablespoons
Tahini paste, 4 teaspoons
All-natural Nayonaise soy-based sandwich spread, 2 tablespoons

Seeds and nuts

Pumpkin seeds, 2 tablespoons
Sunflower seeds, 2 tablespoons
Flaxseeds, 2 tablespoons
Sesame seeds, 2 tablespoons
12 whole almonds
12 whole cashews
Pistachios in the shell, ¼ cup
Shelled hazelnuts, 2 tablespoons
12 mixed nuts
20 peanuts
8 pecan halves
8 walnut halves
Black walnuts, 2 tablespoons
Soy nuts, 1¾ tablespoons

Olives

16 large black olives
20 green olives
10 Kalamata olives

Other fats

Avocado, 4 tablespoons
Prepared pesto, 4 teaspoons

Dividends

Here are some examples of everyday dividends, which are 15 to 20 calories per serving, along with some more healthful alternatives. You can have 3 to 4 dividends every day.

Everyday Foods	The Healthier Alternative
Beverages/Morning Dividends	
16 ounces Propel fitness water	
4 ounces vegetable or tomato juice	
2 tablespoons 2% milk or non-fat evaporated milk (can be used as cream in coffee)	
2 ounces skim milk	
1.5 ounces 1% milk	
4 teaspoons nonfat dry milk powder	
1 tablespoon nondairy liquid creamer	1 tablespoon organic half-and-half
	1 tablespoon soymilk creamer
2 teaspoons nondairy powdered creamer	
1 teaspoon white granulated sugar	1 teaspoon brown sugar
1 sugar cube	
2 teaspoons powdered sugar	
1 teaspoon honey	

Everyday Foods

Sweet Treats

2 tablespoons light or non-fat
   whipped topping

2 sugarless hard candies

1 sugar-free Popsicle

2 tablespoons sugar-free jam or jelly

1 tablespoon low-sugar jam or jelly

2 tablespoons sugar-free syrup

2 sugar-free, fat-free meringues

2 teaspoons marshmallow fluff

1 teaspoon semisweet chocolate
   chunks or mini-morsels

Snacks

5 cocktail olives

1½ large dill pickles

3 pieces Laughing Cow light gourmet cheese bites

1 tablespoon hummus

Condiments and Other Additions

1 tablespoon fat-free cream cheese

2 teaspoons grated Parmesan cheese

1 egg white

1 tablespoon non-fat mayonnaise

1 teaspoon reduced-fat mayonnaise

2 tablespoons light margarine

The Healthier Alternative

2 tablespoons Natural by Nature
   whipped cream

1 all-natural (no-sugar-added) fruit juice
   freezer pop

2 teaspoons organic no-sugar-added fruit
   spread

2 teaspoons organic spreadable fruit
   (containing no more than 7 grams total
   carbohydrates per 1 tablespoon serving)

2 teaspoons organic juice-sweetened apple
   butter

1 teaspoon organic dried fig spread

1 teaspoon organic tart cherry butter

2 teaspoons organic raspberry or French
   vanilla syrup

2 teaspoons low-fat soy Parmesan

1 teaspoon reduced-fat margarine

1 teaspoon light butter

Nonstick cooking spray (3-second spray)

2 teaspoons sour cream

1 tablespoon light sour cream

2 tablespoons non-fat sour cream

1 tablespoon non-fat Miracle Whip

1 teaspoon reduced-fat Miracle Whip   1 tablespoon Vegenaise

1 tablespoon fat-free salad dressing   2 tablespoons Up Country Organics organic

                                              fat-free balsamic dressing

                                    1 tablespoon Annie's Naturals no-fat organic

                                      yogurt with dill dressing

7 classic-cut croutons

3 restaurant-style croutons

3 tablespoons salsa

2 tablespoons sauerkraut

1 tablespoon Worcestershire sauce

2 tablespoons cooking wine

2 tablespoons capers

1 tablespoon lite soy sauce

1 cup prepared (using ½ cube) low-   1 cup prepared Kitchen Basics natural

   sodium bouillon or broth, or 1 cup   chicken, vegetable, or beef stock

   prepared (using ½ cube) (high-

   sodium) bouillon, broth, or consommé

1 teaspoon fish sauce

1 tablespoon stir-fry sauce

1 tablespoon soy-ginger sauce

1 tablespoon teriyaki sauce (should contain about

   15 calories per tablespoon)

1 tablespoon hoisin sauce

Freebies

Enjoy the following foods liberally—they are all 0 to 5 calories per serving.

Beverages
Water
Club soda
Seltzer or sparkling mineral water
Tonic water (sugar free)
Decaf coffee (limit regular coffee to 1 to 2 cups a day)
Decaf teas
Unsweetened iced tea
Other sugar-free diet drink mixes

Condiments
Horseradish
Mustard
Lemon juice or lime juice
Herbs and spices
Tabasco or other hot pepper sauce

Index